FOUNDATIONS OF LIFESTYLE MEDICINE

The Lifestyle Medicine Board Review Manual

3rd Edition

by **John Kelly, MD, MPH, LM Specialist**
and **Jeni Shull Clayton, MD, MPH, DipABLM**

Made possible through generous support from Ardmore Institute of Health

Ardmore Institute of Health

Published by the American College of Lifestyle Medicine

AMERICAN COLLEGE OF Lifestyle Medicine

LifestyleMedicine.org

The American College of Lifestyle Medicine (ACLM) is the medical professional association for physicians and other professionals dedicated to clinical and worksite practice of Lifestyle Medicine as the foundation of a transformed and sustainable health care system. ACLM is a galvanizing force for change. ACLM addresses the need for quality, evidence-based education and certification as well as advocates for its members in their individual practices and in their collective mission to nationally and globally promote Lifestyle Medicine as the first and optimal treatment option. ACLM members are united in their desire to eradicate the root causes of chronic disease. Rather than disease management, Lifestyle Medicine clinicians specialize in health restoration.

education@lifestylemedicine.org

Vision

A world in which all physicians and allied health professionals have been trained and certified in evidence-based lifestyle medicine, integrating healthful behaviors into their own lives, while incorporating a lifestyle medicine-first approach to treating root causes of lifestyle-related diseases into their clinical practices.

Early stages → ~~CBT~~ Motivational

Later " → CBT.

All Stages → + Psychology.

TABLE OF CONTENTS

Lead Authors 1

Acknowledgements 3

Section 1 Introduction to Lifestyle Medicine 5

Section 2 Fundamentals of Health Behavior Change 25

Section 3 Key Clinical Processes in Lifestyle Medicine 57

Section 4 The Role of Physician Health and the Physician's Personal Health 93

Section 5 Nutrition Science, Assessment, and Prescription 103

Section 6 Physical Activity Science and Prescription 183

Section 7 Emotional and Mental Well-Being, Assessment, and Interventions 233

Section 8 Sleep Health Science and Interventions 267

Section 9 Fundamentals of Tobacco Cessation and Managing Risky Alcohol Use 295

Section 10 The Role of Connectedness and Positive Psychology 321

Key Articles Summaries of Key Lifestyle Medicine Studies 335

Appendix Overweight and Obesity 361

Index 369

LEAD AUTHORS

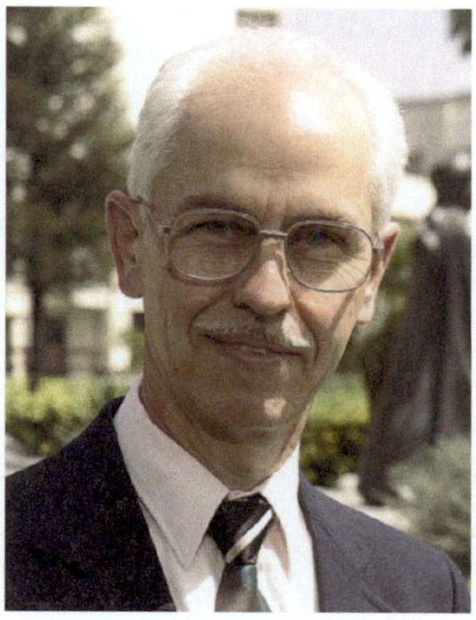

JOHN KELLY, MD, MPH, LM SPECIALIST

Dr. Kelly completed his undergraduate studies in Biochemistry and Molecular Biology, graduating *summa cum laude* as a McMurran Scholar. He completed the Dual MD/MPH Degree Program at Loma Linda University in Epidemiology with honors. He is trained in Preventive and Lifestyle Medicine, and has done private and government-funded research in lifestyle medicine. He was founding President of the American College of Lifestyle Medicine (ACLM), co-authored ACLM's Official Board Review Course in Lifestyle Medicine, co-chairs ACLM's Expert Panel, and serves as adjunct faculty at Loma Linda University. He currently teaches lifestyle medicine nationally using leading-edge intensive lifestyle medicine training programs.

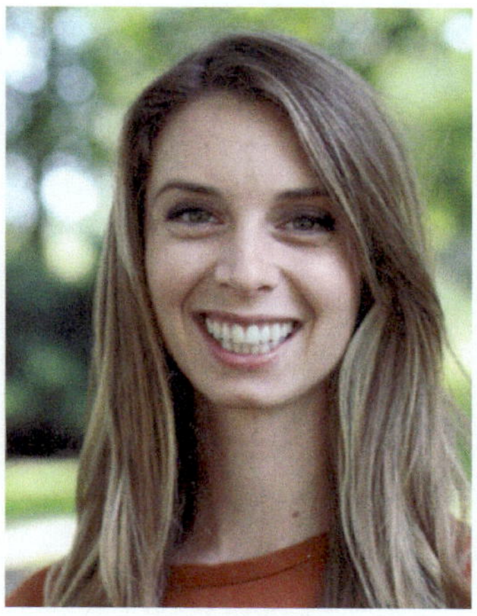

JENI SHULL CLAYTON, MD, MPH, DipABLM

Jeni Shull Clayton is a Family and Preventive Medicine Physician and a Diplomat of the American and International Board of Lifestyle Medicine. Dr. Clayton graduated from Indiana University School of Medicine. She attended Loma Linda University's Family and Preventive Medicine residency, served as chief resident and completed her Master's in Population Health. She was awarded Resident Teacher of the Year and the Will Alexander Whole Person Care Award. Under Dr. John Kelly, founder of the ACLM, she became the first Lifestyle Medicine Fellow at the Black Hills Health and Education Center. She has co-authored the *Foundations of Lifestyle Medicine Board Review Manual* and Course with Dr. Kelly and ACLM. Currently, she serves as the medical director of Well Life by Schneck in Seymour, Indiana. Dr. Clayton recently got married and enjoys hiking with her new husband, cooking, and spending time with her family.

ACKNOWLEDGEMENTS

This third edition of the Lifestyle Medicine Board Review for both the American and the International Board of Lifestyle Medicine Certification Exams is the product of a collective, determined effort involving many leaders and pioneers in lifestyle medicine. It draws upon much that has been done before, building particularly upon the Lifestyle Medicine Core Competencies (LMCC) and related materials. The authors want to especially thank those who contributed to that work, including Liana Lianov, MD, MPH, FACPM, FACLM, DipABLM, and Mark Johnson, MD, MPH, who authored the 2010 JAMA article that first put the LMCC in medical literature. Special thanks, too, to those who developed the LMCC online course which presents much of the material in this Course in a didactic manner.

The authors extend their sincere appreciation to the esteemed members of the expert Editorial Panel who made important contributions that helped fill gaps and shape the final product. This panel included Michael Greger, MD, DipABLM, Hans Diehl, DrHSc, MPH, Jonathan Bonnet, MD, MPH, CAQSM, FAAFP, FACLM, DipABLM, Marc Braman, MD, MPH, Scott Stoll, MD, David Drozek, DO, FACLM, DipABLM, and Brenda Davis, RD. Another major contributor was the Education Committee of the American College of Lifestyle Medicine, led by Brenda Rea, MD, DrPH, PT, RD, FACLM, DipABLM, Jeni Shull Clayton, MD, MPH, DipABLM, and Michelle Tollefson, MD, FACOG, DipABLM, FACLM, and formerly led by Cate Collings, MD, FACC, MS, DipABLM. The authors wish to express their gratitude for the committee's effort and support. The authors would like to acknowledge, with special thanks, the original review question contributors, including Robert Bonacci, MD, DipABLM, Janani Krishnaswami, MD, MPH, DipABLM, Elizabeth Swenor, DO, MA, DipABLM, Roselynn Krantz, MD, MS, DipABLM, Natalie Gentile, MD, DipABLM, Cono Badalamenti, MD, MHSA, DipABLM, David Baker, MD, DipABLM, Helen Kinsey, MD, DipABLM, Paul Washburn, MD, MPH, DipABLM, Jon Bonnet, MD, MPH, CAQSM, FAAFP, FACLM, DipABLM, David Drozek, DO, FACLM, DipABLM, Hans Diehl, DrHSc, and Michele Bichko, DNP, MS, DipACLM. They would also like to thank Micaela Karlsen, PhD, and Kathy Pollard, MS, for efforts in updating the key article section built upon the foundational contributions of Amit Algotar, MD, PhD, MPH. Others, too numerous to name individually, also made significant contributions, among them Susan Benigas, Executive Director of the American College of Lifestyle Medicine, Paulina Shetty, MS, RDN, DipACLM, Senior Director of Education, Katie Hughes, Senior Project Manager, Heather Klein, Instructional Design Manager, Kathy Pollard, MS, Research Projects Manager, Kaitlyn Pauly, MS, RDN, DipACLM, Deputy Director, Senior Director of Engagement and Administration, Leslie Casey, Senior Director of Marketing, Molly Pinera, Associate Director of Marketing and Social Media, Kathie Garbe, Editor, Rikki Campbell Ogden/pixiedesign, Graphic Designer. Thank you, thank you, to each one! While the authors worked long and hard to make this course all it could be, they simply could never have done it without the contributions and support of so many others. This heartfelt gratitude is extended, as well, to the Ardmore Institute of Health, which provided seed funding that enabled this vision to be brought to fruition.

It is the authors' intent for this Course to not only enable clinicians to quickly master the core competencies and pass their certification exam, but also to serve as a reference in the practice of lifestyle medicine and for teaching lifestyle medicine to students, residents, and fellows. The authors intend to build upon this edition in future editions that will continue to serve this two-fold purpose.

With the ardent hope and belief that lifestyle medicine must become the foundation of a transformed and sustainable system of healthcare delivery, thank you for your commitment to educating and equipping yourself to become champions for change in ushering in the future of healthcare.

CONTRIBUTING AUTHORS

Kayli Anderson, MS, RDN, ACSM-EP, DipACLM

Jonathan Bonnet, MD, MPH, CAQSM, FAAFP, FACLM, DipABLM

Stephen Carek, MD, CAQSM, DipABLM

Jeni Shull Clayton, MD, MPH, DipABLM

Param Dedhia, MD

Micaela Karlsen, PhD, MSPH

John Kelly, MD, MPH, LM Specialist

Jessica Matthews, DBH, MS, NBC-HWC, DipACLM

Simon Matthews, FASLM, MHlthSci, DipIBLM, MAPS, NBC-HWC

Gia Merlo, MD, MBA, DipABLM

Neil Nedley, MD

Jill R. Selzle, PA-C, MPAS, RVT, DipACLM

SECTION 1
Introduction to Lifestyle Medicine

Objective 1 Define lifestyle medicine and describe the unique role of lifestyle medicine in health care 6

Objective 2 Describe the lifestyle medicine core competencies as identified by a national consensus panel 8

Objective 3 Describe the importance of lifestyle medicine in treating the nation's lifestyle disease burden. 9

Objective 4 Summarize the role of behavioral determinants of positive health outcomes 10

Objective 5 Interpret the scientific evidence that demonstrates the association of risk conditions (from unhealthy behaviors) as key to health outcomes 12

Objective 6 Compare and contrast to other fields of health and medicine 16

Objective 7 Indicate the place and priority of lifestyle medicine in the spectrum of treatment options for chronic (lifestyle-related) diseases 18

Objective 8 Describe the efficacy of lifestyle medicine and its impact on disease pathophysiology 18

Section 1 Glossary 20

Section 1 Review Questions 21

Section 1 Review Questions Answers and Summaries 22

Section 1 References. 23

OBJECTIVE 1

Define lifestyle medicine and describe the unique role of lifestyle medicine in health care

1) Definitions of lifestyle medicine from leading organizations and texts in the field

a) American College of Lifestyle Medicine[1]

1. Lifestyle medicine is the use of evidence-based lifestyle therapeutic interventions—including a whole food plant-based eating pattern, regular physical activity, restorative sleep, stress management, avoidance of risky substances, and positive social connection—as a primary modality, delivered by clinicians trained and certified in this specialty, to prevent, treat, and often reverse chronic disease.
   a. Note: a whole food plant-based diet consists of mostly food from plants (such as whole-grains, vegetables, fruits, beans, and legumes) with little to no animal products (such as dairy, meat, and eggs).

b) 2018 Lifestyle Medicine Core Competencies[2]

1. Lifestyle medicine offers a unique approach that leverages a whole food plant-based diet, physical activity, sleep, emotional well-being, and avoiding risky substances to not only prevent, but also treat and reverse lifestyle-related diseases.

c) *Lifestyle Medicine*, by Garry Egger[3]

1. Lifestyle medicine is the application of medical, behavioral, motivational, and environmental principles to the management of lifestyle-related health problems in a clinical setting. Teaching self-care and self-management are important elements of lifestyle medicine.

2) Intensive Therapeutic Lifestyle Change (ITLC) treatment programs

a) ITLC programs encourage drastic changes in one's daily routine, including sleep habits, diet, physical activity, and stress management. The program is usually administered in a group setting, and it always involves a multi-modality team. Multi-modality teams may include a provider, pharmacist, registered dietitian, certified health coach, condition management nurse, or physical therapist, among others. Typically, ITLC programs include in-person outpatient visits that last approximately 60 minutes, and those visits occur 1–3 times per week for 8–18 weeks. ITLC programs may also be residential programs that are generally 7–21 days long. Shorter ITLC immersion programs also exist and generally last 3–10 days.[4]

b) The methods of ITLC programs are evidence-based and shown to work with accepted research methods. Notable published ITLC programs include the Pritikin program, Ornish program, and the Diehl CHIP (Coronary Health Improvement Project) program.[5,6,7,8,9]

c) ITLC programs can produce the essential induction phase that is needed in order for people to make the dramatic lifestyle changes that are necessary for treating severe disease, supporting and helping the patient experience health improvements first-hand in their own bodies without requiring much engagement of the patient's motivation or self-efficacy, and transforming a patient's concept of what is possible with lifestyle change. Ideally, an induction phase precedes the maintenance and support phases in lifestyle change.[10,11,12]

3) History of lifestyle medicine

a) Pioneers of lifestyle medicine

1. Hippocrates: Often quoted as saying, "Let your food be your medicine, and your medicine be your food." This statement is consistent with Hippocrates' general philosophy and practice, although the best evidence indicates that the statement is actually not from him. He was, however, an advocate of teaching a healthful diet and being physically active to avoid and combat disease.[13]
2. Thomas Edison: "The doctor of the future will give no medicine but will interest his patients in the care of the human frame, in diet and in the cause and prevention of disease."[14]
3. Nathan Pritikin Longevity Center (1970s): A residential health care center that used nutrition, exercise, and education to treat and reverse heart disease.
4. John McDougall Program (1970s): Residential health care programs using an unlimited whole food plant-based diet, stress reduction, and exercise to treat and reverse disease.
5. Dean Ornish Preventive Medicine Research Center (1980s): The Lifestyle Heart Trial showed regression of cardiac stenosis at 1 year and continued improvement at 5 years through a low-fat vegetarian diet, stress management, exercise, and smoking cessation in a small group setting, and emphasizing positive psychology and connectedness.[7,8]
6. Caldwell B. Esselstyn Jr. Cleveland Clinic (1990s): Began a greater than 20-year longitudinal study about arresting and reversing heart disease in critically ill patients.[10]
7. Hans Diehl CHIP, now called Complete Health Improvement Program (1990s): An outpatient intensive lifestyle change program that encourages a whole food plant-based diet and exercise to prevent, treat, and reverse lifestyle-related chronic disease.[5,9,15]
8. The World Health Organization (WHO) (1990): The WHO inaugural report on "Diet, nutrition, and the prevention of chronic diseases" was written to address how poor diet quality and excess calories are related to the rise in chronic disease. It included nutrient guidance on the optimal intake of fats, proteins, carbohydrates, and salt.[16]
9. James Rippe *Lifestyle Medicine* (1990s): The first comprehensive medical text focused on lifestyle medicine.[17]

b) American College of Lifestyle Medicine (ACLM)

1. The organization was founded in early 2004 by John Kelly, MD, MPH, of Loma Linda University, in collaboration with a small group of visionary physicians. The American Medical Association Foundation awarded Dr. Kelly the Excellence in Medicine Award in 2004 for his leadership in establishing the ACLM, and in 2016 Dr. Kelly was honored with the inaugural Lifestyle Medicine Trailblazer Award.
2. Presidents have included Drs. John Kelly, Marc Braman, Wayne Dysinger, Liana Lianov, David Katz, George Guthrie, Dexter Shurney, and Cate Collings.
3. Over the past six years, since 2014, ACLM has experienced exponential growth in membership, increasing nearly 900% to what is now over 5,800 members.

c) The "Physician competencies for prescribing lifestyle medicine" article was published in the *Journal of the American Medical Association* in 2010. This was a landmark article, the first to describe the competencies necessary for a physician to practice primary care–based lifestyle medicine.[2] It was composed by a blue-ribbon panel of lifestyle medicine experts from multiple disciplines and organizations, including the American College of Preventive Medicine (ACPM) and the ACLM. Liana Lianov and Mark Johnson were the lead authors. (Note: A blue ribbon panel is a group of exceptional individuals who are asked to help answer a question based on their expertise, experience, or authority).[18]

d) American Board of Lifestyle Medicine (ABLM)

1. The board was organized by a group of ACLM leaders in 2016 to develop a credible Lifestyle Medicine Certification Exam and process. The ACLM leaders were Drs. Wayne Dysinger, David Ferriss, Liana Lianov, Eddie Phillips, and Dexter Shurney. Flash forward 3 years, and, in 2020, more than 1,230 sat for the ABLM exam.
2. The inaugural Lifestyle Medicine Certification Exam was offered at ACLM's Lifestyle Medicine 2017 conference in Tucson, Arizona.
3. Lifestyle medicine certification includes an ABLM certification for Lifestyle Medicine diplomat for MDs and DOs, and a separate ACLM certification for others (PhD, PsyD, etc.).

e) International Board of Lifestyle Medicine (IBLM)

1. This board was organized in 2016 by a group of ACLM and ABLM leaders to provide a credible certification exam process for International lifestyle medicine clinicians.
2. The IBLM exam is consistent with the ABLM exam to ensure core lifestyle medicine knowledge and skills and global standardization of the field.
3. IBLM exams are now being offered worldwide multiple times each year.

OBJECTIVE 2

Describe the lifestyle medicine core competencies as identified by a national consensus panel

1) Physician competencies for prescribing lifestyle medicine[2]

a) Leadership

1. Leaders should promote healthy behaviors as foundational to medical care, disease prevention, and health promotion. This may include actions such as giving presentations at grand rounds or local community events, or informing politicians of the need to adopt and promote healthy lifestyle changes.
2. Strive to practice healthy personal behaviors.
3. Create environments that support healthy behaviors at school, work, and home.

b) Knowledge

1. Know the evidence that specific lifestyle changes can have on patients' health outcomes, including:
    a. The effect of smoking cessation on lung conditions, lung cancer, and other health conditions
    b. The effect of exercise on the occurrence and recurrence of breast cancer.
    c. The effect of fitness on heart attack or stroke survival
    d. The effects of a plant-based diet, including reduced blood pressure, lowered lipids, prostate cancer regression, among others
2. Describe ways that physician engagement with patients and families can have a positive effect on patients' health behaviors.

c) Assessment skills

1. Assess the social, psychological, and biological predispositions of patients' behaviors and the resulting health outcomes.
2. Assess patient and family readiness, willingness, and ability to make health behavior changes. In other words, know the stage-of-change level for various changes.

3. Perform a history and physical exam specific to a patient's lifestyle-related health status, including lifestyle "vital signs" such as tobacco use, alcohol consumption, diet, physical activity, body mass index, stress level, sleep, and emotional well-being. Order and interpret tests to screen, diagnose, and monitor lifestyle-related diseases.

d) Management skills

1. Use nationally recognized practice guidelines to assist patients in self-managing their health behaviors and lifestyles (e.g., US Preventive Services Task Force guidelines for smoking cessation).
2. Establish effective relationships with patients and families to affect and sustain behavioral change using evidence-based counseling methods, tools, and follow-up.
3. Collaborate with patients and their families to develop evidence-based, achievable, and specific written action plans, such as lifestyle prescriptions.
4. Help patients manage and sustain healthy lifestyle practices and refer patients to other health care professionals as needed for lifestyle-related conditions. This may include referring to office-based and/or community-based lifestyle education and intervention programs.

e) Office and community support

1. Be able to practice in an interdisciplinary team of health care providers and support a team approach (e.g., physician, dietitian, coach, etc.).
2. Develop and apply office systems and practices that support lifestyle medical care. This includes things like decision support technology, such as proactive electronic medical records and health risk assessment tools, which can bring to attention at-risk behaviors and patients.
3. Measure processes and outcomes to improve the quality of lifestyle interventions in individuals and groups of patients. (Tracking outcomes is a part of good lifestyle medicine practices).
4. Use appropriate community referral resources that support the implementation of healthy lifestyles. This should include intensive "induction-phase" intervention programs when indicated in order to transform self-efficacy and goal setting.

OBJECTIVE 3

Describe the importance of lifestyle medicine in treating the nation's lifestyle disease burden

1) **Leading health organizations have recognized that the nation's burden of disease will not improve without lifestyle interventions.**

2) **The Healthy People initiative is a government program that provides science-based, 10-year national objectives for improving the health of all Americans. Leading health indicators of Healthy People 2020[19]:**

a) Physical activity

b) Overweight and obesity

c) Tobacco use

d) Substance abuse

e) Responsible sexual behavior

f) Mental health

g) Injury and violence

h) Environmental quality

i) Immunization

j) Access to health care

3) **The first and current *National Prevention Strategy: America's Plan for Better Health And Wellness*, was compiled in 2011. It was a key component of the Affordable Care Act, which was overseen by the Surgeon General, Dr. Regina Benjamin. The idea was to create a strategy to change America's health care system from a predominantly sick care model to one that is focused on wellness and disease prevention.[20]**

a) The strategy includes health care providers conducting lifestyle modification services, such as:
    1. Physical activity assessments and counseling
    2. Obesity screening and nutrition counseling
    3. Screening and counseling for excessive alcohol use
    4. Tobacco cessation services

4) **"The National Strategy for Quality Improvement in Health Care" report was submitted to Congress in 2011 by the US Department of Health and Human Services. The report recommended national strategic priorities that included a focus on these lifestyle factors[21]:**

a) Promote the most effective prevention and treatment practices for the leading causes of mortality, starting with cardiovascular disease.

b) Engage each person and family as partners in their health care.

c) Work with communities to promote wide use of best practices to enable healthy living.

OBJECTIVE 4

Summarize the role of behavioral determinants of positive health outcomes

1) **Lifestyle practices and health habits are the most important determinants of positive health outcomes. Improving unhealthy behaviors is foundational to effective medical care, disease prevention, and health promotion. Two key elements for improving health behaviors and outcomes are[2]:**

a) A trusting relationship between physician and patient.

b) Patient support from a multidisciplinary team, loved ones, and the greater community.

2) **The social, psychological, and biological predispositions of patients' behaviors and the resulting health outcomes[2]:**

a) Table 1.1 shows leading causes of death from lifestyle-related conditions. Predominantly lifestyle-related medical conditions are seen in primary care (80% according to Bodai, 2018).[22]
    1. Obesity
    2. Metabolic syndrome
    3. Hypertension

4. Cardiovascular disease
5. Dyslipidemia
6. Arthritis
7. Diabetes
8. Osteoporosis

Table 1.1 The 10 Leading Causes of Death in the US are Significantly Lifestyle-Related (2015)[23]

1	Heart disease	655,381	23.1%
2	Cancer	599,274	21.1%
3	Accidents (unintentional injuries)	167,127	5.9%
4	Chronic lower respiratory diseases	159,486	5.6%
5	Stroke (cerebrovascular diseases)	147,810	5.2%
6	Alzheimer's disease	122,019	4.3%
7	Diabetes	84,946	3.0%
8	Influenza and pneumonia	59,120	2.1%
9	Nephritis, nephrotic syndrome, nephrosis	51,386	1.8%
10	Intentional self-harm (suicide)	48,443	1.7%

b) 80% of all premature deaths are attributable to three factors[24,25]:
   1. Tobacco use
   2. Poor diet
   3. Lack of physical activity

c) Few patients have sufficient healthy behaviors.[26]
   1. Only 3% had healthy levels of all four health behaviors:
      a. Non-smoking 76%
      b. Healthy weight (BMI <25) 40%
      c. Five fruits and veggies per day 23%
      d. Regular physical activity 22%
   2. About 1 out of 7 people still smoke.[27]
   3. About 3 out of 4 people are eating a diet low in fruits and vegetables.[28]
   4. About 4 out of 5 do not get enough physical activity.[19]

d) Unhealthy patient lifestyles persist even after medical problems arise.
   1. 11% of patients with diabetes follow accepted dietary guidelines for saturated fat.[29]
   2. 8% of patients with heart disease continue to smoke.[30,31]

e) Determinants of health include:
   1. Adverse childhood events[32,33]
      a. The more adverse childhood events a person has experienced, the higher the risk for adverse health outcomes, such as poor self-rated health, functional limitations, mental illness and self-harm, drug and alcohol abuse, diabetes, cancer, respiratory disease, and heart attacks.
   2. Genetic and epigenetic predispositions
      a. Experts estimate that DNA sequence (genes) explain ~10% variance in health status and epigenetics (gene switches) explain ~70–90% of variance in health.

b. A 2005 study, "Epigenetic differences arise during the lifetime of monozygotic twins," indicated that environmental factors, not genetic factors, were the main determinant of epigenetic variance.[34] The study looked at monozygous twins who share the same DNA sequence at conception. The largest variance in DNA methylation (a type of epigenetic change) in those twins occurred with time and when their lives were more different (that is, when they spent less time together; for instance, if they grew up in different homes and had different medical histories).

3. Health literacy[35]
    a. People with higher education have higher health literacy rates.
    b. Those with low health literacy have higher rates of hospital admissions and physician visits. They have less knowledge and poorer management of serious health conditions such as HIV/AIDs, asthma, or diabetes.
4. Local environmental conditions
    a. Air pollution
    b. Secondhand smoke
    c. Water supply
    d. Food deserts
    e. War, famine, earthquakes, and other natural disasters

f) Socioeconomic status

1. Lower socioeconomic status correlates with poorer health regardless of country studied.[36,37,38]
2. Racial minorities receive lower-quality care and have less access to interventions.[39]
3. Among socioeconomic factors, higher education is the best predictor of good health.[37,40]

g) Disparities in health outcomes and health care result from different underlying rates of illness that occur because of[39]:

1. Genetic predisposition
2. Local environmental conditions
3. Poorer care
4. Poor lifestyle choices
5. Different care-seeking behaviors
6. Linguistic barriers
7. Lack of trust in health care providers

OBJECTIVE 5

Interpret the scientific evidence that demonstrates the association of risk conditions (from unhealthy behaviors) as key to health outcomes

1) Interheart Study[41]

a) This was a standardized case control study about acute myocardial infarction (AMI) risk factors. The study evaluated all patients who were admitted to a cardiac care or equivalent unit for their first myocardial infarction. Data was gathered from participating centers in 52 countries.

b) The study identified nine significant worldwide risk factors for AMIs. The risk factors were similar across gender, race/ethnicity, and physical location. They included: smoking, lipids, hypertension, diabetes, obesity, diet, physical inactivity, alcohol consumption, and psychosocial factors.

c) Five of the factors identified (smoking, lipids, hypertension, diabetes, and obesity) accounted for 80% of the population-attributable risk for AMI.

d) Nine risk factors accounted for more than 90% attributable risk percent of AMI risk in men and 94% in women.

e) Psychosocial risk factors are seldom given the priority they deserve (e.g., stress, mental illness, isolation, and addictions). This study found that psychological risk factors were comparable to the effect of high blood pressure and abdominal obesity (population attributable risk of 33%).

2) InterSTROKE Study[42]

a) This was a prospective case-control study used to determine stroke risk factors based on data from 32 countries.

b) Ten significant risk factors worldwide were identified for strokes: hypertension, current smoking, abdominal obesity, unhealthy diet, physical inactivity, diabetes, alcohol intake, psychological stress, depression, cardiac causes, and abnormal lipids.

c) Those 10 lifestyle-related risk factors were associated with 90% of the risk of stroke in men and women of all ages.

3) Chicago Heart Association Detection Project in Industry[43]:

a) The project showed that risk of heart disease is determined by the number of cardiac risk factors a person has. It also showed an association between people who were lower risk in middle age (meaning they had fewer risk factors present at that life stage), with a better quality of life at older ages, and with lower Medicare costs.

b) Men at low risk had less than 2/3 total charges ($1,615 less than the control population).

c) Women at low risk had less than 1/2 total charges ($1,885 less than the control population).

4) Making the six changes in Table 1.2 can reduce risk of heart disease by as much as 90–95%[44]

Table 1.2 Lifestyle Changes to Reduce Risk of Heart Disease

Lifestyle Change	% Reduction In Risk Of Heart Disease
1. 50% decrease in total cholesterol	50%
2. 6 mmHg decrease in diastolic pressure	16% (42% reduction in stroke risk)
3. Smoking cessation	50% risk of sudden heart attack
4. Maintain ideal body weight and waist size	35–55%
5. ≥150 minutes per week of moderate exercise	35–55%
6. ≥5 servings of fruits and vegetables per day	20–25%

5) Framingham Heart Study[45]

a) The study looked at the lifetime risk for atherosclerotic cardiovascular disease in people who were free of cardiovascular disease at age 50 and found that:

1. Men with optimal risk status had a 5% lifetime risk of atherosclerotic cardiovascular disease versus men with two or more risk factors, who had a 69% lifetime risk.
2. Women with optimal risk status had an 8% lifetime risk versus women with two or more risk factors, who had a 50% lifetime risk.

b) Men and women with optimal risk status had a median life expectancy of about 10 years longer than people with two or more risk factors at age 50 (11+ years for men, 8+ years for women).

6) Multiple Risk Factor Intervention Trial (MRFIT) Study[46,47]

a) People with low-risk factor status had:

1. 73–85% lower risk for cardiovascular disease mortality
2. 40–60% lower total mortality rate
3. 6–10 years greater life expectancy

7) Nurses' Health Study[48]

a) This prospective study looked at the relative risk for coronary heart disease over 14 years in 84,129 women.

b) The study identified five health factors associated with a lower risk of coronary heart disease:

1. Absence of smoking
2. BMI <25 kg/m^2
3. Physically active 30 minutes per day
4. Moderate alcohol consumption (5–30 grams or 0.2–1 ounce per day)
5. A healthy diet score.
    a. For this study, diet scores were based on the intake of three key items: dietary intake of cereal fiber, marine omega-3 fatty acids, and folate. Diet scores were then categorized into one of five quintiles from most healthy, or highest intake of the three key items, to least healthy. Women who ate in the upper 40%, or the top two quintiles, were considered to have a healthy diet score.

c) When all five factors above were present versus none, there was an 82% lower risk of coronary heart disease, as shown in Table 1.3.

Table 1.3 Health Factors that Lower Risk of Coronary Heart Disease

Group	% Women	# CV Events	RR	95% CI	PAR	95% CI
3 low-risk factors: • Diet score in the upper 40% • Nonsmoking • Moderate-vigorous exercise ≥30 min/day	12.7%	106	0.46	0.37–0.55	51%	42–60%
4 low-risk factors: • 3 + BMI <25 kg/m^2	7.2%	44	0.38	0.28–0.51	60%	47–70%
5 low-risk factors: • 4 + Alcohol ≥5g per day	3.1%	12	0.25	0.14–0.44	74%	55–86%

CV=cardiovascular, RR=relative risk, PAR=population attributable risk, CI=confidence interval, BMI=body mass index

8) **Three large prospective studies—The Nurses' Health Study (described above), Nurses' Health Study 2, and Health Professionals Follow-Up Study—analyzed the effects of healthful versus unhealthful plant-based diets and risk of coronary heart disease.**[49]

- **a)** The study included more than 4,833,042 total person-years of follow-up and documented 8,631 cases of coronary heart disease.
- **b)** The pooled multivariate analyses found that higher adherence to a healthy plant-based diet was independently inversely associated with coronary heart disease (hazard ratio [HR] comparing extreme deciles: 0.92; 95% CI: 0.83 to 1.01; p trend = 0.003).
- **c)** The healthier the plant-based diet (less processed, more whole foods), the stronger the inverse association with coronary heart disease (HR: 0.75; 95% CI: 0.68 to 0.83; p trend <0.001).
- **d)** Conversely, an unhealthy plant-based diet was positively associated with coronary heart disease (HR: 1.32; 95% CI: 1.20 to 1.46; p trend <0.001).

9) **Adventist Health Study 2**[50]

- **a)** The study found a reduced risk of mortality in people consuming a total vegetarian diet versus a non-vegetarian diet from (Figure 1.1):

1.	All-causes	HR = 0.85
2.	Ischemic heart disease	HR = 0.90
3.	Cardiovascular disease	HR = 0.91
4.	Cancer	HR = 0.92
5.	Other causes	HR = 0.74

Figure 1.1 Mortality for Diet-types in AHS-2

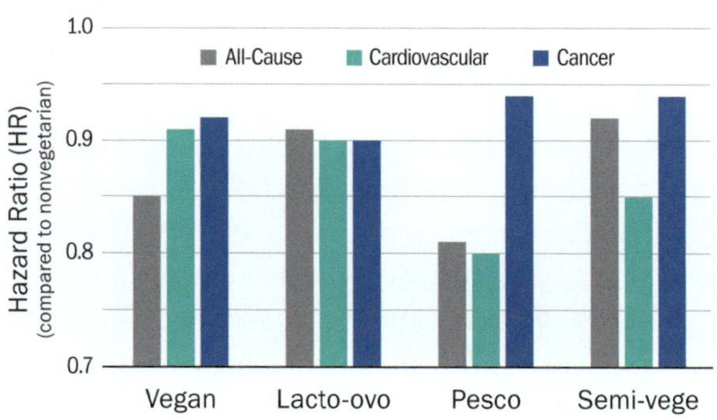

- **b)** The study also found a linear relationship between a total vegetarian diet versus a non-vegetarian diet. Having a total vegetarian diet was associated with a lower BMI and with lower odds of having diabetes, hypertension, or metabolic syndrome.[51]

Table 1.4 Relationship Between BMI and diet

Condition	Vegan	Nonvegetarian
1. Higher BMI	23.6 ± 4.4	28.8 ± 6.3
2. Diabetes	OR = 0.51 (0.40 to 0.66)	
3. Hypertension	OR = 0.37 (0.19 to 0.74)	
4. METs	OR = 0.44 (0.30 to 0.64)	

OR=Odds Ratio

10) The Lyon Diet Heart Study[52]

a) This study looked at secondary prevention of coronary heart disease with a Mediterranean diet vs. the American Heart Association Step 1 diet.

   1. Of those eating the Mediterranean diet, the protective effects of the Mediterranean dietary pattern were maintained for 4 years following a study subject's first heart attack.
   2. Survival analyses are shown below in Figure 1.2:

Figure 1.2 Lyon Diet Heart Study Results

A.

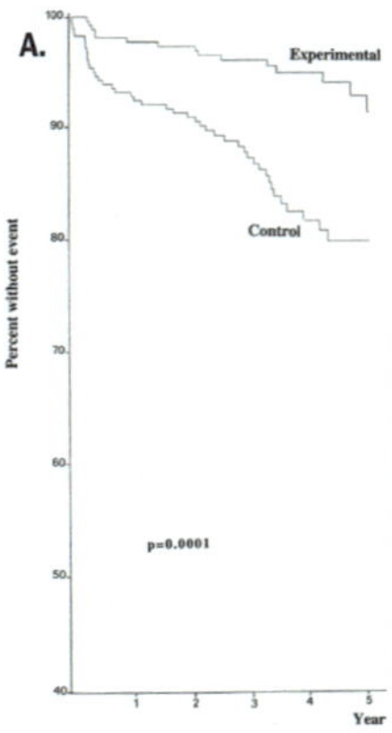

Figure A. Cumulative survival without nonfatal myocardial infarction (CO 1) among experimental (Mediterranean group) patients and control subjects.

B.

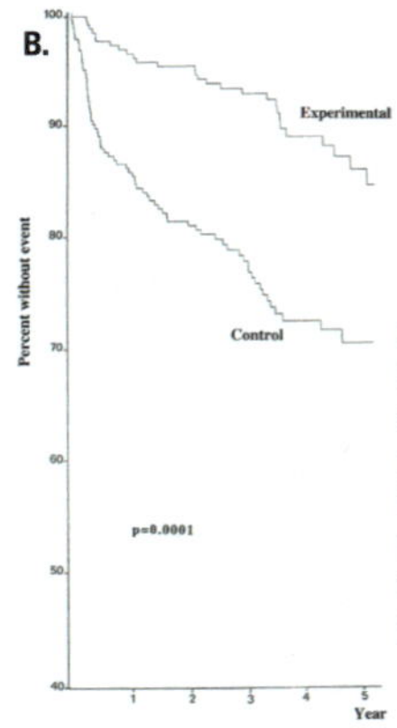

Figure B. Cumulative survival without nonfatal infarction and without major secondary end points (CO 2).

C.

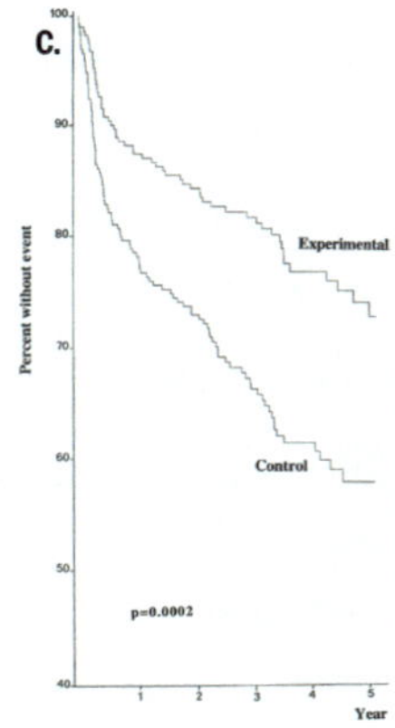

Figure C. Cumulative survival without nonfatal infarction, without major secondary end points, and without minor secondary end points (CO 3).

OBJECTIVE 6

Compare and contrast to other fields of health and medicine

1) Lifestyle medicine

a) Lifestyle medicine is a distinct field of medicine aimed at "treating the cause" of most of our modern diseases with the strongest evidence-based modalities available. Since most modern diseases are caused by lifestyle, lifestyle changes must be part of the cure. Although portions of lifestyle medicine (especially nutrition and physical activity), are included in other fields of medicine, lifestyle medicine is distinct because lifestyle change is prescribed as the first line and most important therapy for disease treatment and reversal. Evidence-based medications and other modalities are used, but only to supplement changes in lifestyle.

   1. Lifestyle medicine requires patient engagement and responsibility for treatment outcomes.
   2. Treatments are long-term.
   3. The provider acts as both medical expert and coach.
   4. Unlike most non-lifestyle medical services, lifestyle medicine saves costs.

b) Lifestyle medicine elements and intervention modalities include:

   1. Predominantly whole food plant-based diet
   2. Physical activity
   3. Stress management and emotional wellness
   4. Sleep
   5. Smoking cessation and avoiding risky substance abuse
   6. Positive psychology and connectedness

2) **Complementary and alternative medicine**

   a) This is an approach to medical care that is not currently considered part of conventional medicine. It uses complementary (together with conventional medicine) and/or alternative (in place of conventional medicine) treatments that historically have not been well-researched.

   b) Evidence-based complementary modalities are appropriate and should be utilized, whereas non-evidence-based alternative treatments should be excluded.

3) **Integrative medicine**

   a) This field of medicine addresses the patient's whole-person needs (physical, social, emotional, mental, environmental, and spiritual) through a combination of conventional, complementary, and alternative medicine.

   b) By definition it "integrates" experience-based complementary and alternative medicine methods with evidence-based conventional methods. Some see this as a strength, while others view it as weakening the practice of conventional evidence-based medicine.

4) **Functional medicine**

   a) This practice of medicine focuses on the physiologic and biochemical functions of the body (from cells to organ systems) and investigates the balance and processes of cellular metabolism, digestive function, detoxification, and control of oxidative stress.

   b) It tends to emphasize testing of various hormones and metabolites in the body that are not well-proven or generally accepted within evidence-based medicine and, thus, is still somewhat controversial.

5) **Mind-body medicine**

   a) Mind-body medicine investigates the interactions between the body and mind—behaviorally, emotionally, mentally, socially, and spiritually. It treats with modalities like relaxation, hypnosis, visual imagery, meditation, yoga, biofeedback, spirituality, and tai chi, among others.

   b) Some mind-body medicine is very solidly evidence-based, while other aspects are still unproven.

6) **Preventive medicine**

   a) This field includes all aspects of morbidity and mortality prevention for the general public, meaning it oversees the field of public health.

   b) It emphasizes population-based interventions, which include immunizations, screening, and protection from bioterrorism.

7) **Conventional medicine**

   a) In conventional medicine, medications or surgical interventions are often the highest level of care and "end" of treatment. Disease is thought to occur from exposure to a pathogen, environmental factor, or genetic predisposition. Treatments may be acute for targeting pathogens, or they may be long-term for controlling disease and/or risk factors that can reduce or degrade long-term primary and secondary outcomes.

   b) In conventional medicine's disease-focused approach, patients are the recipients of care, and other than complying with the treatment, they are not required to make significant changes. Providers are considered responsible for care and outcomes, while the patient is a passive receiver of medical services.

Notes on Disease Reversal

- The definition of "disease reversal" remains quite controversial. Some feel genuine disease reversal or cure may only be achieved with acute infectious processes, like bacterial pneumonia or strep throat; whereas others believe lifelong remission such as that which occurs after successful cancer treatment, resolution of diabetes after bariatric surgery, or intensive lifestyle change, may also be considered a cure from the disease.[53]
- In this manual, disease reversal is defined as: All laboratory markers or diagnostic tests of a disease are within normal range, without current use of any medications, and no present signs or symptoms of disease.
- "Control" of a chronic disease describes improvement in laboratory markers and diagnostic testing to accepted standard levels but without complete normalization of laboratory markers or diagnostic testing. This may be achieved with or without the current use of medication or medical interventions.

OBJECTIVE 7

Indicate the place and priority of lifestyle medicine in the spectrum of treatment options for chronic (lifestyle-related) diseases

OBJECTIVE 8

Describe the efficacy of lifestyle medicine and its impact on disease pathophysiology

1) **Lifestyle medicine is a foundational part of medical care. It offers effective prevention and treatment, provides people with more control over their health, and is essential for disease reversal.**[2]
   a) Lifestyle medicine decreases reliance on medication and therefore reduces medication side effects.
      1. For example, Sarathi and colleagues studied Asian youth who were newly diagnosed with type 2 diabetes and found that intensive lifestyle therapy alone, or in combination with metformin if hemoglobin A1c was greater than 9.0%, could be used to achieve reversal or partial remission of diabetes within 3 months and maintain it during the 2-year follow up.[54]
   b) It is more effective. Lifestyle was almost twice as effective as metformin in the Diabetes Prevention Program[55] and exercise was 26% more effective than PTCA in CAD patients.[56]
   c) It offers safer control of some biological markers than some medications (Jenkin's Portfolio Diet offered equivalent cholesterol control without the concerning side-effects that were seen with the use of a low-dose statin medication).[57]
2) **Effective use of lifestyle medicine can lower health care costs and make the health care system more sustainable, as demonstrated by the following studies:**
   a) Results from the Diabetes Prevention Program and the Diabetes Prevention Program Outcomes Study[58]
   b) Effectiveness of program modification strategies of the Diabetes Prevention Program[59]

c) The results published in "CHIP Lifestyle Program at Vanderbilt University Demonstrates an Early ROI for a Diabetic Cohort in a Workplace Setting"[59]

3) **Health care financing in the United States**

   a) Health care costs continue to climb, and the system is quickly becoming unstable and unsustainable, complicated by health care repeals and replacements.

   b) Employers and the government have become the main payers in health insurance costs, destroying self-balancing marketplace forces.

   c) Direct-to-consumer marketing is legal in the United States and is increasing the demand for pharmaceuticals and interventions.

   d) America is ill-prepared to embrace lifestyle medicine, as almost all reimbursement incentives are misaligned.

4) **Conventional health care influences**

   a) The prevalent belief is that pharmaceuticals, supplements, and biochemical treatments are the key to health and longevity.

   b) The internet has become a new modality for sharing health information through websites, communities, and electronic patient portals. Overall, the field of medicine has not fully embraced this new technology, and patient communication and education are still mainly provided through old operating systems, such as paper documents and charting, telephone calls, and in-person meetings.

SECTION 1 GLOSSARY

Disease reversal: all laboratory markers or diagnostic tests are within normal range without current use of any medications and without present signs or symptoms of the disease.

Intensive therapeutic lifestyle change (ITLC) programs: treatment programs that encourage dramatic changes in one's daily routine, including habits around sleep, diet, physical activity, and stress management. The program is usually administered in a group setting, and it always involves a multi-modality, multidisciplinary team.

Plant-based diet: a plant-based diet consists mostly of food from plants (such as whole-grains, vegetables, fruits, beans, and legumes), with little to no animal products (such as dairy, meat, and eggs).

SECTION 1 REVIEW QUESTIONS

1. **Which of the following refers to a discipline other than lifestyle medicine?**
   - **A.** Assisting patients in enhancing their diets with whole foods, incorporating physical activity and emotional well-being practices, and avoiding risky substances. Medications are used as an adjunct.
   - **B.** Evidence-based reversal, treatment, and prevention of chronic diseases related to lifestyle and behaviors.
   - **C.** Holistic approaches to balance core functional processes, control oxidative stresses at a cellular level, and promote detoxification.
   - **D.** Collaborative techniques that apply medical, behavioral, motivational, and environmental principles to encourage patients to adopt and sustain healthy behavior changes.

2. **Which statement best describes the core competencies for prescribing lifestyle medicine, as identified by the 2010 national consensus panel?**
   - **A.** The use of an interdisciplinary team, such as a coach, dietitian, and physician, is counterproductive in creating the office and community support needed for sustained behavior change.
   - **B.** The core competencies were created to help medical specialists prescribe interventions that promote healthy lifestyle practices.
   - **C.** Leadership is one of the key areas of the competencies and focuses on leading teams to better diagnose chronic conditions and implement standard of care treatments.
   - **D.** Quality improvement projects, such as measuring interventions, tracking outcomes, and implementing process improvements, are part of the practice of lifestyle medicine physicians.

3. **This ability is required by providers in the practice of lifestyle medicine:**
   - **A.** Ignore national guidelines in lifestyle prescriptions.
   - **B.** Make no referrals to community resources or other health professionals.
   - **C.** Recognize the interactions between the mind, body, and behavior, and prescribe appropriate biofeedback techniques.
   - **D.** Expand vital signs to include tobacco use, sleep, stress, and emotional well-being.

4. **Lifestyle medicine and conventional medicine differ in their approach to patient care. Which statement most correctly compares lifestyle medicine and conventional medicine?**
   - **A.** In conventional medicine, the patient is an active partner in care. Whereas, in lifestyle medicine, the patient is a passive recipient.
   - **B.** Conventional medicine treatments are always acute, whereas lifestyle medicine treatments are always long term.
   - **C.** Risk factors and causes are treated in conventional medicine, while the effects of disease are treated with lifestyle medicine.
   - **D.** Patients are not required to make big changes in health behaviors in conventional medicine. However, in lifestyle medicine, patients are asked to move toward substantial behavior changes.

5. **Regarding adverse drug reactions, which one of the following is correct?**
   - **A.** They seldom occur with appropriate use.
   - **B.** They are a small proportion of the causes of death in the US, ranking lower than pulmonary disease, diabetes, AIDS, pneumonia, accidents, and motor vehicle accidents.
   - **C.** There are fewer than 2,000 serious reactions per year.
   - **D.** The total cost of adverse drug reactions is greater than that of cardiovascular disease or diabetes.

SECTION 1 REVIEW QUESTION ANSWERS AND SUMMARIES

1. **Answer: C.** Functional medicine is defined as a holistic approach that is used to balance core functional processes in the body, such as cellular metabolism, control of oxidative stress, detoxification, and digestive function. Evidence-based interventions that use a whole food plant-based diet, physical activity, emotional well-being, and risky substance avoidance are foundational interventions used in lifestyle medicine to prevent, treat, and reverse disease. Medications and supplements are adjuncts to these lifestyle changes. Lifestyle medicine requires persistent treatment with medical, behavioral, motivational, and environmental principles to help individuals adopt and sustain healthy behavior changes.

2. **Answer: D.** An interdisciplinary team is considered imperative to effectively produce and sustain lifestyle change. The core competencies for prescribing lifestyle medicine were created to guide primary care providers, although those competencies can also be applied to most specialties. Certainly, physicians should implement processes to diagnose and treat chronic conditions with excellence, but leadership in lifestyle medicine involves much more, including an emphasis on disease prevention, community advocacy, and the creation of personal and professional environments of health. Tracking performance measures is one of the competencies for lifestyle medicine physicians.

3. **Answer: D.** A lifestyle medicine physician should asses tobacco use, sleep, stress, and emotional well-being. One should be able to assess the social, psychological, and biological predispositions that drive a patient's behavior and the resulting health outcomes, but prescribing biofeedback is not the appropriate lifestyle intervention.

4. **Answer: D.** In conventional medicine patients are not generally required to make big changes in health behaviors, whereas in lifestyle medicine, patients are asked to make substantial lifestyle changes. In the conventional medicine approach, the responsibility for health care falls mainly on the provider, and the patient is a passive recipient. The change required by patients revolves mainly around being compliant with medications and medical interventions, which are generally viewed as the highest level of care. However, in lifestyle medicine, the responsibility for health remains with the patients. They must be active participants in their health care in order to make substantial changes necessary to treat the unhealthy lifestyle behaviors that are the cause of most chronic diseases.

5. **Answer: D.** The total cost is greater than cardiovascular disease or diabetes.[60] They are estimated to be between the fourth and sixth leading cause of death in the US, ranking higher than Alzheimer's disease, diabetes, AIDS, pneumonia, accidents, and motor vehicle accidents.[61]

SECTION 1 REFERENCES

1. American College of Lifestyle Medicine. What is lifestyle medicine? 2015; https://www.lifestylemedicine.org/ACLM/Lifestyle_Medicine/What_is_Lifestyle_Medicine/ACLM/About/What_is_Lifestyle_Medicine_/Lifestyle_Medicine.aspx?hkey=26f3eb6b-8294-4a63-83de-35d429c3bb88. Accessed May 21, 2018.
2. Lianov L., Johnson M. Physician competencies for prescribing lifestyle medicine. *JAMA*. 2010;304(2):202-203.
3. Egger G., Binns A., Rossner, S. *Lifestyle Medicine: Managing Diseases of Lifestyle in the 21st Century*. New York, NY: McGraw-Hill; 2010.
4. Kelly J.H. High Intensity therapeutic lifestyle change. In: Rippe J., ed. *Lifestyle Medicine*. 3rd ed. Boca Raton, FL: CRC Press; 2019:Chapter 87.
5. Rankin P., Morton D. P., Diehl H., Gobble J., Morey P., Chang E. Effectiveness of a volunteer-delivered lifestyle modification program for reducing cardiovascular disease risk factors. *Am J Cardiol.* 2012;109(1):82-86.
6. Barnard R. J., Lattimore L., Holly R. G., Cherny S., Pritikin N. Response of non-insulin-dependent diabetic patients to an intensive program of diet and exercise. *Diabetes Care.* 1982;5(4):370-374.
7. Ornish D., Scherwitz L. W., Billings J. H., et al. Intensive lifestyle changes for reversal of coronary heart disease. *JAMA*. 1998;280(23):2001-2007. http://jamanetwork.com/journals/jama/fullarticle/188274.
8. Ornish D., Brown S. E., Scherwitz L. W., et al. Can lifestyle changes reverse coronary heart disease? The Lifestyle Heart Trial. *Lancet.* 1990;336(8708):129-133.
9. Diehl H. A. Coronary risk reduction through intensive community-based lifestyle intervention: the Coronary Health Improvement Project (CHIP) experience. *Am J Cardiol.* 1998;82(10b):83t-87t.
10. Esselstyn C. B. Jr., Gendy G., Doyle J., Golubic M., Roizen M. F. A way to reverse CAD? *J Fam Pract*. 2014;63(7):356-364b.
11. Esselstyn C. B. Jr. In cholesterol lowering, moderation kills. *Cleve Clin J Med*. 2000;67(8):560-564.
12. Guthrie G. Definition of lifestyle medicine. In: Rippe J., ed. *Lifestyle Medicine*. 3rd ed. Boca Raton, FL: CRC Press; 2019:Chapter 82.
13. Cardenas D. Let not thy food be confused with thy medicine: the Hippocratic misquotation. *ESPEN J*. 2013;8(6):e260-e262. https://doi.org/10.1016/j.clnme.2013.10.002.
14. Evidence in Motion. The doctor of the future. June 5, 2017; https://evidenceinmotion.com/the-doctor-of-the-future. Accessed December 10, 2020.
15. Thieszen C. L., Merrill R. M., Aldana S. G., et al. The Coronary Health Improvement Project (CHIP) for lowering weight and improving psychosocial health. *Psychol Rep*. 2011;109(1):338-352.
16. World Health Organization. Diet, nutrition, and the prevention of chronic diseases. 1990. Updated 2003. https://www.who.int/news/item/23-04-2003-fao-who-launch-expert-report-on-diet-nutrition-and-prevention-of-chronic-diseases.
17. Rippe J. M. *Lifestyle Medicine*. 2nd ed. Boca Raton, FL: CRC Press; 2013:1638.
18. Wikipedia. Blue-ribbon committee. Updated July, 2020; https://en.wikipedia.org/wiki/Blue-ribbon_committee. Accessed December 10, 2020.
19. US Department of Health and Human Services. Healthy people: 2018. Published May 18, 2018; https://www.healthypeople.gov/. Accessed 2018.
20. US Department of Health and Human Services Office of the Surgeon General. *National Prevention Strategy: America's Plan for Better Health and Wellness*. Washington, DC; National Prevention Council; 2011.
21. US Department of Health and Human Services. Report to Congress: *National Strategy for Quality Improvement in Health Care*. Washington, DC; US Department of Health and Human Services; 2011. https://www.ahrq.gov/sites/default/files/wysiwyg/workingforquality/nqs2011annlrpt.pdf.
22. Bodai B. I., Nakata T. E., Wong W. T., et al. Lifestyle medicine: a brief review of its dramatic impact on health and survival. *Perm J*. 2018;22:17-025. https://pubmed.ncbi.nlm.nih.gov/29035175.
23. Centers for Disease Control and Prevention. *Mortality in the United States, 2018 NCHS Data Brief No. 355*. January, 2020. https://www.cdc.gov/nchs/products/databriefs/db355.htm. Accessed December, 2020.
24. Mokdad A. H., Marks J. S., Stroup D. F., Gerberding J. L. Actual causes of death in the United States, 2000. *JAMA*. 2004;291(10):1238-1245.
25. Danaei G., Ding E. L., Mozaffarian D., et al. The preventable causes of death in the United States: comparative risk assessment of dietary, lifestyle, and metabolic risk factors. *PLoS Med*. 2009;6(4):e1000058.
26. Reeves M. J., Rafferty A. P. Healthy lifestyle characteristics among adults in the United States, 2000. *Arch Intern Med*. 2005;165(8):854-857.
27. Jamal A., Phillips E., Gentzke A. S., et al. Current cigarette smoking among adults - United States, 2016. *MMWR Morb Mortal Wkly Rep*. 2018;67(2):53-59.
28. HHS and USDA release new dietary guidelines to encourage healthy eating patterns to prevent chronic diseases. News release. January 7, 2016. Office of Disease Prevention and Health Promotion. https://health.gov/news-archive/blog/2016/01/press-release/index.html. Accessed 2018.
29. Oza-Frank R., Cheng Y. J., Narayan K. M., Gregg E. W. Trends in nutrient intake among adults with diabetes in the United States: 1988-2004. *J Am Diet Assoc*. 2009;109(7):1173-1178.
30. Soni A., Walter K., Ward S. M., Jones H. Geratology rehabilitation units are not just for stroke. *BMJ*. 2007;334(7586):170.
31. Mohamedali B., Shroff A. Impact of smoking status on cardiovascular outcomes following percutaneous coronary intervention. *Clin Cardiol*. 2013;36(7):372-377.

32. Hughes K., Bellis M. A., Hardcastle K. A., et al. The effect of multiple adverse childhood experiences on health: a systematic review and meta-analysis. *Lancet Public Health*. 2017;2(8):e356-e366.
33. Monnat S. M., Chandler R. F. Long term physical health consequences of adverse childhood experiences. *Sociol Q*. 2015;56(4):723-752.
34. Fraga M. F., Ballestar E., Paz M. F., et al. Epigenetic differences arise during the lifetime of monozygotic twins. *Proc Nat Acad Sci USA*. 2005;102(30):10604-10609.
35. Vernon J. A., Trujillo, A., Rosenbaum, S., DeBuono, B. *Low Health Literacy: Implications for National Health Policy*. Department of Health Policy, School of Public Health and Health Services, The George Washington University; 2007. https://hsrc.himmelfarb.gwu.edu/cgi/viewcontent.cgi?article=1173&context=sphhs_policy_facpubs.
36. Marmot M. The influence of income on health: views of an epidemiologist. *Health Aff (Millwood)*. 2002;21(2):31-46.
37. Chen E. Why socioeconomic status affects the health of children: a psychosocial perspective. *Curr Dir Psychol Sci*. 2004;13(3):112-115
38. Marmot M. G., Shipley M. J., Rose G. Inequalities in death–specific explanations of a general pattern? *Lancet*. 1984;1(8384):1003-1006.
39. Katz D. L., Elmore J. G., Wild D., et al. *Jekel's Epidemiology, Biostatistics, Preventive Medicine, and Public Health*. New York, NY: Elsevier Health Sciences; 2013.
40. Winkleby M. A., Fortmann S. P., Rockhill B. Trends in cardiovascular disease risk factors by educational level: the Stanford Five-City Project. *Prev Med*. 1992;21(5):592-601.
41. Yusuf S., Hawken S., Ounpuu S., et al. Effect of potentially modifiable risk factors associated with myocardial infarction in 52 countries (the INTERHEART study): case-control study. *Lancet*. 2004;364(9438):937-952.
42. O'Donnell M. J., Chin S. L., Rangarajan S., et al. Global and regional effects of potentially modifiable risk factors associated with acute stroke in 32 countries (INTERSTROKE): a case-control study. *Lancet*. 2016;388(10046):761-775
43. Daviglus M. L., Liu K., Yan L. L., et al. Body mass index in middle age and health-related quality of life in older age: the Chicago heart association detection project in industry study. *Arch Intern Med*. 2003;163(20):2448-2455.
44. Lloyd-Jones D. M., Dyer A. R., Wang R., Daviglus M. L., Greenland P. Risk factor burden in middle age and lifetime risks for cardiovascular and non-cardiovascular death (Chicago Heart Association Detection Project in Industry). *Am J Cardiol*. 2007;99(4):535-540. https://pubmed.ncbi.nlm.nih.gov/17293199.
45. Lloyd-Jones D. M., Leip E. P., Larson M. G., et al. Prediction of lifetime risk for cardiovascular disease by risk factor burden at 50 years of age. *Circulation*. 2006;113(6):791-798.
46. Multiple risk factor intervention trial. Risk factor changes and mortality results. Multiple Risk Factor Intervention Trial Research Group. *JAMA*. 1982;248(12):1465-1477.
47. Stamler J., Daviglus M. L., Garside D. B., Dyer A. R., Greenland P., Neaton J. D. Relationship of baseline serum cholesterol levels in 3 large cohorts of younger men to long-term coronary, cardiovascular, and all-cause mortality and to longevity. *JAMA*. 2000;284(3):311-318.
48. Stampfer M. J., Hu F. B., Manson J. E., Rimm E. B., Willett W. C. Primary prevention of coronary heart disease in women through diet and lifestyle. *N Engl J Med*. 2000;343(1):16-22.
49. Satija A., Bhupathiraju S. N., Spiegelman D., et al. Healthful and unhealthful plant-based diets and the risk of coronary heart disease in US adults. *J Am Coll Cardiol*. 2017;70(4):411-422.
50. Orlich M. J., Singh P. N., Sabate J., et al. Vegetarian dietary patterns and mortality in Adventist Health Study 2. *JAMA Intern Med*. 2013;173(13):1230-1238.
51. Orlich M. J., Fraser G. E. Vegetarian diets in the Adventist Health Study 2: a review of initial published findings. *Am J Clin Nutr*. 2014;100 Suppl 1(1):353S-358S. https://pubmed.ncbi.nlm.nih.gov/24898223.
52. de Lorgeril M., Salen P., Martin J. L. Mediterranean diet, traditional risk factors and the rate of cardiovascular complications after myocardial infarction: final report of the Lyon Diet Heart Study. *Circulation*. 1999;99(6):779-785. http://dx.doi.org/10.1161/01.CIR.99.6.779.
53. Buse J. B., Caprio S., Cefalu W. T., et al. How do we define cure of diabetes? *Diabetes Care*. 2009;32(11):2133-2135.
54. Sarathi V., Kolly A., Chaithanya H. B., Dwarakanath C. S. High rates of diabetes reversal in newly diagnosed Asian Indian young adults with type 2 diabetes mellitus with intensive lifestyle therapy. *J Nat Sci Biol Med*. 2017;8(1):60-63.
55. Knowler W. C., Barrett-Connor E., Fowler S. E., et al. Reduction in the incidence of type 2 diabetes with lifestyle intervention or metformin. *N Engl J Med*. 2002;346(6):393-403.
56. Hambrecht R., Walther C., Möbius-Winkler S., et al. Percutaneous coronary angioplasty compared with exercise training in patients with stable coronary artery disease: a randomized trial. *Circulation*. 2004;109(11):1371-1378.
57. Jenkins D. J., Kendall C. W., Marchie A., et al. Effects of a dietary portfolio of cholesterol-lowering foods vs lovastatin on serum lipids and C-reactive protein. *JAMA*. 2003;290(4):502-510.
58. Herman W. H. The cost-effectiveness of diabetes prevention: results from the Diabetes Prevention Program and the Diabetes Prevention Program Outcomes Study. *Clin Diabetes Endocrinol*. 2015;1:9.
59. Shurney D., Hyde S., Hulsey K., Elam R., Cooper A., Groves J. CHIP lifestyle program at Vanderbilt University demonstrates an early ROI for a diabetic cohort in a workplace setting: a case study. *J Manag Care Med*. 2012;15:5-15.
60. Lazarou J., Pomeranz B. H., Corey P. N. Incidence of adverse drug reactions in hospitalized patients: a meta-analysis of prospective studies. *JAMA*. 1998;279(15):1200-1205.
61. Davies E. C., Green C. F., Mottram D. R., Pirmohamed M. Adverse drug reactions in hospitals: a narrative review. *Curr Drug Saf*. 2007;2(1):79-87.

SECTION 2
Fundamentals of Health Behavior Change

Objective 1 Demonstrate the key elements of conducting patient-readiness assessments and stage-matched responses **27**

Objective 2 Describe the process of building effective relationships with patients **27**

Objective 3 Apply motivational interviewing, cognitive behavioral techniques, and positive psychology techniques to the behavior change process **29**

Objective 4 Develop a written action plan based on the treatment prescription adjusted for the appropriate stage of change **33**

Objective 5 Demonstrate use of readiness, importance, and confidence scales **35**

Objective 6 Describe strategies for helping patients maintain healthy behaviors. **37**

Objective 7 Differentiate at least three health behavior change theories and their potential application to practice **37**

Objective 8 Identify two key constructs for effective, sustainable self-management **40**

Objective 9 List components of relapse prevention planning **41**

Objective 10 Describe the process of follow-up for ongoing lifestyle change progress, including building patient self-efficacy **42**

Objective 11 Describe the 5 A's and how to incorporate them into the office visit **43**

Objective 12 Cite the evidence base for effective coaching that promotes health behavior change and improves health outcomes. **44**

Objective 13 Describe how to create relationships with patients which foster their personal growth. **45**

Objective 14 Describe how effective coaching and creating positive relationships with patients impacts the role of self-motivation and self-confidence in successful health behavior change **45**

Objective 15 Describe the main stages of the coaching process **46**

Objective 16 List the coaching questions for each stage of change **47**

Section 2 Glossary **49**

Section 2 Review Questions **50**

Section 2 Review Questions Answers and Summaries **53**

Section 2 References **55**

OBJECTIVE 1

Demonstrate the key elements of conducting patient-readiness assessments and stage-matched responses

1) Assess the patient's readiness to change.

- **a)** Transtheoretical model-stages of change[1,2]
  1. Precontemplation
     - a. Lack of awareness of the need to change a problem health behavior
     - b. Not planning on making a change in the foreseeable future (usually defined as the next 6 months)
     - c. "I don't need to change," or, "I can't change."
  2. Contemplation
     - a. Considering making a change in the next 6 months
     - b. Ambivalent about change (weighing the pros and cons)
     - c. "I may change."
  3. Preparation
     - a. Aware of the need to make a health behavior change
     - b. Preparing to make a change within the next month
     - c. "I will change."
  4. Action
     - a. Started making specific changes but have not yet hit a target goal or engaged in the behavior for 6 months
     - b. "I am changing."
  5. Maintenance
     - a. Goal behavior is achieved, and behavior is sustained for more than 6 months
     - b. "I have been making a change for more than 6 months."
  6. Termination
     - a. Has no temptation to return to previous unhealthy behavior
     - b. "I won't return to my old habit."

2) Nonadherence

- **a)** Nonadherence describes the behavior of not following through with prescribed treatment(s).[3]
  1. This behavior accounts for the large discrepancy between prescribed treatment and the number of patients who follow through with that treatment.
  2. The rate of nonadherence for chronic illness medication regimens is 50–80%.[4]

OBJECTIVE 2

Describe the process of building effective relationships with patients

1) Providers have distinct roles as "experts" and as "coaches" who support patients in the process of enacting and sustaining behavioral change.

a) The "expert" role: Conducting medical assessments, making specific recommendations, and prescribing treatments.

b) The "coach" role: Using a collaborative communication style positioning patients in their own care.

2) **Establish effective patient-provider relationships.**

a) Assess the readiness level for change (from the transtheoretical model stages of change).

b) Offer stage-matched brief intervention ("offer" is used rather than "perform" or "conduct" because the change must have patient buy-in and ideally be the patient's idea).

c) Empower patients; help them make the change successfully.

d) Create an inclusive environment: To establish a positive and productive patient-provider relationship, providers must utilize inclusive language that makes patients feel comfortable and valued.

3) **Utilizing people-first language is a way to respect and honor patients instead of defining them by a disease, condition, or disorder. Using this language helps to ensure a safe and supportive environment in which patients are more inclined to discuss health behaviors.**

a) For example, it is more respectful to say "a patient with diabetes" as opposed to "a diabetic," or "a patient with obesity" as opposed to "an obese patient."

b) People-first language should be used when speaking directly to patients and when speaking about patients with other professionals within the care team.

4) **Additional care should be taken when discussing weight and lifestyle interventions in the office[5,6]**

a) Most people with obesity have made numerous prior attempts to lose weight. Acknowledge their previous efforts and investment in health.

b) The cause of obesity is complex, and the treatment is ongoing.

c) The treatment of obesity is a sensitive and personal topic. Ask permission to check the patient's weight, and then check their weight in private. Additionally, discussing weight should never be done as a way to humiliate, blame, shame, degrade, or characterize people.

d) Utilizing the skills of motivational interviewing (see Objective 3, #1) can be helpful in discussing lifestyle changes in a way that enhances patient self-efficacy and demonstrates the provider's commitment to being a trusted partner in the behavior change journey.[6]

e) Further information for clinicians may be found in guidelines for the management of overweight and obesity in adults.[7]

5) **Collaborate with qualified health and wellness coaches for additional patient support.**

a) The National Board for Health & Wellness Coaching (NBHWC), in partnership with the National Board of Medical Examiners, provides national board certification for health and wellness coaches.

b) NBHWC maintains a directory of national board-certified health & wellness coaches (NBC-HWC) to help providers identify, collaborate with, and refer to qualified coaches. The latter can provide additional support to patients in the behavior change journey.

OBJECTIVE 3

Apply motivational interviewing, cognitive behavioral techniques, and positive psychology techniques to the behavior change process

1) Motivational interviewing (MI)[8,9,10]

- **a)** Most helpful in the precontemplation and contemplation stages
- **b)** Four general principles of MI are:
  1. Expressing empathy and showing an understanding of the patient and their situation.
  2. Support self-efficacy, which is the patient's confidence in their ability to succeed.
  3. Roll with resistance, you can avoid or deflect resistance by remaining nonjudgmental, listening well, and encouraging the patient to continue to share.
  4. Show the discrepancy between where the patient is and what the patient wants. Hold this up to the patient, without being judgmental, to allow the patient to draw their own conclusions.
- **c)** Four core skills of MI are:
  1. Open-ended questions: questions that cannot be answered with a one- or two-word response.
     - a. Open-ended questions invite the patient to provide more thoughtful, narrative-like responses, which allows the patient and provider to collaboratively explore the patient's needs, expectations, experiences, feelings, ideas, and priorities.
     - b. Open-ended questions often begin with the word "what" or "how," or they may begin with a phrase such as "tell me more" to invite the patient to elaborate on something that has been shared.
  2. Affirmations: genuine statements that accentuate a patient's strengths, intentions, or effort. Unlike praise or compliments, affirmations seek to enhance patient self-efficacy by recognizing the patient's strengths, intentions, or efforts.
     - a. The most effective affirmations use the word "you" rather than "I" to support patients in creating a more positive perception of their abilities and efforts and recognize and leverage their own strengths.
  3. Reflections: actively listening and intentionally offering a statement that conveys interest and empathy while also seeking to understand what the patient is saying to guide the conversation forward.
     - a. The type and depth of reflections can vary (see Objective 15, 2.b).
  4. Summaries: provide a recap of what the patient has shared.
     - a. A summary can be given at the end of a visit and during the visit to transition from one topic to another.

2) Cognitive behavioral therapy (CBT)[11]

- **a)** CBT is most useful during the preparation, action, and maintenance stages.
- **b)** CBT assists with problem-solving and a deeper understanding of underlying challenges.
- **c)** Behavioral health specialists generally perform CBT, however, providers can apply basic principles using a "coach" approach.

1. Before beginning CBT with a patient, go through the following four steps
   a. Hear your internal dialogue: What are you thinking?
   b. Analyze your internal dialogue: Identify which cognitive distortions are present.
   c. Reconstruct your thinking: Write factual statements to replace distorted thinking.
   a. Practice: Because realistic thinking does not come naturally, the more you practice, the easier it eliminates distorted thinking.

d) The basic principles of CBT that all providers can apply include recognizing and reframing nonproductive thinking, empowering patients to be more aware of underlying beliefs and emotions, and working through the ABCDE model of behavioral change, discussed later in this objective.

1. Recognize and reframe nonproductive thinking.
   a. Be aware of the different types of nonproductive thinking, also known as cognitive distortions.
      (1) Examples of 10 common cognitive distortions and reframed thoughts are:[12]
         (a) All-or-nothing thinking: There is no "in-between." It's entirely one way or the other.
            1. Distortion: "I haven't accomplished anything with my life since I've been in graduate school."
            2. Reframed: "The fact that I'm almost done with graduate school is a huge accomplishment in and of itself, and I can be proud of that."
         (b) Overgeneralization: Using limited factual evidence to hold a firm belief that is not true.
            1. Distortion: "He never washes the dishes!"
            2. Reframed: "While it may not be as often as I like, he does occasionally wash the dishes."
         (c) Mental filter: Singling out one aspect of a situation to the complete exclusion of others that should be considered.
            1. Distortion: "My boss' review was full of criticism."
            2. Reframed: "My boss gave me some positive feedback with areas to improve."
         (d) Mind reading: Having the certainty of knowing what another person is thinking without having to ask.
            1. Distortion: "I know my partner thinks I did a terrible job on that presentation!"
            2. Reframed: "Though my partner looked stern, I do not know if it was related to my presentation."
         (e) Fortune telling: Knowing that if THIS happens, THAT will definitely occur.
            1. Distortion: "I will probably just mess up and make a fool of myself."
            2. Reframed: "I will do my best and be grateful for the opportunity to try."
         (f) Magnification/minimization: Majoring in minors and minoring in majors. Priorities are mixed up or irrational.
            1. Distortion: "I haven't accomplished anything with my life since I've been in medical school."
            2. Reframed: "The fact that I'm almost done with medical school is a huge accomplishment in and of itself. I didn't need to get married or have an amazing job to prove that I am accomplishing things with my life."

(g) Personalization and blame: You or others are totally responsible for the good or bad that happens to you.

   1. Distortion: "That jerk just cut me off and made me spill my coffee; they just ruined my day!"
   2. Reframed: "They may not have been looking, or perhaps there is a family emergency. Whatever the reason, they didn't do it to make me mad."

(h) Emotional reasoning: Your feelings don't lie.

   1. Distortion: "I feel like an idiot, so I really must be one."
   2. Reframed: "It feels like I can't do this, but everybody feels this at times."

(i) Labeling/mislabeling: Habitually defining ourselves or others with a descriptive term.

   1. Distortion: "I'm such a disorganized person!"
   2. Reframed: "I could improve my organization skills."

(j) Disqualifying the positive: Acknowledging the good, appearing to be objective, but believing the good side has no value.

   1. Distortion: "Giving up caffeine may have benefits, but those benefits will be worthless since I might have a headache for a few days."
   2. Reframed: "Giving up caffeine will have a short-lasting downside, but the benefits will be worth the effort.

2. Reframe nonproductive thinking.

   a. Assist the patient in becoming more aware of their emotions. Help the patient understand that by being more conscious of the nonproductive thoughts that lead to negative emotions, they can consciously choose different thoughts that may lead to positive emotions and ongoing behavior.

   b. Address "nonproductive" thoughts.

      (1) In an exploratory way, ask whether the patient's thoughts affect their behavior. Examine the evidence for and against nonproductive thoughts.
      (2) Elicit the patient's ideas about possible thoughts that lead to nonproductive emotions and might be getting in the way of behavior change.
      (3) The provider may reflect a patient's statement (e.g., "I noticed you said, 'I have tried everything, what's the point?'").
      (4) Ask the patient how they might see the situation differently. Is there a more neutral position? Has the patient indeed tried everything?
      (5) Help the patient substitute more realistic interpretations in the place of nonproductive thinking.
      (6) Ask the patient for ideas about language, or "self-talk," that can be used during difficult moments to support oneself and improve emotions about the change. For example, if a patient is trying to quit smoking but finds himself desiring a cigarette, he could remember to say to himself, "I know this is hard right now, but I can do this. These feelings will pass. I can relax in another way."
      (7) Give the patient a "homework" assignment to practice new thinking strategies and more effective problem solving.

(8) Assist the patient in becoming more aware of their emotions. Help the patient understand that by being more conscious of the nonproductive thoughts that lead to negative emotions, they can consciously choose different thoughts that may lead to positive emotions.

3. Reframe thoughts and self-talk to support behavior change.
   a. Teach the patient that adjusting thoughts can lead to a change in emotions, which can change ongoing behavior.
   b. Examples of reframing thoughts:
      (1) Patient thoughts: "Walking helps me stay in shape and lose weight, but I can't walk outside if the weather is not right, if I'm too tired, or if my spouse can't walk with me."
      (2) Reasonable thoughts: "These are excuses. I can go to the mall and walk if the weather is not right or use the treadmill we have at home. When I'm tired, walking could give me more energy. My walking is not dependent upon my spouse coming with me."
4. Recognize underlying beliefs that can interfere with behavior change.
   a. Unproductive thought processes can keep patients from making positive and lasting health behavior changes.
      (1) These underlying beliefs reinforce negative thoughts and feelings and alter how patients see events, leading to a chronically negative and unproductive view of themselves and life.
   b. To counter unproductive thought processes, Dr. Albert Ellis developed a mnemonic device to help patients identify and reframe nonproductive thinking.[13] This mnemonic—ABCDE—serves as a helpful framework for patients and providers working together to catch, check, challenge, and change irrational beliefs.[14]
      (1) Work through the ABCDE method of behavioral change with the patient by asking:
         A: What Action or event occurred?
         B: What Beliefs do you have about what happened?
         C: What are the Consequences of those beliefs? How does that make you feel?
         D: How can you Dispute those beliefs that seem to be distorted or unhealthy?
         E: What Effect does this new way of thinking have on how you feel and how you will move forward?

3) Positive psychology (see Section 10 for more details on positive psychology)

a) Positive psychology principles should be utilized in all stages of change.

b) Benefits of positive psychology:

1. Builds patient's confidence
2. Emphasizes patient's current skills and abilities
3. Reinforces autonomy and self-efficacy, which are keys to sustainable self-management
4. Emphasizes the patient's strengths and positive actions:
   a. What did the patient achieve?
   b. What successes were achieved with each step?
5. Enhances resiliency and helps undo negative feelings
6. Increases the positivity of the patient-provider interaction

c) The ability to flourish as a human depends on one's fundamental ability to experience positive emotions like affection, love, enjoyment, happiness, playfulness, contentment, and satisfaction.[5]

4) **Social support**

   a) Enlist support from the patient's social circles.

      1. Engage family and friends with whom the patient has a positive relationship to support the patient's autonomy, accountability, and self-efficacy.
      2. Support groups: sports team, club, class, workplace, and faith-based or social networks (including social media).
      3. Behavior change "working" groups:

         a. Peer modeling strategies: Pair individuals with others who have already succeeded in making the desired change. For example, Alcoholics Anonymous uses peer modeling.

         b. Peer to peer programs: Peers encourage and help each other troubleshoot scenarios that are difficult to overcome. Group classes are an example of peer-to-peer programs.

   b) Encourage patients to use their current social support team maximally.

   c) Refer the patient to relevant community resources.

   d) Ask the patient to complete an analysis of their support network (see Table 2.1 Support Analysis Tool below)

Table 2.1 Support Analysis Tool

Current Support Network	Support Needs		
	Ride to farmer's market	Sharing progress with someone doing a similar plan	Childcare during workouts
Family			
Friend			
Social Group			

OBJECTIVE 4

Develop a written action plan based on the treatment prescription adjusted for the appropriate stage of change

1) **Key considerations for providers**

   a) Assist patients in moving from their current stage of change to the next stage.

   b) Identify and adapt assessments and interventions to the patient's literacy level and cultural background.

   c) Create a written action plan based on the results of the patient's readiness to change, the patient's perceived level of importance to make change, and the patient's confidence that change can be accomplished.

   d) Follow up with the patient after the action plan is implemented to support ongoing lifestyle change.

   e) For every change that is being made and coached, a readiness level should be assessed.

2) **Stage-matched interventions (Table 2.2)**[15]

Table 2.2 Stage-Matched Interventions		
Stage	**Patient**	**Provider**
Precontemplation	"I am not thinking about making a change at all now or within the next 6 months."	Discuss health risks associated with specific behaviors (e.g., smoking and lung cancer) and highlight benefits associated with behavior change.
Contemplation	"I am thinking about making a change within the next 6 months."	Personalize health risks, weigh risks and benefits, and highlight the impact on personal goals (e.g., highlight smoking and risk of heart attack if the patient has a family history of heart disease).
Preparation	"I am preparing to make a change within the next month."	Assist with commitment, plan specific change(s), and discuss ways to modify their environment.
Action	"I have started a change within the last 6 months. I have not hit the target change goal or have not hit it consistently for 6 months."	Structure the plan, identify sources of frequent barriers to behavior change, identify social support, problem-solve obstacles, use CBT, and reframe unhealthy thought patterns (e.g., "I can't walk in winter" changes to "I can dress for the weather.").
Maintenance	"I have been successfully making the target change for more than 6 months."	Discuss coping strategies to mitigate stress and continue reinforcement as well as CBT.

3) Prescription versus action plan

a) Lifestyle prescriptions

1. Prescriptions are brief, clear instructions for care or treatment pertaining to an individual patient.
2. A lifestyle medicine prescription describes the action or behavior change in the full extent necessary to treat or prevent.
3. An example would be a prescription for 150 minutes of moderate physical activity a week.

b) Action plan

1. The lifestyle prescription is adjusted and personalized for the patient's ability, readiness, and confidence.
2. An example action plan: Start with walking 5 minutes a day for 5 days a week, increasing as tolerated up to the recommended amount of 150 minutes per week.
3. Creating action plans
   a. Collaborate with the patient to develop evidence-based, achievable, specific, and written action plans.
   b. Review the action plan during the visit or with a team member who can do this with the patient.
   c. Emphasize the importance of writing the plan down, not just talking about it.
   d. Keep a copy of the action plan in the patient's medical chart.
   e. Work with your team to follow up on the patient's progress.
   f. Encourage digital apps or other methods of self-monitoring to track progress.

4) Step-by-step collaboration with the patient for developing the action plan

a) Explain your role as "expert" and "coach," and agree on an agenda as part of collaborative care. For example:

1. "My role as your doctor is to present a diagnosis and offer the lifestyle and medication prescriptions that can help you. I need your help to identify the areas where you are ready and willing to commit to making changes. We can use a readiness assessment exercise if this is helpful for you to identify those areas. My goal today is for you to commit to making lifestyle changes of your choice and for us to develop your wellness plan. Does that sound agreeable to you? How confident are you that you will master this change(s) in the next 3 to 6 months?"

b) Share diagnosis and potential outcomes if no lifestyle or conventional medical treatments are initiated.

c) Describe lifestyle prescription (list behaviors) and potential outcomes when lifestyle behaviors are mastered.

d) Identify current areas of progress and use positive psychology to support and encourage the patient's changes and progress.
   1. Ask: "Which of the areas that I've recommended have you mastered, or are you working on now?"
   2. Listen intently, reflect, and summarize to show understanding.
   3. Affirm the patient's strengths and progress.

e) Identify new areas for action.
   1. "How do you feel about your situation?"
   2. "Which health behaviors are you ready and willing to work on now?"
   3. The provider should then assess readiness to change and provide stage-matched interventions.

OBJECTIVE 5

Demonstrate use of readiness, importance, and confidence scales

1) **Identify the patient's confidence and importance level for each area of change.**
   a) The provider can ask: "On a scale of 0 to 10, how confident are you that you will master this/these areas in the next 3 to 6 months?"
   b) To help assess readiness to change, a patient's perception of how important it is to make the behavioral change can be measured during the early stages of the change process.

2) **Score confidence and importance levels (see Table 2.3).**
   a) If the score is above 7, the patient is more likely to accomplish their goal.
   b) If the score is 7 or below, help the patient identify ways to increase importance or confidence levels.
      1. Consider asking: "What will it take to get your confidence (or importance) level to an 8 to 10 level?"
      2. Inquire why they chose that number and not a lower one. This exercise may help illicit statements that reflect a patient's desire or importance to change.

Table 2.3 Readiness, Importance, and Confidence scales

	Confidence	Importance
Precontemplation	0–3/10	0–3/10
Contemplative	4–6/10	4–6/10
Preparation	7/10	7/10
Action	8–9/10	8–9/10
Maintenance (or Action)	10/10	10/10

10-point Confidence and Importance Scales (0 = low, 10 = high) correlated with transtheoretical model of stages of change

c) Ask the patient to summarize their goals, what resources they need, and how they will stay focused on their goal.

d) Make sure goals follow the SMART goal format.

1. SMART goals:[16]
    a. Specific (identify the exact behavior to be addressed)
    b. Measurable (how one will know when the goal is reached)
    c. Attainable (the goal is achievable and can be accomplished)
    d. Relevant (the goal is in alignment with the specific behavior change)
    e. Timebound (the timeframe for achieving that goal)
2. Ask the patient what benefits of this behavior change they value the most.
3. Ask what would help the patient stay on track with these changes.
4. Create reasonable strategies to overcome an identified obstacle.
5. Connect the patient with available programs or referrals to support their efforts.
6. Confirm the patient's commitment to the action plan.
    a. Have the patient sign and date the action plan. "We've got a deal!"
    b. Give the patient a form for an action plan and ask them to complete it during the visit or before leaving.
    c. Keep a copy of the action plan and follow up during the next visit (see Table 2.4 and Table 2.5 for more).

Table 2.4 Sample Action Plan (lifestyle prescription of 150 minutes of exercise/week)

What	walk
How much/intensity	at a pace that I can still speak or converse
How long	for 10 minutes
How often	three times a week
With whom	my neighbor, spouse, or dog
Where	around the neighborhood
When	in the evenings
Support system	my spouse can help remind me to walk
Biggest barrier	feeling tired at the end of the day
Solution to barrier	remind me that walking will increase my energy
Confidence level	8/10

Table 2.5 Resources for Action Plans

1. Rollnick S., Mason P., Butler C. *Health Behavior Change: A Guide for Practitioners*, 2002
2. Rollnick S., Miller W., Butler C. *Motivational Interviewing in Health Care: Helping Patient Change Behavior*, 2007
3. Moore M. *Coaching Psychology Manual*, 2009

OBJECTIVE 6

Describe strategies for helping patients maintain healthy behaviors

1) Step-by-step maintenance of an action plan

- **a)** During subsequent visits:
  1. Reiterate the provider's role in supporting the patient's efforts to improve health and work on their action plan.
  2. Review and update the diagnosis and lifestyle recommendations.
  3. Review the patient's action plan from the prior visit.
     - a. Ask the patient first to discuss their successes and then their challenges.
     - b. Then, ask the patient to summarize their overall experience.
  4. Listen intently, reflect, and summarize to show understanding.
  5. Use positive psychology and affirm the patient's strengths and any progress made.
     - a. Ask the patient:
       - (1) "What benefits have you gained from the changes you've made?"
       - (2) "What have you learned from the challenging areas?"
       - (3) "How do you feel about your situation?"
     - b. Finish with: "Which of the behavioral goals are you ready and willing to master by the time of our next visit in 3–6 months?"
     - c. Summarize and clarify the new goals just like the initial goal: Create a new action plan, list resources and challenges, ask about the confidence level to complete that goal, probe what it will take to increase confidence, summarize, confirm the patient's new commitment, and keep a copy of the new action plan.

OBJECTIVE 7

Differentiate at least three health behavior change theories and their potential application to practice

1) Health behavior change models and theories and potential application to practice

- **a)** Health belief model (HBM)[11,17]
  1. A theoretical model that proposes that personal beliefs or perceptions mostly influence health behavior. Since the 1950s, HBM has primarily been used to explain and predict behavior in adopting disease prevention strategies or complying with early disease detection screening. The HBM model explains that before seeking preventive measures or adopting a specific health behavior, people must believe there is a threat to their health and that there is a preventive measure that is accessible and low risk. This preventive measure (health behavior change) will help them successfully avoid the health threat in the future.
  2. The process for behavioral change is described in Table 2.6.

Table 2.6 Six Key Constructs	
1. Perceived susceptibility	One's subjective perception of the risk of acquiring or being susceptible to a health threat.
2. Perceived severity	One's subjective feelings about the seriousness of having the health threat (contracting the disease or leaving it untreated). Perceived severity includes feelings on potential health outcomes like death or disability, and social outcomes like relationships and activities.
3. Perceived benefit	One's beliefs about the effectiveness of measures available to avoid, reduce, or treat the health threat.
4. Perceived barriers	One's perception of the negative aspects or obstacles that may impede adopting a health behavior or preventive measure.
5. Cues to action	Events or stimuli that prompt action in adopting behavior change or a preventive measure.
6. Self-efficacy	One's confidence in their ability to act and succeed in completing the behavior change or adopting the preventive measure.

b) Theory of planned behavior[11,17]

1. The theory of planned behavior evolved from the theory of reasoned action. This theory helps explain the intention to engage in healthy behavior and how engaging in that healthy behavior is influenced by one's beliefs and attitudes about the risks, benefits, and capability of achieving the desired health outcome. The theory helps predict the likelihood of engaging in a specific behavior over which one has control at a particular time and place. Behavioral achievement is based on motivation (intention) and ability (behavioral control).
2. The theory uses six main constructs to represent one's actual control over behavior collectively.
   a. Attitude: the positive or negative evaluation of a behavior of interest and its outcomes
   b. Behavioral intention: the motivational factors for a behavior of interest; the most important factor in predicting behavior
   c. Subjective norms: one's perception of the beliefs of others (peers and people of importance) concerning the behavior and whether they approve or disapprove
   d. Social norms: customary codes or standards of behavior in a group of people
   e. Perceived power: one's perceived control over factors that may help or impede performing the behavior of interest
   f. Perceived behavioral control: one's perception about the ease or difficulty in completing the behavior of interest and the control to accomplish it. This perception changes with different surroundings

c) Social cognitive theory[11,17]

1. Social cognitive theory evolved from social learning theory. This theory explains that behavior does not occur in isolation but rather is a product of the influence that personal factors, environment, and human behavior exert on one another. Credible role models are important in producing behavior change in a population.
   a. Reciprocal determinism: the person, the behavior, and the environment all influence each other in a dynamic and reciprocal fashion
   b. Behavioral capability: possessing the knowledge and skill to complete a behavior
   c. Observational learning (modeling): people do not just learn from their own experiences but also the experiences of others

d. Reinforcements: behaviors are maintained or omitted due to internal and external social reinforcements

e. Expectations: anticipating consequences that will encourage or discourage behavior change, these consequences are often driven by prior experiences

f. Self-efficacy: the level of confidence to successfully perform a behavior; influenced by one's behavioral capability and environmental facilitators or inhibitors

d) Transtheoretical model (TTM)[11,17]

1. TTM originally developed to help patients with smoking cessation, integrates key constructs of various psychological theories. This model has been expanded to describe the process of change for other health behaviors. TTM recognizes that behavior change is a process that unfolds over time through a series of stages in which different interventions are more effective. It is important to recognize that behavior change is an individualized, non-linear process (Figure 2.1). Patients may skip stages, move quickly between them, or stay in one phase for an extended period.

Figure 2.1 Transtheoretical Model

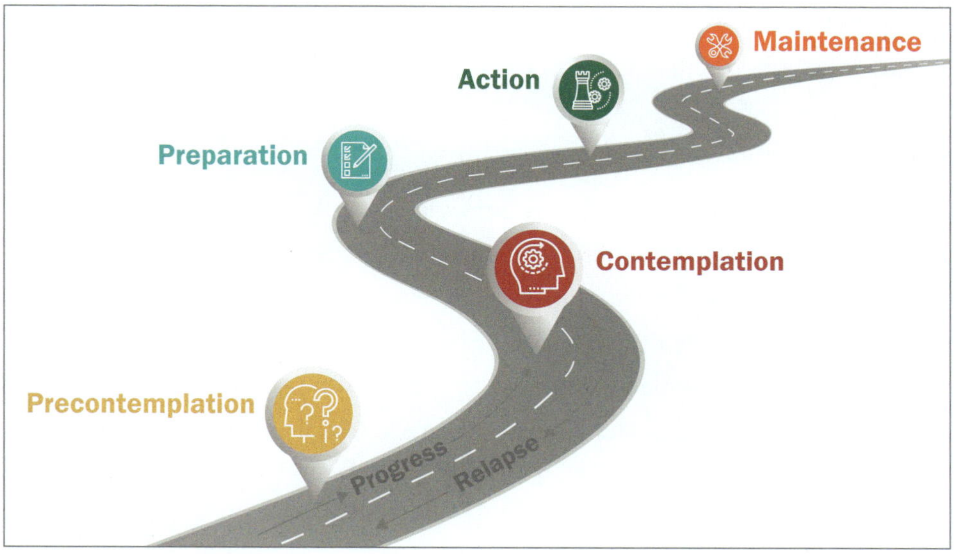

2. Stages of change

a. Precontemplation: the patient is not ready for change and does not intend to take action in the foreseeable future (typically described as within the next 6 months)

b. Contemplation: the patient is considering making a change in their behavior within the next 6 months

c. Preparation: the patient has determined that behavior change is beneficial and intends to take action within the next month

d. Action: the patient has enacted a specific health behavior change but has been doing so for less than 6 months

e. Maintenance: the patient has sustained the health behavior change for at least 6 months

f. Termination: the patient is no longer tempted to return to their old unhealthy behavior. This stage is included in the original model, but often only the five main stages are presented

e) Self-determination theory[18,19]

  1. A key theory in coaching psychology focuses on the belief that individuals are naturally motivated to pursue activities and goals in which they are interested or from which they believe they will obtain some benefit. This type of motivation, known as autonomous motivation, leads to sustained motivation and successful health behavior change.
  2. According to the theory, the three primary psychological needs that influence motivation are autonomy, competence, and relatedness.

f) Other models[11,17]

  1. Precaution adoption model: similar to the transtheoretical model with seven stages ranging from unawareness to maintenance; however, this model describes linear change instead of cyclical change, as people cannot go backward in stages and become "unaware" again.
  2. Diffusion of innovation theory: describes the adoption of a new idea or behavior across a population identified as innovators, early adopters, early majority, late majority, and laggards.

2) Common components of health behavior models and theories include:

- **a)** Beliefs about risks and benefits
- **b)** Motivation
- **c)** Self-efficacy
- **d)** Environmental influence (e.g., social norms)

3) Health behavior is influenced by various factors including:[17]

- **a)** Intrapersonal: knowledge, attitudes, beliefs, and personality
- **b)** Interpersonal: influence of family, friends, peers, and health providers
- **c)** Institutional: rules, regulations, and policies
- **d)** Community factors: social networks, social norms in one's circle, and built environments
- **e)** Public policy: local, state, and federal policies and laws that regulate action for disease prevention, detection, control, and management (e.g., calories listed on menus or laws regarding where you can smoke)

OBJECTIVE 8

Identify two key constructs for effective, sustainable self-management

1) Cognitive behavioral techniques: These are especially useful when the patient is dealing with feelings of outside pressures, failures, or being out of control.

2) Social support strategies

- **a)** When social support is present, people have better long-term success with weight loss.[20]
- **b)** For patients with overweight or obesity, group support can provide additional incentives for weight loss beyond what individuals do on their own. This may be due to accountability, friendly competition, and encouragement.[20]

3) Community and employee programs

4) **Support with digital technology (e.g., apps, wearable devices, etc.), telehealth (video/phone counseling), or "high-tech/high-touch" (a combination of digital and live counseling)**
   a) Behavior contracts[21] note that the evidence on general patient contracts is inconclusive
   b) If behavior contracts are being used:
      1. Clarify terminology with the patient, so they understand these are not actual "contracts" but instead are aids in behavior change.
      2. Clarify the patient's goals (e.g., is the contract an acknowledgment of clinic policies or criteria for medication?).
      3. Treat the "contract" as part of the therapeutic process and as a mode of helping the patient set and meet her goals.
      4. Offer resources alongside the contract to help the patient meet her goals.
   c) Contracts can help provide accountability and assist with self-monitoring.

5) **Focus on skill power, not willpower[22]**
   a) Create an external system and guidelines for the patient until their new behaviors become the default choice.
   b) Long-term success combines skill power and willpower.

OBJECTIVE 9

List components of relapse prevention planning

1) **Relapse prevention planning**
   a) Definitions
      1. "Lapse" is a short-term period when an action plan is not followed.
         a. A lapse is easier to address because the unhealthy behavior is a temporary "slip" and has not yet become a habit again.
      2. "Relapse" is a sustained period when an action plan is not adhered to.
         a. Addressing relapse is similar to the steps in forming a "new action plan."
         b. The patient and provider must address thoughts and emotions that can arise from a potential feeling of failure.
         c. Relapse is more challenging to address because the unhealthy action has become a habit again, and now there are psychological implications of not meeting the initial goal.
   b) Relapse prevention plans should be designed for each ongoing behavior change.
      1. Relapse prevention planning was originally used in an alcohol use disorder model, but the principles are useful for all behavior changes.
      2. These plans assess potential triggers for lapses and situations that may lead to ongoing lapses.
      3. Relapse prevention plan addresses the following:
         a. When might a lapse occur?
         b. Under what circumstances?
         c. With whom?
         d. How to notice a lapse before it becomes a relapse?
         e. Who to turn to during a lapse? Relapse?

c) Relapse prevention tools (also see Table 2.7)
    1. Identify relapse prevention support (family, friends, social and faith groups, etc.).
        a. Establish a relapse reminder and a back-up plan (e.g., the patient will contact the physician's office in 3 weeks to check in, a family member will go with the patient to the party to make sure he does not drink, etc.).

Table 2.7 Resources for clinicians on relapse prevention
1. Leahy R.L. *Cognitive Behavioral Techniques: A Practitioner's Guide*, 2003.
2. Larimer M.E., Palmer R.S., Marlatt A. Relapse Prevention: an overview of marlatt's cognitive behavioral model. *Alcohol Res and health*. 1999; 23(2):151-160.

OBJECTIVE 10

Describe the process of follow-up for ongoing lifestyle change progress, including building patient self-efficacy

1) **Follow up in-person, by phone, or by digital medium.**
    a) Build a supportive relationship, listen, affirm the patient's perspective and situation, and emphasize their self-efficacy. Remember that the patient is in the driver's seat, but, as providers, we assist the patient by keeping them accountable, with their permission.
    b) Focus on the specific patient action plan.
    c) If the patient's plan is achieved:
        1. Congratulate the patient on their progress.
        2. Ask about barriers that arose and what problem solving was used. This is important for creating confidence to meet future goals.
        3. Check the patient's progress against the ideal lifestyle prescription (e.g., the patient is now exercising 40 minutes per week, but the ideal lifestyle goal is 150 minutes of exercise per week).
    d) If the patient's plan is not achieved:
        1. Discuss and congratulate them on any progress they have made (despite not achieving the goal).
        2. Discuss barriers and co-create solutions.
    e) Develop a revised action plan that the patient has more than 7/10 confidence they can achieve.
    f) Establish accountability and support.
        1. Check in with the patient more frequently.
        2. Connect the patient with resources, support groups, (i.e., Alcoholics Anonymous or a community exercise group), and other professionals who can help, (i.e., a national board-certified health and wellness coach [NBC-HWC]).
    g) Encourage digital apps, social media, or other methods of self-monitoring for tracking and support.

OBJECTIVE 11

Describe the 5 A's and how to incorporate them into the office visit

1) Understand the 5 A's (Figure 2.2) and how to incorporate them into the office visit.[6,23,24]

Figure 2.2 The 5 A's

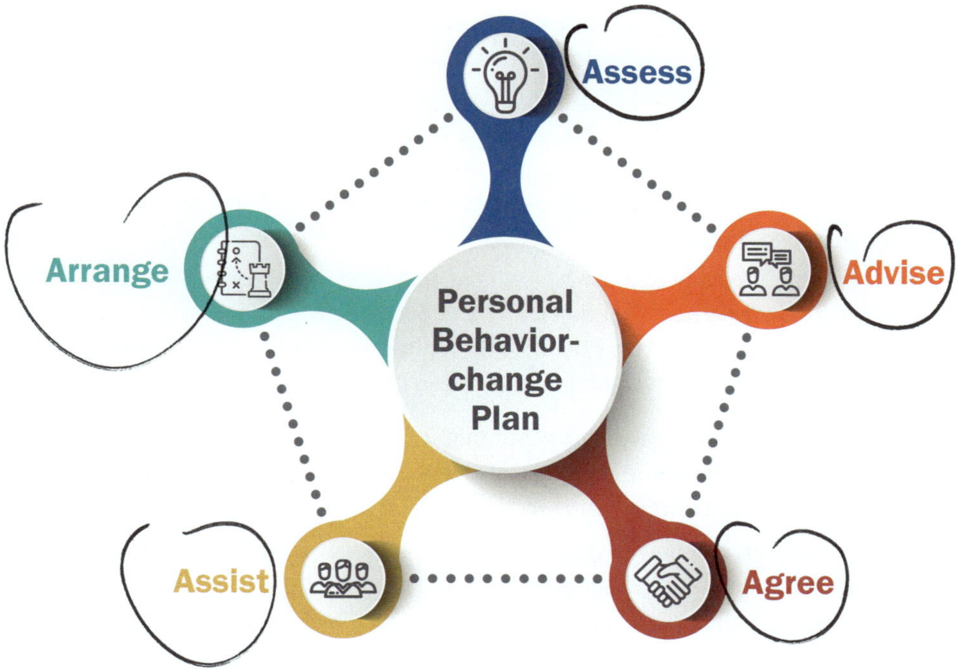

- **a)** Assess practices in the context of health risks.
- **b)** Advise changing practices with clear, specific, and personalized advice for behavior change.
- **c)** Agree on the focus of counseling and treatment based on the patient's interest and willingness to change and collaboratively set specific goals.
- **d)** Assist the patient in achieving goals to change practices.
  1. Address motivational barriers via counseling and self-help techniques.
  2. Determine whether the patient needs additional information or help.
  3. Refer the patient to a dietitian or other resources as needed.
- **e)** Arrange for regular follow up and support.
- **f)** The 5 A's were conceived to:
  1. Guide a brief approach to health behavior counseling
  2. Improve patient motivation and intention to change behavior (they have been shown to improve motivation for weight loss)[24]
  3. Provide a patient-centered approach to care
  4. Encourage internal motivation for change
  5. Use a collaborative approach (patient-provider interaction that is crucial for success)

OBJECTIVE 12

Cite the evidence base for effective coaching that promotes health behavior change and improves health outcomes

1) **A rapidly growing body of evidence shows coaching supports health behavior change and improves health outcomes.**
   a) A 2017 systematic review published in the *American Journal of Lifestyle Medicine* provides a comprehensive and organized compendium of health and wellness coaching literature using a defined set of inclusion criteria based on an operationalized definition of health and wellness coaching.[25]
      1. In 2019, a supplement by the same group was also published in the *American Journal of Lifestyle Medicine*, in which another 104 peer-reviewed health coaching–related journal articles were added to the compendium.[26]
      2. The most consistent effects of health and wellness coaching were observed in both exercise and nutrition behavior.[25] In addition, health coaching has shown to improved health outcomes for patients with diabetes and obesity. Improvements were seen in hemoglobin A1c (HbA1c) and reductions in weight and body mass index (BMI).[26,27]
2) **A systematic review of 35 studies of interventions that might alter the patient-provider clinical interaction found several simple and some complex interventions that could change the clinical interaction and possible health outcomes.[28]**
   a) Three main categories of interventions were applied in the studies to change the clinical interaction between the patient and practitioner:
      1. Intervention 1: Activating the patient by helping them take a more active role. The provider encouraged the patient's questions and elicited their concerns.
      2. Intervention 2: Enhancing the provider's approach. The provider improved their approach by paying more attention to the patient's emotion, changing their consultation style to match the patient's personality, or providing more information to the patient in advance or during the consultation.
      3. Intervention 3: A combination of both activating the patient and enhancing the provider's approach.
   b) Results
      1. Twenty-two of 30 trials (73%) showed that the interventions did alter the patient-provider clinical interaction.
      2. Health outcomes were positively affected in 11 out of 25 trials (44%) and negatively affected in 5 of 25 studies (20%).
      3. Overall, health outcomes were poorly assessed, and the evidence on a specific consultation style is inconclusive due to few studies specifically examining this.
      4. When the provider's approach was enhanced, it led to greater collaboration in the provider-patient relationship. Strategies with collaboration during the consultation appeared to have more positive outcomes.
3) **Physicians with high empathy scores from their patients were more likely to achieve good HbA1c control than those with low empathy scores (56% versus 40%).[29]**

4) **Ten-hour provider training on empathy skills can achieve similar empathy results as those providers who have had longer training on empathy. The 10-hour training results in positive effects on the consultation process and the patient's perception of the provider's attentiveness.**[30]

5) **Health outcomes for hypertension, glucose levels, and functional status are related to the patient-provider relationship.**[31]

OBJECTIVE 13

Describe how to create relationships with patients which foster their personal growth

OBJECTIVE 14

Describe how effective coaching and creating positive relationships with patients impacts the role of self-motivation and self-confidence in successful health behavior change

1) **Self-motivation and self-confidence**
   - **a)** Self-motivation is also known as autonomous or internal motivation.
     1. This motivation comes from within a person in contrast to external motivation produced by one's environment. It's based on one's needs, perceived benefits of behavior, values, vision, purpose, and meaning in life.
     2. Coaching can help connect one's deeper values, meaning, and purpose to desired health behavior to help increase autonomous motivation.
   - **b)** Self-confidence
     1. Self-confidence is the trust a person has in their reasoning, capabilities, and qualities.
     2. Self-confidence can be increased by eliciting positive emotions, leveraging one's strengths, developing a robust support system, providing appropriate education at each step of the journey to increase knowledge and skills, and improving self-efficacy.
   - **c)** Self-motivation and self-confidence play essential roles in developing self-efficacy.
     1. Self-efficacy is the level of a person's confidence to perform a behavior successfully. Confidence is influenced by one's behavioral capability and environmental facilitators or inhibitors. Self-efficacy is at the core of successful health behavior change, just like successful sports performance.[32]

2) **Strategies to foster self-motivation and self-confidence**
   - **a)** Hold the possibility that the patient can commit to change and master change.
     1. Understand that even "baby steps" build self-esteem and momentum.
   - **b)** Clear one's mind of "noise" in order to listen to the patient with full attention.[33]
   - **c)** Be empathetic, adopting a warm, caring, accepting, open, and compassionate attitude.
   - **d)** Focus on and affirm the positive as much as possible.
     1. Look for opportunities to highlight the patient's positive intentions, actions, and strengths.
     2. Look for ways to increase confidence in her ability to change.

e) Share personal or other anonymous examples where disclosure would be beneficial to the patient.

f) Encourage the patient to take charge, decide on, and commit to a wellness plan.

g) View obstacles and setbacks as necessary parts of behavior change and the path to success.
   1. Use these challenges to look for underlying learning opportunities.

h) Look for teachable moments.
   1. A time of challenge or transition (e.g., after a heart attack or a diagnosis with a chronic disease) may be an important opportunity to encourage lifestyle change. These times are called teachable moments.
   2. Be aware that physicians often underestimate the importance and power of these moments and the impact they can have on health behavior change.

OBJECTIVE 15

Describe the main stages of the coaching process

1) The main steps of the coaching process include:

a) Helping patients develop awareness, establish self-determined goals, create an action plan, and implement accountability and self-monitoring systems to support continuous behavior change.[34]

b) Coaching plays an important role in relationship building, goal setting, action planning, problem-solving, and increasing self-efficacy.[35]

c) Match the patient's readiness to change with the prescribed treatment, as this may help with adherence

d) Emphasize working on areas where the patient will see quick success with little to some effort.
   1. Focus on changes that will make a meaningful difference to the patient, which can also be done relatively easily.
   2. Begin with small but important successes and build upon them.

2) Developing awareness and assisting with analysis of a patient's current health behaviors and their desired future health through reflections

a) Open-ended questions are an effective way to support patients in discovering what is possible to move forward with in terms of their health.

b) As previously noted, reflections are commonly used in coaching. Coaches will make reflective statements to the patient using the same phrases or a summary of what the patient stated. Reflections help the patient create connections, tap into emotions, and bring awareness to what has been vocalized.
   1. Types of reflections
      a. Simple reflections are a paraphrase or restatement of what the patient has said without added opinion or interpretation.
      b. Amplified reflections provide an accurate, direct, and more exaggerated form of the patient's statement to evoke statements of the desired change.
      c. Double-sided reflections are reflections that reveal more than one perspective at the same time. This could be a comparison of a patient's verbalized readiness to change with a contrasting statement of resistance.

c) There are other types of reflective strategies that can also be used, especially if a patient's language sounds resistant to change.

1. Shifting focus is an approach to redirect attention from a statement of resistance to a new area in an attempt to create more space for change talk.
2. Reframing is another approach that invites the patient to consider a different perspective of what is being described.

OBJECTIVE 16

List the coaching questions for each stage of change

1) Stage-matched interventions for the transtheoretical model stages of change

a) If the patient is not yet making a change:

1. Ask: "Are you considering making a change in [X behavior]?"
   a. If the patient says "no," they are in the precontemplation stage.
      (1) Provide information about diseases, risks associated with maintaining the status quo, and the benefits of healthy behavior.
      (2) You may ask: "Did you know that [X behavior] is one of the leading causes of [Y result]?"
      (3) To honor the patient's autonomy, you may consider asking an open-ended question such as: "How will you know when it is time to think about making a change?"
   b. If the patient says "yes," you can determine the timeframe for behavior change to occur.
      (1) Ask: "Are you considering a change in the next month or before your next visit?"
         (a) If the patient says "no," they are in the contemplation stage.
            1. Encourage patient to evaluate the benefits of changing as well as the perceived barriers to changing.
            2. Provide resources and information.
            3. Encourage problem-solving.
         (b) If the patient says "yes," they are in the preparation stage.
            1. Co-create an action plan.
            2. Ask the patient to write it down.
            3. Assess the patient's confidence level.
            4. Make a note of it in the chart.
            5. Schedule and perform follow-up.

b) If the patient is experimenting with a change:

1. If action has been taken, but the patient has not yet met their goal or engaged in the behavior consistently, they are still in the preparation stage.
   a. Help the patient develop or refine their action plan (see "preparation phase" above).
2. If the patient meets their goal but is not yet 6 months into change, the patient is in the action stage.
   a. Be aware that the patient is extremely vulnerable to relapse in this phase.
   b. Structure a plan.
   c. Problem-solve through obstacles. Ask: "What is giving you the most challenge?"

    d. Reframe unhealthy thought patterns utilizing cognitive behavioral techniques.
    e. Establish systems of accountability and self-monitoring.
    f. Enlist help from social support. Ask: "How can your support network better help you?"
3. If the patient meets their goal and has sustained the behavior change for more than 6 months, the patient is in the maintenance stage.
    a. Reinforce the behavior change and continue to build autonomous motivation.
    b. Use cognitive behavioral techniques and other problem-solving strategies.

SECTION 2 GLOSSARY

Coaching: the process of empowering patients to develop the knowledge, skills, resources, and confidence to enact and sustain lifestyle changes to achieve their self-directed health goals.

Double-sided reflection: a type of reflective response highlighting the patient's reasons for and against behavior change.

Lapse: a short-term period where an action plan for change is not being followed.

Reframing: reflective strategy invites the patient to consider a different perspective and a more positive interpretation of the situation.

Relapse: when a person has previously made a positive change but now, for a sustained period, has not been maintaining that change.

Transtheoretical model: a model of behavior change that recognizes that change is a process that unfolds over time through a series of stages.

SECTION 2 REVIEW QUESTIONS

1. During a follow-up visit, a 31-year-old patient with obesity shares that she has been consuming more vegetables and whole-grains for the past 2 weeks, resulting in feeling more energized and her clothes fitting more comfortably. Upon recognizing and celebrating her progress, the patient appears discouraged and says, "I've lost weight initially with the other diets I've tried, but then I gain it right back. I know that's going to happen this time, too." Which of the following is the best response to support the woman in reframing this nonproductive thinking?

A. "Besides gaining all the weight right back, what are some other possible outcomes of your health changes?"

B. "Who will be your support system this time?"

C. "How important is it to you to lose weight?"

D. "What would be a good next step toward long-term weight loss?"

2. During a previous visit, a 49-year-old patient with cardiovascular disease developed an action plan to pack a lunch for work 3 days a week. In reviewing this action plan, the patient states that he has not been able to adhere to his plan because his wife recently started a new job, and he's now in charge of getting the kids ready for school in the morning. He shares that there were a couple of days over the last month where he was able to pack a healthy lunch, which helped him feel more focused and energized at work. But he's just too busy to prepare food for himself given his new household responsibilities. Which of the following is the best example of a double-sided reflection based on what the patient has shared?

A. "You don't have time to pack a lunch and, when you eat healthy, you feel more energized during the workday."

B. "It sounds like even though you tried you weren't able to follow through on the goal you set for yourself."

C. "You have a number of responsibilities that are making it challenging for you to follow through on your goal."

D. "It might not be the right time to take on this particular goal. Is there something else you'd like to focus on?"

3. During an initial visit with a patient recently diagnosed with type 2 diabetes, the physical activity as a vital sign tool indicates that she is not currently meeting the established physical activity guidelines. Using 5A's framework for coaching patients toward health behavior change, which of the following is the best next step in helping the patient increase her physical activity?

A. Assist the patient in identifying specific strategies to increase physical activity, such as attending group fitness classes.

B. Advise the patient on the current physical activity guidelines and the benefits of regular exercise in the treatment and reversal of type 2 diabetes.

C. Agree to co-create an exercise prescription that includes specific activities that are in alignment with the patient's current fitness level.

D. Arrange for a referral to a qualified exercise professional to devise a specific exercise plan to help the patient reach her personal health goals.

4. **For the last 4 months, a 52-year-old patient with anxiety and chronic pain has successfully adhered to her plan of practicing yoga 30 minutes per day, 4 days a week before work. According to the transtheoretical model of behavior change, which of the following best describes the patient's current stage of change?**
   - **A.** Contemplation
   - **B.** Preparation
   - **C.** Action
   - **D.** Maintenance

5. **During an initial consultation, a 24-year-old patient with hypertension and obesity states she would like to focus on managing her stress. Which of the following responses best exemplifies a "coach" role in helping the patient with her desired behavior change?**
   - **A.** "How helpful do you think it would be to try meditation using an app?"
   - **B.** "I recommend practicing yoga, as many patients find it helpful in managing stress."
   - **C.** "Did you know that research shows chronic stress can lead to weight gain?"
   - **D.** "What are your top three reasons for wanting to manage your stress?"

6. **During an initial visit, a 68-year-old patient with osteoarthritis expresses interest in increasing her physical activity through pool-based workouts. She is very motivated to make this change and has even started researching water fitness classes in her area. She scores a 9/10 in confidence in making the change. Which of the following is the best example of a well-defined SMART goal to guide this patient's personalized action plan for the next month?**
   - **A.** Attend water fitness classes in the morning to decrease joint pain and stiffness.
   - **B.** Attend a 45-minute class at the local community center to improve health and fitness.
   - **C.** Attend a 45-minute water fitness class twice per week at the local community center.
   - **D.** Attend classes at the local community center most days of the week.

7. **After a recent myocardial infarction, a 56-year-old patient is referred by his cardiologist, who then recommends that he quit smoking. When asked on a scale of 1 to 10 how important it is to quit smoking, the patient responds with a score of 3/10. He says he "feels fine now," and mentions that smoking helps him relax after work. Based on the information provided, the man is in which of the following stages of change?**
   - **A.** Precontemplation
   - **B.** Contemplation
   - **C.** Preparation
   - **D.** Action

8. **A 33-year-old patient with endometriosis shares that she regularly drinks three to four glasses of wine at night after work. After reading a magazine about the adverse effects of alcohol consumption on reproductive health, she has decided that she is ready to stop drinking since she and her husband would like to start a family soon. Which of the following constructs of the health belief model best describes the woman's decision to quit drinking?**
   - **A.** Stimulus control
   - **B.** Cues to action
   - **C.** Social learning
   - **D.** Counter conditioning

9. **A 50-year-old man with prostate cancer is interested in eating healthier and, specifically, consuming more plant-based meals. In developing an action plan, it is determined the patient will dedicate 30 minutes per day, 5 days a week, after work to cooking a plant-based dinner with his wife, who will help to keep him accountable. Although he mentions feeling tired after work as a potential barrier, the patient states that a solution to this barrier will be to record the local news and watch it after dinner. Watching TV right after work tends to decrease his motivation to cook. Which of the following is the most appropriate question to ask the patient to support him in developing a complete action plan?**

   A. "I'm curious, how do you think your dietary choices have affected your health?"

   B. "In reflecting back, what has your relationship with food been like over the years?"

   C. "On a scale of 0 to 10, what is your confidence level in completing this action plan?"

   D. "What do you foresee being the biggest challenge when it comes to cooking?"

10. **During a follow-up appointment, a patient's action plan to walk during lunch with her coworker for 20 minutes, 4 days per week, is reviewed. The patient reports that, for the past month, she has consistently walked twice a week; however, she is frustrated that she did not achieve the goal she set for herself. Which of the following would be the best first step to build patient self-efficacy to support ongoing lifestyle change progress?**

   A. Revise the action plan to something more realistic.

   B. Encourage the patient to establish a system of accountability.

   C. Discuss and affirm the progress the patient has made thus far.

   D. Reflect the patient's frustrations of not meeting the established goal.

SECTION 2 REVIEW QUESTION ANSWERS AND SUMMARIES

1. **Answer: A.** The patient's statement about knowing she will gain all her weight right back is a type of nonproductive thinking known as fortune-telling. It occurs when a patient attempts to predict the future, typically foreseeing a negative outcome arbitrarily. To help reframe nonproductive thinking, a provider can ask the patient how she might see the situation differently. This can help the patient replace nonproductive thinking with more realistic and positive perspectives to support behavior change and create the possibility for future improvement.

2. **Answer: A.** As outlined in motivational interviewing, a double-sided reflection acknowledges sustain talk ("I don't have time to pack a lunch") and pairs it with expressed change talk ("I feel more energized and focused when I eat healthy"), exploring the patient's ambivalence by highlighting reasons he has given both for and against change.

3. **Answer: B.** After determining the patient's physical activity level using the physical activity as a vital sign tool ('Assess'), the next step in the 5A's of behavior change is to provide relevant information to the patient, such as recommended physical activity guidelines and the benefits of regular exercise in the treatment and reversal of type 2 diabetes ('Advise').

4. **Answer: C.** According to the transtheoretical model of behavior change, individuals are in the action stage of change when they have made specific, intentional lifestyle changes but have not yet maintained their target behavior for 6 months or more.

5. **Answer: D.** It is important to note that providers have distinct roles as "experts" and as "coaches" when helping patients initiate and sustain health behavior changes. The "expert approach" positions the provider as an authority figure and educator who solves problems and prescribes treatment. The "coach approach" positions the provider as a partner and facilitator of change who fosters possibilities and co-discovers answers with the patient. Asking an open-ended question helps connect the patient's deeper values to the desired health behavior change, increasing autonomous motivation.

6. **Answer: C.** SMART is an acronym for the specific components that make goals most effective: specific, measurable, attainable, relevant, and timebound. Given that the action plan being developed is specifically for the next month (timebound), the best example of a well-defined SMART goal would be to "attend a 45-minute water fitness class twice per week at the local community center." This goal is specific (identifies the exact behavior of a water fitness class held at the local community center), measurable (45 minutes per day, 2 days per week), attainable (in alignment with patient's ability, readiness, and confidence), and relevant (aligned with patient's area of focus on increasing physical activity through pool-based workouts).

7. **Answer: A.** Patients in the precontemplation stage of change are not thinking about making a change at all now or within the next 6 months. The patients in this stage of change are not currently interested in changing, so the level of readiness and importance is generally quite low (0–3/10).

8. **Answer: B.** As outlined in the health belief model, cues to action are events or stimuli that prompt a patient to change their behavior. Examples of cues to action may include but are not limited to mass media content, social marketing, and health education.

9. **Answer: C.** As part of developing an action plan, in addition to creating SMART goals and inquiring about social support, barriers, and strategies for overcoming obstacles, it is also important to gauge the patient's confidence and commitment to completing the action plan. One effective approach, particularly in the early stages of change, is to ask a scaling question in which the patient scores their confidence, importance, or readiness level on a scale of 0 to 10.

10. **Answer: C.** Despite not achieving the specific goal outlined in the patient's action plan, it is beneficial during the follow-up process to first discuss and affirm the progress the patient has made to increase patient self-efficacy. The patient and provider can then discuss specific barriers that arose and devise solutions to overcome these obstacles to support ongoing progress in the specified area of lifestyle change.

SECTION 2 REFERENCES

1. Prochaska J. O., Norcross J. C., DiClemente C. C. *Changing for Good: A Revolutionary Six-Stage Program for Overcoming Bad Habits and Moving Your Life Positively Forward.* New York, NY: Quill; 2010.
2. Prochaska J. O., Velicer W. F. The transtheoretical model of health behavior change. *Am J Health Promot.* 1997;12(1):38-48.
3. Hugtenburg J. G., Timmers L., Elders P. J., Vervloet M., van Dijk L. Definitions, variants, and causes of nonadherence with medication: a challenge for tailored interventions. *Patient Prefer Adherence.* 2013;7:675-682.
4. Middleton K. R., Anton S. D., Perri M. G. Long-term adherence to health behavior change. *Am J Lifestyle Med.* 2013;7(6):395-404.
5. Fredrickson B. L. The role of positive emotions in positive psychology. The broaden-and-build theory of positive emotions. *Am Psychol.* 2001;56(3):218-226.
6. Rippe J. M. *Lifestyle Medicine.* 2nd ed. Boca Raton, FL: CRC Press; 2013:1638.
7. Jensen M. D., Ryan D. H., Apovian C. M., et al. 2013 AHA/ACC/TOS guideline for the management of overweight and obesity in adults: a report of the American College of Cardiology/American Heart Association Task Force on Practice Guidelines and The Obesity Society. *Circulation*. 2014;129(25 Suppl 2):S102-138.
8. Miller W. R., Moyers T. B. Motivational interviewing and the clinical science of Carl Rogers. *J Consult Clin Psychol.* 2017;85(8):757-766.
9. Miller W.R., Rollnick, S. Motivational Interviewing: Helping People to Change. 3rd ed. Guilford Press; 2013.
10. Miller W. R., Rollnick S. Ten things that motivational interviewing is not. *Behav Cogn Psychother.* 2009;37(2):129-140.
11. W. LaMorte. Behavioral change models. September 9, 2019; http://sphweb.bumc.bu.edu/otlt/MPH-Modules/SB/BehavioralChangeTheories/index.html.
12. C. Ackerman. Cognitive distortions: when your brain lies to you. October 31, 2020. https://positivepsychology.com/cognitive-distortions.
13. Ellis A. Rational psychotherapy. J Gen Psychol. 1958;59(1):35-49. https://doi.org/10.1080/00221309.1958.9710170.
14. Ellis A., Dryden W. *The Practice of Rational-Emotive Therapy (RET)*. New York, NY: Springer Publishing; 1987.
15. Raihan N., Cogburn M. Stages of Change Theory. Treasure Island, FL; StatPearls Publishing; 2021. https://www.ncbi.nlm.nih.gov/books/NBK556005/.
16. verywellmind. SMART goals for lifestyle change. December 15, 2020. https://www.verywellmind.com/smart-goals-for-lifestyle-change-2224097.
17. Hayden J. *Introduction to Health Behavior Theory*. 3rd ed. Burlington, VT: Jones & Bartlett Learning; 2019.
18. Deci Edward L., Ryan Richard M. The "What" and "Why" of Goal Pursuits: Human Needs and the Self-Determination of Behavior. *Psychological Inquiry*. 2000;11(4):227-268. https://doi.org/10.1207/S15327965PLI1104_01.
19. Deci E. L., Eghrari H., Patrick B. C., Leone D. R. Facilitating internalization: the self-determination theory perspective. *J Pers.* 1994;62(1):119-142.
20. Wing R. R., Jeffery R. W. Benefits of recruiting participants with friends and increasing social support for weight loss and maintenance. *J Consult Clin Psychol.* 1999;67(1):132-138.
21. Volk M. L., Lieber S. R., Kim S. Y., Ubel P. A., Schneider C. E. Contracts with patients in clinical practice. *Lancet.* 2012;379(9810):7-9.
22. Katz D. L., Colino S. Disease-Proof: The Remarkable Truth about What Makes Us Well. Waterville, ME: Thorndike Press; 2014.
23. Whitlock E. P., Orleans C. T., Pender N., Allan J. Evaluating primary care behavioral counseling interventions: an evidence-based approach. *Am J Prev Med.* 2002;22(4):267-284.
24. Substance Abuse and Mental Health Services Administration. About screening, brief intervention, and referral to treatment (SBIRT). June 4th, 2015. https://www.samhsa.gov/sbirt/about. Accessed September 6th, 2017.
25. Sforzo G. A., Kaye M. P., Todorova I., et al. Compendium of the health and wellness coaching literature. *Am J Lifestyle Med.* 2018;12(6):436-447.
26. Sforzo G. A., Kaye M. P., Harenberg S., et al. Compendium of health and wellness coaching: 2019 addendum. *Am J Lifestyle Med.* 2020;14(2):155-168.
27. Jay M., Gillespie C., Schlair S., Sherman S., Kalet A. Physicians' use of the 5As in counseling obese patients: is the quality of counseling associated with patients' motivation and intention to lose weight? *BMC Health Serv Res.* 2010;10:159.
28. Griffin S. J., Kinmonth A. L., Veltman M. W., Gillard S., Grant J., Stewart M. Effect on health-related outcomes of interventions to alter the interaction between patients and practitioners: a systematic review of trials. *Ann Fam Med.* 2004;2(6):595-608.
29. Hojat M., Louis D. Z., Markham F. W., Wender R., Rabinowitz C., Gonnella J. S. Physicians' empathy and clinical outcomes for diabetic patients. *Acad Med*. 2011;86(3):359-364.
30. Dwamena F., Holmes-Rovner M., Gaulden C. M., et al. Interventions for providers to promote a patient-centred approach in clinical consultations. *Cochrane Database Syst Rev.* 2012;12:CD003267.
31. Kaplan S. H., Greenfield S., Ware J. E. Jr. Assessing the effects of physician-patient interactions on the outcomes of chronic disease. *Med Care.* 1989;27(3 Suppl):S110-127.
32. A. Bandura. *Self-Efficacy: The Exercise of Control.* New York, NY: W.H. Freeman; 1997.
33. Rollnick S., Mason P., Butler C. *Health Behavior Change,* A Guide for Practitioners. London, UK: Churchill Livingstone, 1999.
34. Strober D. S., Grant A. M. Evidence-Based Coaching. Hoboken, NJ: John Wiley & Sons; 2006.
35. Moore M., Jackson E., Tschannen-Moran B. Coaching Psychology Manual. 2nd ed. Philadelphia: Wolters Kluwer; 2016.

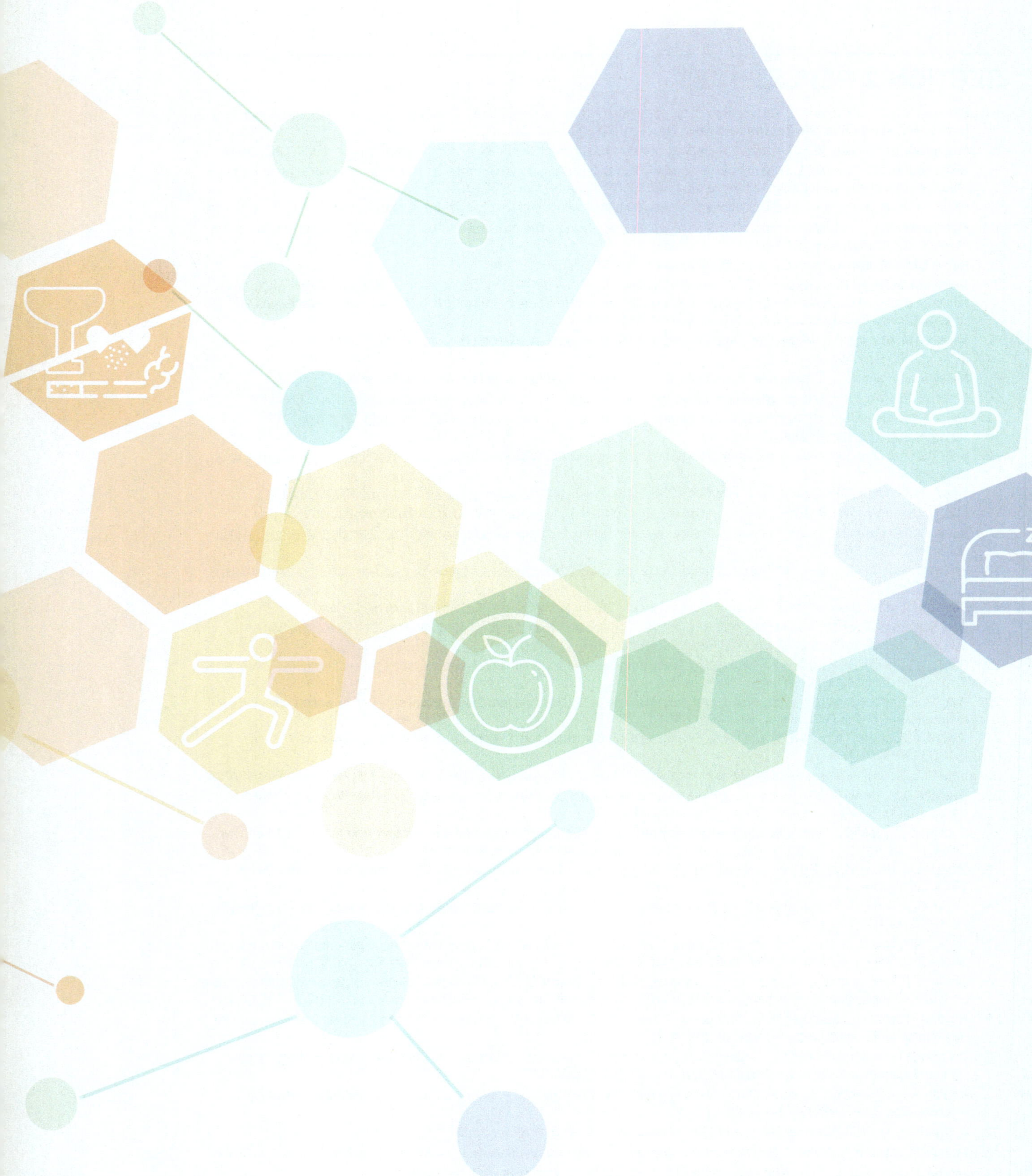

SECTION 3
Key Clinical Processes in Lifestyle Medicine

Objective 1 List the components of a patient history and physical with an emphasis on lifestyle related factors 59

Objective 2 Describe the screening and diagnostic tests that are relevant to lifestyle-related diseases 66

Objective 3 Describe how to interpret the laboratory testing for diabetes using evidence-based national guidelines 67

Objective 4 Cite strategies for effective office systems and office tools for tracking screening frequency and test results, and for proactively prompting follow-up 68

Objective 5 Describe strategies for a clinical practice to obtain information about local community resources and strategies for designing an office flow that assures consistent and up-to-date referrals 70

Objective 6 Describe how to create and sustain clinical lifestyle medicine interventions through a network of health care professionals and services 71

Objective 7 Describe the key strategies for leveraging an interdisciplinary team to enhance health behavior change interventions 72

Objective 8 List at least three resources that support healthy lifestyles/lifestyle change that are available nationally 73

Objective 9 Describe how group visits can optimize office visits to support lifestyle modification 74

Objective 10 Cite the evidence for collaborative and chronic care models on improved lifestyle outcomes by use of allied health professionals 75

Objective 11 Cite examples of team implementation from demonstrated chronic care models 76

Objective 12 Describe the chronic care model components and how they can be implemented to support lifestyle modification 77

Objective 13 Describe successful primary care and office-based models for lifestyle modification, such as the "Prescription for Health" model. **80**

Objective 14 Describe the process for health care service quality improvement with applications for lifestyle interventions, such as the Plan-Do-Study-Act (PDSA) cycles. **81**

Section 3 Glossary **84**

Section 3 Review Questions **85**

Section 3 Review Question Answers and Summaries **87**

Section 3 References. **89**

OBJECTIVE 1

List the components of a patient history and physical with an emphasis on lifestyle related factors

1) **A lifestyle medicine history and physical exam involves:**
   a) Vital signs
   b) Risk factor assessment
   c) Physical exam
   d) Lab work and interpretation
   e) Diagnosis and management
   f) Collaborative care and referrals

2) **Vital signs**
   a) Lifestyle medicine vital signs as discussed in the *Journal of the American Medical Association* 2010 article, "Physician competencies for prescribing lifestyle medicine," include physical activity, diet, stress, sleep, emotional well-being, tobacco use, alcohol consumption, and body mass index (BMI).[1]
   b) The vital signs above should not be considered standards; they should be used to create regular check-ins about every major healthy lifestyle component. More research needs to be done for these vital signs to become standardized.
   c) Physical activity vital sign
      1. Physical activity is an important vital sign because it is an aspect of daily total energy expenditure (TEE) over which people have control. Other sources of calorie expenditure, such as from rest and the thermic effect from food, can change with increased muscle mass or types of food but may take longer to see or have a smaller impact.
         a. Components of TEE
            (1) Resting energy expenditure = 60 to 75% of TEE
            (2) Physical activity = 15 to >30% of TEE
            (3) Diet induced thermogenesis = 10% of TEE
      2. The physical activity vital sign is easily and quickly measured using the two-item exercise vital sign.[2]
         a. "How many days a week do you engage in moderate to strenuous exercise, such as a brisk walk?"
         b. "On average, how many minutes per day do you exercise at this level?"
         c. This information is considered a valid measure for classifying inactive, insufficiently active, or sufficiently active levels of exercise, based on recommendations from the physical activity guidelines.[3,4]
         d. The two-item exercise vital sign provides general information about cardiovascular exercise but does not address strength and resistance exercises, balance, or flexibility exercises.
      3. Strength training is usually assessed separately.
         a. It's important to assess strength training because it can increase resting energy expenditure, improve activities of daily living, and reduce the risk for falls, especially in the elderly.

b. Ask: "How many days a week do you engage in strength training or resistance exercises?"

d) Diet vital sign

1. It's important to assess diet as a vital sign since chronic disease and being overweight or obese are all directly correlated with poor diet. It's important to assess for these risk factors.
2. Assess for the presence of whole foods in the patient's diet based on the US Department of Agriculture *Dietary Guidelines for Americans, 2020–2025.*[5] It is better to assess for whole foods or eating patterns rather than isolated nutrients. Looking at specific nutrients is complicated, possibly misleading, and generally not necessary.
   a. Typical shortfall nutrients are vitamins A, D, E, C, folate, calcium, magnesium, fiber, and potassium.
   b. The key food groups important in providing these nutrients are mainly found in vegetables, fruits, whole-grains, beans and legumes, and low-fat dairy products.
   c. Ask: "How many servings of vegetables do you generally have in a day?" Repeat the question with fruits, whole-grains, beans and legumes, nuts and seeds, herbs and spices, and then low-fat dairy products.
3. Note that people who are not meeting the recommended servings of healthy foods are likely over-consuming unhealthy foods. If time allows, it may be helpful to understand what foods and food components are being over-consumed (e.g., added sugars including high-fructose corn syrup, cholesterol, refined grains, sodium, saturated fats, and trans fats).
   a. Usually these food components are found in sugar-sweetened beverages; processed and packaged foods with added fat, sugar, and salt; fried foods; and animal products, including high-fat dairy products (milk, cheese), meat, and eggs.
   b. Ask: "How many sugar-sweetened beverages do you have in a day?" Repeat the question with servings of processed and packaged foods, fried foods, high-fat dairy products, meat, and eggs.
   c. Some tools may be helpful in collecting data on dietary intake but may be too time-consuming to use as a vital sign. However, these tools can be used by a dietitian, or in a separate visit. Please see Section 5, Objective 8.2.e), "Dietary assessment."
   d. Short dietary assessments may not be as accurate but may be useful in detecting higher or lower intakes of certain foods for individuals or populations.[6]
      (1) The National Institutes of Health has made several validated screening tools available including the following:
         (a) Dietary Screener Questionnaire (DSQ) in the National Health and Nutritional Examination Survey (NHANES)[7]
         (b) Dietary screeners in National Health Interview Survey (NHIS) Cancer Control Supplements (CCS)[8]
         (c) Dietary screeners in the California Health Interview Survey (CHIS)[9]
         (d) Fruit and Vegetable Intake Screeners in Eating at Americas Table Study (EATS)[10]
         (e) Percentage of Energy from Fat Screener[11]
         (f) Multifactor Screener in Observing Protein and Energy Nutrition (OPEN) study[12]
      (2) The Mediterranean-DASH Diet Intervention for Neurodegenerative Delay (MIND) diet score is a dietary screening tool. A positive score is associated with slower decline in global cognitive score, but findings need to be replicated in an intervention trial.[13,14]
      (3) The SOS-Free (salt/oil/sugar-free) Diet Screener from T. Colin Campbell Center for Nutrition Studies[15]

(a) Foods included

1. Vegetables 10–30+ servings per day

2. Fruits 4–10+ servings per day

3. Whole-grains 0–10+ servings a day

4. Legumes 0–5+ servings a day

5. Nuts and seeds 1 ounce per day

(b) Foods not included

1. Animal products

2. Added sugar, salt, and oil

3. Refined grains

4. Other processed foods

(4) A Short Form Food Frequency Questionnaire (SFFFQ) was shown to be an effective instrument for assessing diet quality amongst primary care patients when compared to an extensive food frequency questionnaire but it did not show significant agreement with a 24-hour telephone-based diet recall.[16]

(5) Assessing diet patterns may become a method of assessing a patient's general nutrition habits.[17,18]

e) Stress vital sign

1. Stress vital signs are important to address, as approximately 70% of visits to a primary care provider are related to stress. Stressed individuals are at a higher risk for many diseases, and they are less likely to engage in healthy habits.[19,20]
2. Stress vital signs can be assessed with a brief questionnaire on perceived stress.[21,22]

a. The perceived stress scale assessment is a 10-item questionnaire that evaluates symptoms of stress on a scale of 0 (never) to 4 (very often) over the past month by asking if patients are:

(1) Upset because of something that happened unexpectedly.

(2) Unable to control the important things in your life.

(3) Felt nervous and stressed.

(4) Felt confident about your ability to handle your personal problems.

(5) Felt that things were going your way.

(6) Could not cope with all the things that you had to do.

(7) Able to control irritations in your life.

(8) Felt that you were on top of things.

(9) Angered because of things that happened that were outside of your control.

(10) Felt difficulties were piling up so high that you could not overcome them.

b. Scoring of the 10-item perceived stress score is as follows:

(1) For the negatively phrased questions (items 1, 2, 3, 6, 9, and 10) the scoring is "never" (0), "almost never" (1), "sometimes" (2), "fairly often" (3), and "very often" (4).

(2) For the positively phrased questions (items 4, 5, 7, and 8) the scoring is reversed and becomes "never" (4), "almost never" (3), "sometimes" (2), "fairly often" (1), and "often" (0).

(3) The higher the score the more perceived stress one is under.

3. A longer length validated stress questionnaire is the "Short Stress State Questionnaire" based on the Dundee Stress State Questionnaire (DSSQ). It is a 24-item assessment assessing 3 aspects of subjective stress, including task engagement, distress, and worry.[23]

f) Sleep vital sign

1. A mini sleep assessment asks about:
    a. Typical weekday hours of sleep
    b. Typical weekend hours of sleep
    c. Perceived sleep quality
2. The Epworth Sleepiness Scale (ESS) is a validated 8-question assessment for daytime sleepiness. The higher the score, the higher a person's average sleep propensity.[24] Nearly all individuals with narcolepsy had elevated ESS scores consistent with moderate to severe excessive daytime sleepiness.[25]

g) Emotional well-being vital sign

1. A quick screening of emotional well-being may be done by asking the patient to rate the following on a scale of 1 (lowest) to 5 (highest):
    a. In most ways, my life is close to my ideal.
    b. I am satisfied with my life.
2. The above two questions come from a slightly longer questionnaire called the Satisfaction with Life Scale (SWLS). It was created to help measure one's satisfaction with life and includes five questions. Testing of this instrument in public health surveys showed responses were overall negatively skewed. Older age, higher levels of education, and higher income were associated with greater subjective well-being. Lower satisfaction with life was associated with identifying as "other" race/ethnicity (in this study meaning not being white, black, or Hispanic), the lowest levels of education, and lower household incomes.[26]
3. Other options may include the 12-Item Short Form (SF-12) or 36-Item Short Form (SF-36) to assess an overall sense of well-being. These resources can be found online at https://www.rand.org/health-care/surveys_tools.html.

h) Tobacco use vital sign

1. Ask the patient about tobacco use (including cigarettes, cigars, chew, and e-cigarettes) and document the status (current user, past user, or never used).
2. If the patient is using tobacco, document the amount of tobacco used and the years of use.
3. The World Health Organization (WHO) offers a guide on tobacco surveillance for those with current or past use of tobacco products. They suggest also screening for secondhand exposure or who a tobacco user may be putting at risk by exposing.[27]

i) Alcohol consumption vital sign

1. If the patient is regularly drinking, screen her at every visit. If not, screen for this once a year at her physical.
2. AUDIT–C (The Alcohol Use Disorders Identification Test–Concise) has three items
    a. Questions, rated 0 (never, low number of occurrences) to 4 (daily, high number of occurrences) are:
        (1) How often do you have a drink containing alcohol?
        (2) How many drinks containing alcohol do you have on a typical day when you are drinking?
        (3) How often do you have six or more drinks on one occasion?

j) BMI vital sign

1. Being overweight or obese has been associated with at least 20 different health conditions, including musculoskeletal disorders, cardiovascular disease, diabetes mellitus, chronic kidney disease, and several cancers. Screening for risk factors and documenting BMI is important for diagnosis and treatment.[28]
2. Calculate BMI in metric: (Body weight in kg) / (height in m)^2
3. Calculate BMI in imperial: (Weight in pounds / (height in inches)^2 x 703
4. BMI designations
   a. Underweight <18.5
   b. Normal 18.5–24.9 (lowest risk ~19–22)
   c. Overweight 25.0–29.9
   d. Obese
      (1) 30.0–34.9 (class I)
      (2) 35.0–39.9 (class 2)
      (3) Extreme obesity ≥40 (class 3)

$$\text{BMI} = \frac{\text{Weight (lbs)}}{[\text{Height (in)}]^2} \times 703$$

$$\text{BMI} = \frac{\text{Weight (kg)}}{[\text{Height (m)}]^2}$$

3) Several forms and tools have been created to assess for multiple lifestyle factors within the same questionnaire.

a) The American College of Lifestyle Medicine, in collaboration with Loma Linda University, offers two lifestyle behavior screening questionnaires on their website available in English and Spanish. These tools are not yet validated.

1. Lifestyle Assessment Short Form is a two-page questionnaire with 14 questions .
2. Lifestyle Assessment Long Form is a 12-page detailed assessment and includes recommended preventive screenings, a section on weight management, and the six pillars of lifestyle medicine.

b) The US Department for Veterans Affairs Whole Health Personal Health Inventory[29]

1. This is a very comprehensive patient self-assessment used to identify environmental, behavioral, or psychosocial issues that could impact the patient's state of health or medical care.

c) The US Army's Global Assessment Tool, also known as the Azimuth test, which assesses a soldier's level of fitness across five domains of life: Physical, Emotional, Social, Spiritual, and Family. [30]

d) The American Heart Association's Life's Simple 7 Questionnaire[31]

1. Created to help assess seven risk factors people can improve through lifestyle changes to achieve improved cardiovascular health.
2. Risk factors assessed include smoking status, physical activity, weight, diet, blood glucose, cholesterol, and blood pressure.
3. If at least five of these factors are in the ideal range, studies have shown this is associated with a 78% reduction in cardiovascular related death compared to those with no factors in ideal range.[32]

4) Risk factor measurement

a) Screening tools are helpful because they bring up the discussion of lifestyle factors sooner rather than later, allowing time for lifestyle interventions.

b) Cardiovascular disease

1. Life's Simple 7 Questionnaire[31]

2. ASCVD Risk Estimator Plus by the American College of Cardiology[33]
    a. The assessment indicates the patient's risk of myocardial infarction in next 10 years.
        (1) This tool was developed based on data from pooled cohorts from non-Hispanic whites and African Americans. It may underestimate cardiovascular risk amongst American Indians, some Asian Americans (south Asian ancestry), and some Hispanics (Puerto Ricans). It may overestimate risks for Asian Americans of east Asian ancestry and some Hispanics (Mexican Americans).
    b. Results apply to adults 20 years to 79 years of age without heart disease.
    c. The assessment considers: age, gender, total cholesterol, high-density lipoprotein (HDL) cholesterol, low-density lipoprotein (LDL) cholesterol, smoking status, diabetes history, and treatment for hypertension, such as use of a statin and/or aspirin therapy.
    d. The results give a 10-year risk evaluation for atherosclerotic cardiovascular disease (ASCVD) as categorized by low-risk, borderline risk, intermediate risk, or high risk.
3. The 2015 MESA (Multi-Ethnic Study of Artherosclerosis) risk score is multi-ethnic and includes a coronary calcium score. It was validated as an accurate measure of 10-year coronary heart disease risk in men and women in a multi-ethnic study (39% non-Hispanic whites, 12% Chinese Americans, 28% African Americans, and 22% Hispanic Americans).[34]
    a. Risk factor calculator can be found online at www.mesa-nhlbi.org/MESACHDRisk/MesaRiskScore/RiskScore.aspx
4. The Reynold's risk score for women considers family history and high sensitivity c-reactive protein, which predicts risk of global cardiovascular disease.[35]
    a. Risk factor calculator can be found online at www.reynoldsriskscore.org
5. Cardiovascular risk factor calculators have been developed and put to use around the world. It may be important to choose a calculator specific to one's region or country for the most accurate assessment.

c) Prediabetes screening test

1. The Centers for Disease Control prediabetes screening test can be found online at Prediabetes Risk Test (https://www.cdc.gov).

d) Diabetes risk assessment

1. American Diabetes Association risk assessment for developing type 2 diabetes
    a. http://main.diabetes.org/dorg/PDFs/risk-test-paper-version.pdf
2. Finnish Diabetes Association, risk assessment for developing type 2 diabetes within 10 years
    a. http://www.idf.org/webdata/docs/FINDRISC_English.pdf
3. Australian government type 2 diabetes risk assessment tool
    a. https://www.health.gov.au/sites/default/files/the-australian-type-2-diabetes-risk-assessment-tool-ausdrisk.pdf

5) Lifestyle medicine physical evaluation and examination

a) Waist circumference

1. There is a higher risk of disease (type 2 diabetes, hypertension, and cardiovascular disease) relative to increased weight and waist circumference.
2. Waist circumference is considered increased if the waist is:
    a. ≥40 inches (≥102 centimeters) for men
    b. ≥35 inches (≥88 centimeters) for women

b) Waist/hip ratio

1. Normal waist to hip standards for men and women are:[36]
    a. ≤0.90 for men
    b. ≤0.85 for women
2. As shown in Table 3.1, ratios above normal are correlated with a substantially increased risk of metabolic complications.[36]
    a. Those of Asian descent are at higher risk of diabetes at lower BMIs compared to whites.[37] Based on this knowledge, the WHO in conjunction with the International Association for Obesity suggested lower-cut off points for BMI in those of Asian descent, leaving it up to countries to create the final definition of overweight or obesity based on the country's risk factors. In the WHO report *Waist Circumference and Waist-Hip Ratio*, 2008, Chinese, Japanese and Korean, or South Asian (or Indian) ethnic groups where analyzed as a homogeneous population under the name "Asians".[38]

Table 3.1 Overweight/Obesity Classification by BMI, Waist Circumference, and Associated Disease Risk

Diagnosis	BMI (kg/m^2)		Comorbidity Risk	Risk of DM2, HTN, CVD (Relative to normal weight & WC)	
	Non-Asian	Asian		Men: <40 in* Women: <35 in*	>40 in >35 in
Underweight	<18.5	<18.5	Low, but other problems		
Normal weight	18.5–24.9	18.5–22.9	Average		
Overweight	25.0–29.9	23–24.9	Increased	Increased	High
Obese class 1	30.0–34.9	≥25	Moderate	High	Very High
Obese class 2	35.0–39.9		Severe	Very High	Very High
Obese class 3—Extreme Obesity	≥40		Very severe	Extremely High	Extremely High

Abbreviations: BMI = body mass index; CVD = cardiovascular disease; HTN = hypertension; DM2 = type 2 diabetes; WC = waist circumference

*35 in = 88 cm; 40 in = 102 cm

Obesity: Preventing and Managing the Global Epidemic a report from the World Health Organization consultation on obesity.[39]

c) Bio-impedance analysis[40]

1. Low accuracy, but this analysis is safe and easy to use in clinic setting.
2. Other methods of body composition testing exist, but may not be feasible to assess in clinic setting or financially viable for patients. These include the BodPod, Omron scale, Dexa Bone scan, and hydrostatic underwater weighing.

d) Pulse

1. Pulse is a nonspecific indicator of possible health problems and potential lack of fitness.
2. Possible lifestyle causes of tachycardia include physical deconditioning, alcohol, or caffeine.

e) Blood pressure

1. Highlights from the *2017 Guideline for the Prevention, Detection, Evaluation, and Management of High Blood Pressure in Adults*,[41] a report from the American College of Cardiology and American Heart Association
    a. 2017 update of standards of blood pressure measurement[41]

(1) Normal blood pressure: <120/<80 mmHg

(2) Elevated blood pressure: systolic 120–129/<80 mmHg

(3) Stage 1: systolic 130–139/80–89 mmHg

(4) Stage 2: systolic ≥140/≥90 mmHg

2. Hypertension increases morbidity and mortality, leading to:[41]
   a. Higher mortality from heart disease, stroke, and other vascular disease.
   b. Higher morbidity from cardiovascular disease incidence, angina, myocardial infarction, heart failure, stroke, peripheral artery disease, and abdominal aortic aneurysm.
3. Prevalence of hypertension increases with age 42.
   a. More than 50% of adults over 60 years old have hypertension.
   b. It's important to screen for hypertension at each periodic visit (every 6 to 12 months).
4. Small reductions in blood pressure can substantially reduce illness burden (Table 3.2).[41,42,43,44,45,46,47]

Table 3.2

Reduction in Blood Pressure (mmHg)	% Reduction in Mortality		
	Stroke	Coronary Heart Disease	Total
2	6	4	3
3	8	5	4
5	14	9	7

Table based on data from the INTERSALT Study, N = 10,079, men and women 20–59 years of age from 32 countries.[46]

f) Measure of fitness[48,49]

g) Fitness testing options (See Section 6 for complete testing information)

1. Step testing for cardiorespiratory fitness
2. Squats, pushups, and sit-ups for muscular endurance
3. Sit and reach test for flexibility
4. Skin calipers to evaluate body composition
5. Note: Muscular strength is difficult to test in a clinic unless weights or the ability to apply a load are available (such as with a bench or squat press). It may be best to refer to a medical fitness professional for this.

OBJECTIVE 2

Describe the screening and diagnostic tests that are relevant to lifestyle-related diseases

1) Complete metabolic panel which includes 14 tests evaluating the health of the kidneys and liver, blood glucose and blood proteins, and electrolyte and acid/base balance.

a) Consider that further testing may be indicated.

2) Complete blood count which includes tests for cell counts and measurements of red blood cells, white blood cells, and platelets.

a) Consider that further testing may be indicated.

3) **Fasting lipids provide information about:**

   a) Total cholesterol (TC)

      1. This test is usually ordered in a lab panel that includes HDL cholesterol and triglycerides (TG), and it's not ordered alone unless it's being used as an indicator for more detailed testing. If TC is less than 150 mg/dL (3.879 mmol/L) the risk of overall heart disease is very low.

   b) LDL cholesterol

      1. Usually calculated by the Friedewald equation: LDL = TC – HDL – (TG*0.2).[50]
      2. The above calculation is not a valid calculation if TG are over 400 (4.516 mmol/L).

   c) HDL cholesterol

      1. Particle size has been shown to help stratify risk; particle density alone does not completely describe the role and function of cholesterol fractions.[51,52]

   d) TG

      1. Elevations are often associated with low HDL and increased girth (waist circumference).

   e) High-sensitivity CRP

      1. A marker of chronic inflammation that is used as a biomarker for cardiovascular disease and that can help determine the risk of developing myocardial infarction in people who have cardiovascular disease or in asymptomatic people who are at risk of developing cardiovascular disease.

4) **Fasting serum glucose, hemoglobin A1c (HbA1c), oral glucose tolerance test, fasting serum insulin, possibly C-peptide, and homeostatic model assessment for insulin resistance (HOMA-IR)**

   a) A stimulated C-peptide measurement may be used to assess endogenous insulin production in order to identify how well beta cells are functioning to meet the demands of insulin production. This test can help determine whether a patient has type 1 diabetes, type 2 diabetes, or something else.

   b) HOMA-IR is an estimate of insulin sensitivity and beta cell function based on the fasting plasma glucose concentrations and fasting plasma insulin or C-peptide measurements.[53,54,55]

5) **Vitamin D (25-hydroxycholecalciferol) is used to diagnose vitamin D deficiency, hypervitaminosis, or to monitor treatment.**

6) **Thyroid stimulating hormone and total and free thyroxine are used to diagnose disorders of the thyroid.**

OBJECTIVE 3

Describe how to interpret the laboratory testing for diabetes using evidence-based national guidelines

1) **Diabetes diagnosis**

   a) Diabetes lab tests include:

      1. HbA1c ≥6.5%, but this identifies 1/3 fewer cases of undiagnosed diabetes than looking at a fasting plasma glucose test or:

         a. Fasting serum glucose ≥126 mg/dL (7.0 mmol/L)

         b. 2-hour postprandial glucose ≥200 mg/dL (11.1 mmol/L) during an oral glucose tolerance test (OGTT)

2. In absence of unequivocal hyperglycemia, the results should be confirmed with repeated testing.

b) Prediabetes lab tests, include:

1. Fasting serum glucose ≥100 mg/dL (5.6 mmol/L) but <126, or:
2. 2-hour serum glucose in the 75 g OGTT of 140–199 mg/dL (7.8–11.0 mmol/L), or:
3. HbA1c of 5.7–6.4%

c) Diabetes testing should be considered in all adults who are overweight or obese (BMI ≥25) with any of the additional risk factors below. If there are no risk factors, begin screening at age 45 and repeat every 3 years.

1. Physical inactivity
2. A first-degree relative has type 2 diabetes
3. High-risk race, including Asian American, Black, Latino, Native American, or Pacific Islander
4. Women who delivered a baby >9 pounds (4.1 kg) or received a diagnosis of gestational diabetes
5. Hypertension with blood pressure ≥140/90 mmHg or on hypertension medications
6. Women with polycystic ovary syndrome
7. Prediabetes
8. Signs of insulin resistance (i.e., acanthus nigricans)
9. History of cardiovascular disease

OBJECTIVE 4

Cite strategies for effective office systems and office tools for tracking screening frequency and test results, and for proactively prompting follow-up

1) Tracking is already a common practice in most clinics to assess progress, high risk patients, and outcomes.

a) Many offices track things such as vital signs, laboratory results, and patient satisfaction scores. This may be a part of meeting quality or performance metrics and tied to financial reimbursement.

b) Primary care clinics typically track information for the Healthcare Effectiveness Data and Information Set (HEDIS), which is one of the most widely used healthcare performance improvement tools. HEDIS rates health plans, programs, and providers on their quality, and the public can review the rating online.[56]

2) In lifestyle medicine, tracking is essential for patient care, treatment analysis, reimbursement, and follow up

a) Tracking lifestyle changes helps patients and financial payers see the effectiveness of a lifestyle intervention improving engagement and commitment.

b) Tracking provides information necessary for quality improvement, such as the evidence for the effectiveness or ineffectiveness of a treatment or treatment program.

c) Tracking is the basis for cost savings analysis.

d) Tracking allows provider team to monitor reimbursement for services rendered.

3) **Electronic medical records (EMRs) can often be helpful in tracking metrics and high-risk patients. It's important to know what the EMR is tracking, how the information is stored and maintained, and if automatic prompts are possible.**

a) Most EMR have some built-in capacity or comply with programs that allow for data extraction. Some tracking programs make it easier to collect information than others.

b) Ideally, the EMR should be used to track high-risk patients or those with uncontrolled chronic conditions.

1. Tracking high-risk patients can be done with reports based off of a diagnosis code, recorded labs such as an elevated hemoglobin A1c, or reported high risk behaviors such as tobacco use.
2. These reports allow for targeted management of these high-risk patients.
3. Some clinics have a condition-management nurse who can help monitor and oversee patients whose medical conditions are not ideally controlled.

c) Some EMRs can also send reminders or automatic prompts to the clinical care team or through the patient portal system for things such as yearly physicals, necessary, lab work, or vaccinations.

d) Be familiar with the capabilities and limitations of an EMR to use it to its full extent.

e) When using an EMR to track lifestyle measures:

1. Know exactly where and how the lifestyle measures will be collected, stored, and maintained.
   a. Have an effective way to extract information from the EMR. Unfortunately, not all EMRs are capable of this and recording manually with a spreadsheet document may be necessary.
   b. Make sure data extracted can be translated into meaningful results to share with others.
   c. Helpful hint: It may be beneficial to start backwards by identifying what information you would like to share with others, then solving what would be needed to do that.

f) Frequency of reporting

1. HEDIS is typically reported on once a year.[56]
2. Lifestyle medicine changes are often tracked more frequently.
   a. If patients are enrolled in an Intensive Therapeutic Lifestyle Change program, lab work and tests may be collected within 1–4 weeks into the program. This may be dependent upon a patient's coverage and ability to follow up.
   b. A potential timeline for collecting lifestyle medicine measurements might be:
      (1) Before the start of lifestyle changes
      (2) 2 to 4 weeks into making changes
      (3) 3 months, 6 months, and 12 months may also be desirable to show sustainability.
      (4) Some patients may not be able to afford to have labs done this frequently, but taking both physical vital signs, lifestyle medicine vital signs, and potentially fitness measurements can be more affordable and still provide useful information about the patient's progress.

4) **Sharing information[57]**

a) Lifestyle medicine is a relatively new specialty and still growing in acceptance in the larger medical community.
   1. For newer lifestyle medicine programs, results should be collected and shared more frequently to make assessments, improvements, and build confidence and rapport.
   2. Once a program is well established, and the results are consistent, reporting may occur after more extended periods.
   3. Reporting over longer periods is generally going to give a more accurate measure of real change as some data may fluctuate with the seasons.

Helpful Tip

Questions to consider when creating office systems for tracking health information:

- What information is tracked already?
- What other information should be collected?
- Why will it be important?
- When and how will the data be collected, stored, and maintained?
- How will this data be translated into something useful to share with others?

OBJECTIVE 5

Describe strategies for a clinical practice to obtain information about local community resources and strategies for designing an office flow that assures consistent and up-to-date referrals

1) **Maintain an up-to-date list of local resources, including worksite wellness programs, to assist patients.**
   a) Designate a team member to serve as the lead coordinator to community services and to maintain an up-to-date list of local and national resources.
   b) The team member should regularly check (at least semi-annually) websites and the contact list for the local health department, hospital, and health systems for information about lifestyle change classes, educational support services, and fees.
   c) The physician/provider should review the list to assure the resources align with lifestyle medicine values and clinic practices.
   d) Providers and staff can direct patients to helpful resources as indicated.
2) **Refer patients to other health professionals and community resources as appropriate and financially feasible (remembering that some patients are not covered by insurance).**

OBJECTIVE 6

Describe how to create and sustain clinical lifestyle medicine interventions through a network of health care professionals and services

1) **Refer patients to other health professionals who ideally are also trained in lifestyle medicine such as:**
   a) Lifestyle medicine specialists, especially for treatment with intensive therapeutic lifestyle therapy change programs
   b) Registered Dietitians
   c) Pharmacists
   d) Physical and Occupational therapists
   e) Nurses
   f) Health educators
   g) Certified exercise physiologists
   h) Fitness trainers
   i) Coaches
   j) Psychologists

2) **Reach out to professionals in the local network to discuss how to mutually support each other's work with an emphasis on the lifestyle medicine approach.**
   a) Prioritize working with lifestyle medicine specialists and lifestyle coaches to assist with lifestyle behavior changes and treatments.

3) **Collaborate with integrative medicine practitioners who usually include some aspects of lifestyle medicine in their practices already.[58] Many integrative medicine providers will already be discussing lifestyle medicine changes with their patients. If you are referring patients, check to make sure those integrative medicine practices align with lifestyle medicine. Integrative medicine practitioners include:**
   a) Acupuncture and Oriental medicine, LAc—masters program, with 2–4 years of training; regulation in 43 states; National Certification Commission for Acupuncture and Oriental Medicine (NCCAOM)
   b) Chiropractic, DC—doctorate program, with 4 years of training; regulation in 50 states; Federation of Chiropractic Licensing Boards (FCLB)
   c) Midwifery, CPM—variable degrees and variable training; licensing or certification in 22 states; North American Registry of Midwives (NARM)
   d) Massage therapy—no degree with 500–1,000 hours of training; regulation in 39 states; National Certification Board for Therapeutic Massage and Bodywork (NCBTMB)
   e) Naturopathic medicine, ND—doctorate program, with 4 years of training; licensing in 15 states; North American Board of Naturopathic Examiners (NABNE)

4) **Online referral resources**
   a) Academy of Nutrition and Dietetics: www.eatright.org
   b) National Association of Nutrition Professionals (holistic nutrition): www.nanp.org
   c) Registered Clinical Exercise Physiologist, Certified Clinical Exercise Physiologist, and Certified Personal Trainer through American College of Sports Medicine: www.acsm.org
   d) US Registry of Exercise Professionals: www.usreps.org
   e) Certified Medical Fitness facilities: www.medicalfitness.org
   f) Personal trainer directory: www.ideafit.com/find-personal-trainer
   g) The Yale-Griffin Prevention Research Center tips for chronic disease prevention: www.yalegriffinprc.org/Programs-Resources/Tips-for-Chronic-Disease-Prevention

---

OBJECTIVE 7

Describe the key strategies for leveraging an interdisciplinary team to enhance health behavior change interventions

1) **Train support staff to:**
   a) Routinely collect lifestyle medicine vital signs (exercise, nutrition, waist circumference, BMI, physical activity, etc.).
   b) Provide basic counseling and instruction (including the importance of various lifestyle factors).
   c) Provide tools and resources (handouts, community resources, websites, and apps).
   d) Help patients identify community resources (where they are and what they provide).
2) **Use a team-based approach.**
   a) Set specific standards and roles for all team members during office visits. Example:
      1. Check-in: administrative or front office staff
      2. Lifestyle vital signs: medical assistant
      3. Pre-visit assessments: medical assistant
      4. Clinical encounter: provider
      5. Coaching for behavioral change: based on availability, could be the provider, medical assistant, wellness coach, registered nurse, or registered dietitian
      6. Check out: administrative or front office staff
      7. Referral follow up: referral coordinator
   b) Hold regular team meetings and use effective communication. It may be beneficial to use Six-Sigma quality management strategies.
3) **The outcomes of interdisciplinary team care for patients should include:**[59]
   a) Advocating for lifestyle modification as a primary modality for chronic disease
   b) Supporting high levels of self-efficacy and self-management in patients
   c) Attaining higher levels of treatment compliance with improved health outcomes
   d) Implementing office work flows to effectively identify and address patients' needs for therapeutic lifestyle change

e) Optimizing patient time for support and offering counseling if applicable

f) Using electronic medical records, websites, and mobile apps that track lifestyle change progress and that prompt lifestyle interventions

g) Using patient registries to identify patients who are in need of intensive lifestyle interventions and referring them on if needed

h) Implementing group visits to provide therapeutic lifestyle change treatments

4) **Effective interdisciplinary teams should be able to demonstrate the following 10 characteristics:**[60]

   a) Positive leadership and management attributes

   b) Communication strategies and structures

   c) Personal rewards, training, and development

   d) Appropriate resources and procedures

   e) Appropriate skill mix

   f) Supportive team climate

   g) Individual characteristics that support interdisciplinary teamwork

   h) Clarity of vision

   i) Quality and outcomes of care

   j) Respecting and understanding roles

OBJECTIVE 8

List at least three resources that support healthy lifestyles/lifestyle change that are available nationally[60]

1) **National Diabetes Education Program:** http://ndep.nih.gov

2) **Centers for Disease Control and Prevention National Diabetes Prevention Program:** www.cdc.gov/diabetes/prevention/

3) **California Smokers' Helpline (1-800-NO-BUTTS):** www.nobutts.org

4) **American Heart Association: www.heart.org (Getting Healthy tab)**

5) **Million Hearts Initiative:** http://millionhearts.hhs.gov/index.html

6) **Human services, referrals, and information:** www.211.org

7) **State or Area Agency on Aging (housing, food, employment, health care, and counseling):** https://aoa.acl. gov/aoa_programs/oaa/How_To_Find/Agencies/find_agencies.aspx

8) **Classes and educational resources offered by local health systems, hospitals, and public health departments**

9) **Local parks and recreation classes and services**

10) **Senior center services**

OBJECTIVE 9

Describe how group visits can optimize office visits to support lifestyle modification[61,62]

1) **Group visits use a team approach to monitor and treat medical conditions.**

2) **Comprehensive group medical visits:**

    a) Provide a supportive group setting for consenting patients with similar concerns

    b) Are billable at individual rates

    c) Focus on chronic disease and can be an important tool in chronic disease population management for a primary care practice and for a community

    d) Require two to four health professionals, including a provider (MD, DO, NP, or PA)

    e) Can still offer personalized care as each patient's unique needs may be addressed individually while maintaining privacy—sometimes through an adjoining exam room

3) **Value of group visits**

    a) Improved access to care

        1. Group visits can reduce wait times for appointments, especially for new patients.
        2. Physicians with a full panel may be able to accommodate more patients.
        3. Physicians may appropriately see more patients more frequently and for a longer period of time to follow up on chronic disease management.
        4. These visits can be a means of reaching out to underserved patients.

    b) Increased patient and provider satisfaction

        1. Provider benefits[63,64]
            a. More efficient use of time, allowing more time to:
                (1) Check patient test results and consultation reports by leveraging existing resources
                (2) Return patient phone calls and emails
                (3) Spend more time practicing proactive, lifestyle, and preventive medicine
                (4) Manage and lead clinical teams
                (5) Collaborate with colleagues
                (6) Coordinate patients' care across a complex care system
            b. Enhances quality, outcomes, and patients' health experiences while containing cost and increasing income
            c. Something different, interesting, and fun
            d. Reduces repetition and allows for more frequent contact and longer amounts of time with each patient
            e. Documentation support can be provided by another staff member
            f. Group support and collaborative care is helpful in managing difficult, time-consuming and psychologically needy patients.
        2. Patients[64]
            a. Have improved adherence to standards of care, improved patient satisfaction, lower hospitalization rates, higher trust in providers, and improved access; for complex and elderly patients, also better monitoring[65,66,67,68,69]

b. Receive greater patient education from group discussions and peer support
c. Experience improved access to the professional skills of a behaviorist/psychologist and/or a nurse, which better addresses psychosocial needs
d. Gain additional choices in their health care treatment options
e. Use peer support

c) Reduces costs, as there's increased efficiency and leveraging of existing resources

1. Among adults with uncontrolled type 2 diabetes, group visits reduced total health care expenditure cost by approximately 30%.[67]
2. Group visits also increases physician productivity.

d) Billable under Medicare when billing criteria are followed

4) Operation of group visits[64]

a) Several different types of group visits exist. Shared medical appointments are often used for chronic disease treatment or perinatal care. Drop-in group medical appointments (DIGMAs), where patients can walk-in and be seen in a group, are used for many types of medical diseases. Physical shared medical appointments are shared medical appointments that include the opportunity for a private physical.

b) Group visits can be heterogeneous with varying ages, genders, and medical conditions or homogeneous with similar group demographics and medical condition

1. The majority of visits are pre-scheduled shared medical appointments and not drop-in group medical appointments.

c) Patients sign a confidentiality release, consenting to:

1. Have their medical information discussed in front of others
2. Agree not to discuss the personal information of others once the group is over

d) Physicians manage, advise, and treat each patient individually, but they do so in front of others (except for brief private discussions and examinations).

e) Education is part of each visit.

OBJECTIVE 10

Cite the evidence for collaborative and chronic care models on improved lifestyle outcomes by use of allied health professionals

1) Interdisciplinary team care is associated with:[59]

a) Higher levels of treatment compliance

b) Improved health outcomes

c) Enhanced patient engagement and chronic disease self-management[70]

d) Increased weight loss after 1 year (compared to standard care), when a provider, dietitian, or both provided educational interventions[71]

1. Doctor (general provider) −2.6 lbs (1.2 kg)
2. Dietitian −12.3 lbs (5.6 kg)
3. Doctor and dietitian team −13.2 lbs (6.0 kg)

2) **Healthy eating activities and lifestyle programs are associated with:**[72]
   a) Weight reduction
   b) Improvements in blood pressure and physical fitness parameters
   c) Maintained behavior changes at 5 months after the program's completion
3) **Training lay health educators is associated with improved implementation of lifestyle interventions.**[58]
   a) This has been successfully completed in rural senior centers.
4) **Lifestyle modification in primary care**[73]
   a) The acceptance and referral to a collaborative or chronic care program from a primary care practice is dependent on the level of facilitation provided by program coordinators. It's important that referrals into the program, regular communication, and follow up are easy and don't take much time for primary care providers.
   b) Having a nurse who is involved and helps coordinate the collaborative or chronic care program is important for sustaining its implementation.

OBJECTIVE 11

Cite examples of team implementation from demonstrated chronic care models

1) **Ornish Spectrum program** (http://deanornish.com/ornish-lifestyle-medicine/)
   a) Intensive cardiac rehab program
   b) The team is collaborative, synergistic, and interdisciplinary, including:
      1. Physician, exercise physiologist, stress management specialist, program director, chef/food services, registered nurse, group support specialist, registered dietitian, administrative assistant, and marketing recruiter
      2. Team roles
         a. Registered nurse
            (1) Educational co-presentation
            (2) Biometrics assessments
            (3) Continuity of care and follow-up for chronic conditions
         b. Exercise physiologist
            (1) Physical Activity Rediness Questionnaire (PAR-Q) assessment
            (2) Individual and group exercise supervision
            (3) Biometric assessment
            (4) Fitness safety and principles presentation
         c. Health coach
            (1) Mechanism for implementation
            (2) Consistent sources of social support throughout change
            (3) Built-in accountability
         d. Stress management specialist
            (1) Introduction to various mind-body techniques

        (2) Group facilitation and support
        (3) Participation with individual and group fitness instruction

    e. Registered dietitian
        (1) One-on-one nutrition counseling
        (2) Group presentation on nutrition guidelines
        (3) Recipe referral

    f. Chef/food services
        (1) Training in food selection and preparation
        (2) Removes barrier of healthy eating

    g. Group support specialist
        (1) Facilitating social dynamic and group growth
        (2) Focus on lifestyle impact of intervention

    h. Administration assistant or medical assistant
        (1) Scheduling, follow-up, referrals, and coordination of materials in the program

    i. Marketing director
        (1) Communication with providers and resources in the community

2) Medical fitness collaboration (http://www.medicalfitness.org/)[74]

a) These are medically supervised, integrated, and outcomes- and accountability-based fitness programs that include:

1. Active and regular medical oversight
2. Qualified and credentialed staff
3. Disease management and clinical integration of programs
4. Individualized exercise prescriptions

b) Programs provide a safe way for patients to transition from a structured clinical treatment setting to a home- or community-based exercise program.

c) Helpful for patients who need medical oversight and counseling for a long-term fitness program

OBJECTIVE 12

Describe the chronic care model components and how they can be implemented to support lifestyle modification

1) *Innovative Care for Chronic Conditions (ICCC)* is a report by the World Health Organization explaining how health care systems can and must update their practices to be able to care for chronic disease at each societal level.[75]

a) Micro level (patient and family)

b) Meso level (health care organization and community)

c) Macro level (policy)

2) Collaborative Care Manager Model by the Agency for Healthcare Research and Quality (AHRQ) is a model showing how the patients, clinical experts, residents, nurse practitioners, and interdisciplinary teams can collaborate in an academic setting to provide care for chronic conditions.[76]

a) Patient
    1. At the center of model and sets goals, develops skills and assumes self-care
b) Nurse practitioner (NP) or physician assistant (PA)
    1. Manages planned visit, updates care process, trains residents, provides intensive care, and engages patients in their care
c) Clinical expert (MD/DO)
    1. Leads team meetings, provides intensified care, trains residents, and assumes accountability
d) Resident
    1. Learns to provide intensive care, undergoes coaching for her own self-care goals, oversees medical care, and learns to work in a team effectively
e) Interdisciplinary care team that includes but is not limited to a pharmacist, nutritionist, social worker, psychologist, podiatrist and ophthalmologist
    1. Works with NP/PA, clinical expert MD/DO, and the resident to coordinate and facilitate patient care

3) **Value-based care**
    a) Provides financial incentives for accountable care organizations, patient-centered medical homes, and similar organizations to achieve standard health goals instead of merely having visits for disease treatment
    b) May provide the support systems that are needed to achieve successful behavior change with lifestyle prescriptions

4) **The Chronic Care Model, created by the MacColl Institute and Ed Wagner, MD, MPH, is a model that is helpful in explaining the involvement of the community and health care system in chronic disease care (Figure 3.1).**[77]
    a) This model is centered on an informed, activated, and engaged patient and a prepared, pro-active primary care practice team. Together, the patient and primary care practice must work under and with the overarching local and national health care system. They must also work with the local community (local gyms, politicians, community centers, organizations, and faith systems). As each of these entities work together, the interactions are more productive, and the patient's health care and treatments improve.

Figure 3.1 The Chronic Care Model

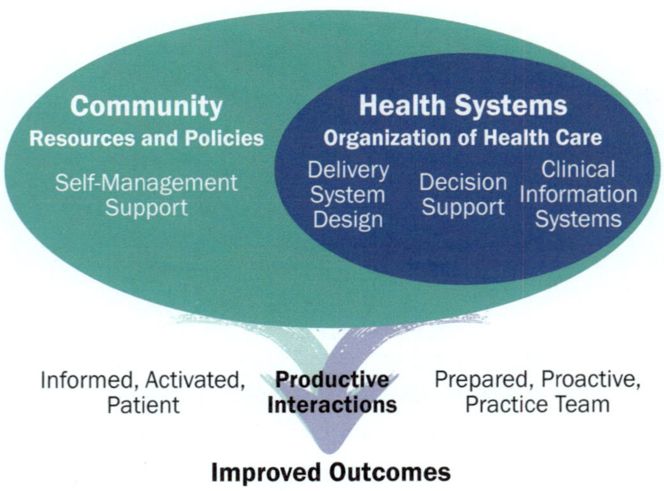

5) **Guidelines fore implementing the Chronic Care Model**[77]

a) Implementing the Chronic Care Model into a local medical practice

1. Seek community-wide coordination between your office and community agencies in caring for patients.
2. Create linkages between the community and the primary care practice.
3. Partner with community organizations and develop formal supportive programs and policies for the local health care system.

b) Health care delivery support

1. Support improvement from the senior leadership on down.
2. Promote strategies aimed at comprehensive system change.
3. Encourage open, systematic handling of errors and quality problems.

c) Self-management support

1. Benefits of self-management
    a. Patients and families cope with the challenges of their illness more effectively.
    b. Patients and families become experts in their own management.
    c. There are reduced complications and symptoms.
    d. It improves patients' overall sense of health and well-being.
2. Emphasize patients' central role in their health care.
3. Systematically assess patients' self-management needs and use peer support groups routinely.
4. Train physicians and staff in behavior change techniques and encourage use of these skills as an integral part of routine care.

d) Delivery system design

1. Implement planned patient care with strategic visits, call reminders, online communication, group visits, contact between visits, and by identifying the missed elements of care.
2. Coordinate care between the patient, office and subspecialists (in an oral and written format).
3. Install an electronic medical record (EMR) with a patient portal for ease of communication among the health team.

e) Decision support

1. Physicians and providers have access to the evidence-based information that is necessary for decision making.
2. Integrate evidence-based guidelines into care through reminders and behavior change methods.
3. Give patients specific personalized goals with a process and recommendations on how to achieve those goals.

f) Clinical information systems are most effective when:

1. Finding timely and useful information is a critical feature of population-based approaches
2. A patient registry or electronic health record has prompts and reminders of needed services
3. Guideline reminders are sent to the care team at the time of a patient encounter
4. Timely, specific performance feedback to providers can be extracted for review and correction of deficiencies

5. Specific treatment targets and goals can be entered in the system for patient self-management and clinical tracking, with the ability to adjust these with medical response and patient feedback

6) **The US Department of Veterans Affairs hospital system has developed a comprehensive, multi-site model of care called the "Whole Health model" of care. Preliminary outcomes have been very promising.[30]**

OBJECTIVE 13

Describe successful primary care and office-based models for lifestyle modification, such as the "Prescription for Health" model

1) **Prescription for Health: http://www.prescriptionforhealth.org**
   a) Prescription for Health is a 6-year initiative funded by the Robert Wood Johnson Foundation in collaboration with the Agency for Healthcare Research and Quality (AHRQ).
   b) The initiative involved 22 primary care, practice-based research networks (PBRNs) that developed, piloted, and evaluated 27 evidence-based strategies to improve delivery and effectiveness of health behavior change services in the field of primary care.
   c) Four health risk behaviors were targeted:
      1. Tobacco use
      2. Risky alcohol use
      3. Unhealthy diet
      4. Lack of physical activity
   d) Results[78,79]
      1. The initial work examined whether primary care offices would be willing and able to address health behavior issues. Findings showed that primary care offices were capable and wanted to address health behavior when funding and support were available through the PBRNs.
      2. The second wave of research revealed that in order to implement health behavior change strategies, a health care delivery model—such as a patient-centered medical home—was important. The research also found that substantial practice redesign needed to occur along with the integration of public health and community resources.
      3. Dozens of studies were published on the findings of the Prescription for Health initiative.
      4. A Prescription for Health toolkit was created, but it's now outdated, and it's no longer accessible: www.prescriptionforhealth.org/results/toolkit.html
      5. AHRQ developed the Electronic Preventive Services Selector (ePSS), which can be used by providers at the time of time of visit for decision support with screening, counseling, and preventive services.[80]
         a. The ePSS is a website and an app based on current US Preventive Services Task Force recommendations. This resource can be found online at: https://www.ahrq.gov/cpi/about/otherwebsites/epss.ahrq.gov/index.html

OBJECTIVE 14

Describe the process for health care service quality improvement with applications for lifestyle interventions, such as the Plan-Do-Study-Act cycles

1) **Quality improvement in health care**

   a) Creating a culture of quality improvement involves ongoing measurement and improvement as well as flexible team members who are open to innovation. Note that team member roles and workflows may need to be adjusted based on measurement results.

2) **Process mapping for analyzing areas of clinical practice that could be improved**

   a) Are the steps done in a standardized way or differently?

   b) Are the steps repeated unnecessarily or out of sequence?

   c) Are there process steps where errors frequently occur?

   d) Map out the current process with the team.

   e) Analyze the process.

      1. Which steps have value? Which ones don't?
      2. Which steps can be removed? Which steps can't?

   f) Create a new process map.

      1. Use the Plan-Do-Study-Act (PDSA) cycle to continue to improve (Figure 3.2).

Figure 3.2 The Plan-Do-Study-Act (PDSA) cycle

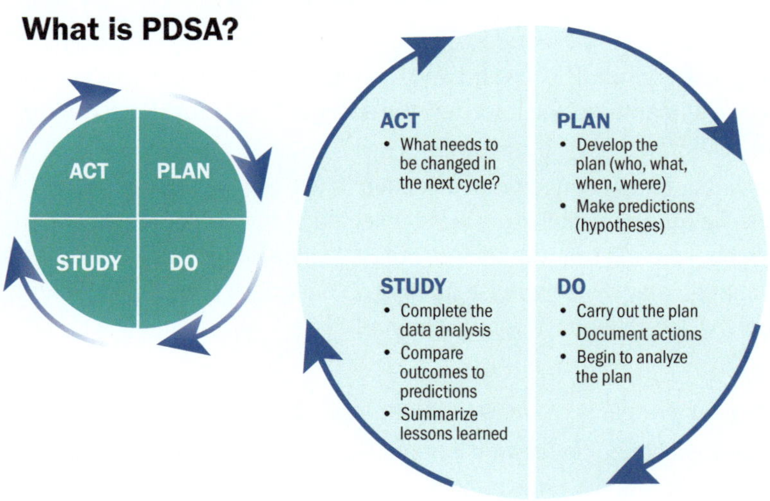

   g) Analyze when something goes wrong or is a near miss.

      1. Root-cause analysis

3) **PDSA cycle**

   a) Small scale improvements over short periods of time that typically require several cycles to create desired change

4) Example: PDSA cycle for capturing lifestyle vital signs

a) Plan

1. Desired improvement is capturing lifestyle vital signs.
2. What change will be tested? Capture data (what) by medical assistant (who) above the regular vital signs in the chart (where) at the beginning of patient visit (when). The provider will double check for information before entering the room (who).
3. What outcome are we looking for? We want 90% of charts to contain the above data (provide some margin for incomplete information or patient refusal).
4. Theory is that having a written prompt (above the regular vital signs) and having the assistant and provider check that data is completed will increase completeness of data.

b) Do

1. Map the process flow.
    a. The patient arrives, checks in at the front office, and then billing/insurance information is exchanged.
    b. The assistant takes the patient to an exam room, and then lifestyle vital signs are captured.
    c. The assistant briefs the physician, and then the physician checks lifestyle and standard vital signs.
    d. The assistant notates data in the chart, and then the physician double-checks the chart for completeness.
2. Carry out the practice change on a small pilot (e.g., complete the process above with every patient 1 day a week).
3. Evaluate the change with qualitative and quantitative data (e.g., collect all charts from that day and enter results [all vitals captured] on a tracking log).

c) Study

1. Review the number of vitals collected and the total number of patients seen. Calculate the completeness percentage, and interview the assistant and provider about the process (pros and cons).
2. Determine what, if any, change or modification to the new process is needed (e.g., only 50% of lifestyle medicine vital signs were collected at the end of the day when a provider was double booked and running behind, but 80% were completed on a less busy day; a proposed change may be to increase staffing on busy days to assist with charting or to avoid double booking, which leads to running behind).

d) Act

1. Adopt testing on a larger scale (collect information 3 days a week).
2. Adapt the method based on lessons learned (e.g., recruit a second assistant to assist in the afternoons to help with the time crunch).
3. Abandon by trying something different (e.g., hand out patient lifestyle medicine questionnaires in the waiting room so they can be completed before the visit and given to the medical assistant at the time of the visit).

5) Root cause analysis

a) Use the root cause analysis tool when something goes wrong or a “near-miss” is experienced.

b) Ask five "whys" to get to root causes.[81]

1. Repeatedly ask "why?" five times, because it generally takes three to five times to get to the root cause of an incident.

c) Ask: "So what?"

1. What is the consequence of something not going as planned? (This question reframes what is important).

d) Draw cause and effect diagrams (Figure 3.3).

1. See the fishbone diagram, for example.
   a. Define the problem and place it at the head of the "fish."
   b. Write the categories leading to the problem as the "bones" (e.g., people, methods, machines, material, environment, measurement system, communications, policies, and patients/customers).

Figure 3.3 Factors Contributing to Defect XXX

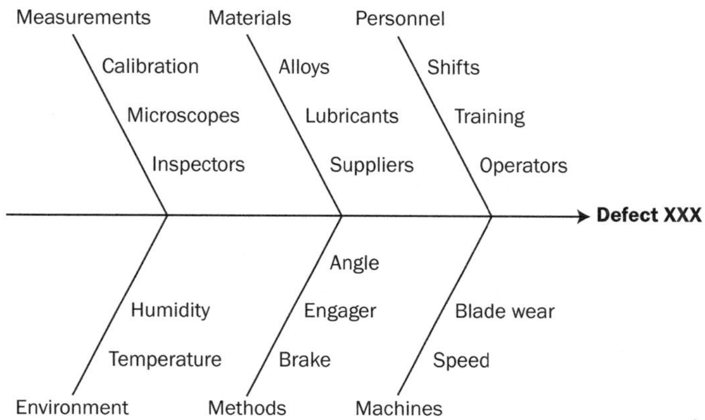

e) Steps for analysis

1. Analyze and discuss with the team: Are there any repeat causes? Is there one main problematic category?
2. Research: Interview team members, conduct patient surveys, and create process maps.
3. Decide to address a few causes: review solutions with team and apply PDSA cycle discussed above.

SECTION 3 GLOSSARY

C-peptide: a stimulated C-peptide measurement may be used to assess endogenous insulin production in order to identify how well beta cells are functioning to meet the demands of insulin production. This test can help determine whether a patient has type 1 diabetes, type 2 diabetes, or something else.

Chronic Care Model: this model is helpful in explaining the involvement of the community and health care system in chronic disease care. The model, developed by Ed Wagner, MD, centers on an informed, activated, and engaged patient and a prepared, pro-active practice team.

Drop-In Group Medical Appointments (DIGMAs): are used for many types of medical diseases. With these appointments, patients can walk-in and be seen in a group.

HOMA-IR: stands for homeostatic model assessment for insulin resistance, which is an estimate of insulin sensitivity and beta cell function based on the fasting plasma glucose concentrations and fasting plasma insulin or C-peptide measurements.[54,55]

Physical Shared Medical Appointments: are shared medical appointments that include the opportunity for a private physical.

Plan-Do-Study-Act (PDSA) cycle: a method for creating change that includes planning, doing, studying, and acting on each incremental change. The method often involves several cycles of small-scale improvements.

Root cause analysis: this tool is used when something goes wrong or a “near-miss” is experienced. Root cause analysis involves repeatedly asking, “why?” to get to the root cause of an incident and then asking, “so what?” to determine the consequence of what occurred and to help reframe what’s important.

Shared Medical Appointments: are often used for chronic disease treatment or perinatal care.

SECTION 3 REVIEW QUESTIONS

1. **What component of a lifestyle medicine visit delineates it most from a primary care visit?**
   A. Discovering and treating the underlying cause of disease as related to sleep, stress, nutrition, substances, physical activity, or relationships
   B. Emphasis on genetic predisposition
   C. Medications are rarely used to treat chronic disease
   D. Assessments exploring future risk of cardiovascular or endocrine diseases

2. **Which patient would be at higher risk of chronic disease?**
   A. A 45-year-old man of south-east Asian descent with a BMI of 22.3.
   B. A 38-year-old woman who gets 9.5 hours of moderate quality sleep most nights
   C. A 23-year-old man who achieves 160 minutes of moderate physical activity a week
   D. A 64-year-old woman with a waist circumference of 36 in (91.5 cm)

3. **Which of the following statements about diabetes diagnosis are true?**
   A. Fasting serum glucose ≥115 mg/dL (6.4 mmol/L) or 1-hour postprandial glucose ≥200 mg/dL (11.1 mmol/L) during an oral glucose tolerance test (OGTT) is diagnostic of diabetes.
   B. Fasting serum glucose ≥126 mg/dL (7.0 mmol/L) or 1-hour postprandial glucose ≥200 mg/dL (11.1 mmol/L) during an oral glucose tolerance test (OGTT) is diagnostic of diabetes.
   C. A 2-hour serum glucose during an oral glucose tolerance test (OGTT) of 140–199 mg/dL (7.8–11.0 mmol/L) is diagnostic of diabetes.
   D. A patient with frequent urination whose random blood sugar in office is 165 mg/dL (9.2 mmol/L).

4. **A physician recently became board certified in lifestyle medicine and would like to develop a lifestyle medicine team in her clinic. Which of the following team members would be most important to seek out to be part of an interdisciplinary team?**
   A. Integrative medicine practitioners, marketing specialist, and a masseuse
   B. Fitness expert, condition management provider, and a chef
   C. Local public health officials and insurers paying for preventive services
   D. Endocrinologist, cardiologists, and gastroenterologists

5. **A physician begins a new collaboration with the local dietitian and physical therapist. The local dietician typically promotes a Mediterranean diet for general health and a ketogenic diet for weight loss. The physical therapist is into body building and maintains a personal fitness blog. They are both very enthusiastic about helping patients with lifestyle changes. Which next step would likely be the most beneficial in treating morbidly obese patients?**
   A. Using the office's marketing specialist to advertise and inform patients of a dietician and physical therapist joining the team for weight-loss counseling.
   B. A meeting between the physician, physical therapist, and dietitian to review the education and lifestyle medicine treatment plans for morbidly obese patients.
   C. Hosting a journal club at the hospital to begin educating other local health care providers on lifestyle medicine.
   D. Routine collection of vital signs (blood pressure, heart rate, respiratory rate, and oxygen saturation) and including these in referral notes.

6. **Which of the following statements about the value of group visits is true?**
   - **A.** Group visits decrease access to care.
   - **B.** Group visits increase patient satisfaction but decrease provider satisfaction.
   - **C.** DIGMAs are drop-in group medical appointments.
   - **D.** Group visits shorten appointment length.

7. **Which of the following is a process for health care service quality improvement with applications for lifestyle interventions?**
   - **A.** Plan-Do-Study-Act (PDSA) cycle.
   - **B.** Value-based care involves financially rewarding institutions for value, not just treatment.
   - **C.** The Agency for Healthcare Research and Quality (AHRQ).
   - **D.** Innovative Care for Chronic Conditions (ICCC).

8. **Examples of team implementation from demonstrated chronic care models include:**
   - **A.** Ornish Spectrum program
   - **B.** Robert Wood Johnson Foundation
   - **C.** Lean Six Sigma
   - **D.** Drop-in group medical appointments

9. **Which statement is true concerning the lifestyle medicine vital signs?**
   - **A.** In the diet vital sign, it is important to assess for specific shortfall nutrients.
   - **B.** Perceived stress level does not need to be screened for at every visit.
   - **C.** The two-item exercise vital sign is a valid measure for classifying inactive, insufficiently active, or sufficiently active levels of exercise.
   - **D.** The Alcohol Use Disorders Identification Test–Concise (AUDIT–C) questionnaire is insufficient to screen for alcohol use disorder at a yearly physical.

10. **The following is an example of a well-written lifestyle prescription:**
    - **A.** The patient has atherosclerosis and should reduce his total fat intake and increase his fruit and vegetable intake to reverse disease.
    - **B.** The patient has obesity and should include 150 minutes of moderate intensity aerobic exercise per week, including two to three times per week of resistance training.
    - **C.** The patient has untreated attention deficit hyperactivity disorder (ADHD) and a high stress job; she should try to complete relaxation techniques, such as mindfulness meditation, more in the future.
    - **D.** The patient has an enlarged prostate with minor urinary difficulty; he should consider adding crushed flax seed to his diet.

SECTION 3 REVIEW QUESTION ANSWERS AND SUMMARIES

1. **Answer: A.** Lifestyle medicine visits do take genetics into account; however, gene DNA sequences likely only play a role in the variance of health around 10% of the time, whereas epigenetics (gene switches) explain 70–90% of the variance in health and are impacted by the environment, mainly one's lifestyle. Lifestyle medicine practitioners will often use medications to treat and prevent disease, however, medications are used as adjunctive therapy until lifestyle behaviors are at an optimal level to treat disease. Both primary care and lifestyle medicine practitioners routinely assess future risk of cardiovascular and endocrine diseases.

2. **Answer: D.** Women with a waist circumference greater than 35 in (88 cm) have an increased risk of chronic disease. A BMI ≥23 in those of Asian descent would be associated with an increased risk of type 2 diabetes. Most people need 7–8 hours of sleep a night; sleeping less than 6 hours a night is associated with an increased risk of cardiovascular disease. Patients who achieve over 150 minutes of physical activity have lower rates of chronic disease.

3. **Answer: B.** HbA1c ≥6.5% or 2-hour postprandial glucose ≥200 mg/dL (11.1 mmol/L) during an oral glucose tolerance test (OGTT) or fasting serum glucose ≥126 mg/dL (7.0 mmol/L) is diagnostic of diabetes. A 2-hour serum glucose during an OGTT of 140–199 mg/dL (7.8–11.0 mmol/L) is diagnostic of prediabetes. Classic symptoms of hyperglycemia such as polyuria, polydipsia, and polyphagia in combination with a random blood sugar of ≥200 mg/dL (11.1 mmol/L) is consistent with a diagnosis of diabetes.

4. **Answer: B.** A good internal team for outpatient lifestyle medicine could include any of the following: advanced practice providers, condition management providers, nursing team, registered dietitian, health coaches, chefs, fitness experts, support staff, and social workers. It is helpful to form collaborative partnerships with specialists so patients get a consistent message and support but this is not essential for a lifestyle medicine practice. Public health officials may be useful for advocating for lifestyle medicine services in the community and insurers who support preventive services may be excellent partners for ensuring appropriate screenings and reimbursement.

5. **Answer: B.** The physician has formed a new collaboration with a registered dietitian and physical therapist, but the three must work together to speak the same message to patients when it comes to the pillars of lifestyle medicine. Of each of the pillars (healthful eating, physical activity, stress management, relationships, sleep, and substance abuse), the message on nutrition often varies the most between providers; yet, it is often the most important factor in the treatment of chronic disease, as people can "out eat" an exercise program or healthy sleep. If the physician is promoting a whole food plant-based diet, the dietitian is instructing a ketogenic diet, and the physical therapist likely promoting a high-protein diet as body builder, patients can become frustrated and confused. The other options may be appropriate but not the most important to address initially.

6. **Answer: C.** Group visits increase access to care. Group visits increase patient and provider satisfaction. DIGMAs are drop-in group medical appointments. The length of group visits exceeds those of traditional appointments, allowing for more time for interaction between the provider and patients.

7. **Answer: A.** Plan-Do-Study-Act (PDSA) cycles are processes that can be used in health care for quality improvement and can be applied to lifestyle interventions. Value-based care involves financially rewarding institutions for value not just treatment. The Agency for Healthcare Research and Quality (AHRQ) is not a process; rather it's an agency of the US Department of Health and Human Services that generates the evidence needed to improve the safety, quality, and access of health care. The Innovative Care for Chronic Conditions (ICCC) is a template, produced by the World Health Organization, that countries can follow to improve chronic disease management.

8. **Answer: A.** The Medical Fitness Collaboration and the Ornish Spectrum program are examples of team implementation from demonstrated chronic care models. The Robert Wood Johnson Foundation is one of the nation's largest public health philanthropies focused solely on health. Lean Six Sigma is a quality improvement process that uses a disciplined, data-driven approach and methodology for eliminating defects (driving toward six standard deviations between the mean and the nearest specification limit). Drop-in group medical appointments are a type of office appointment and not an example of a chronic care model.

9. **Answer: C.** The two-item exercise vital sign has been researched and found to be a valid measure of insufficient to sufficient cardiovascular physical activity. Lifestyle medicine vital signs should not be considered standard vital signs, but rather should be used as 'check-ins' about each major healthy lifestyle component at every visit. More research needs to be done before these vital signs can become standards. Since nutrients come in "food packages," it's better to assess for whole foods rather than particular nutrients. Perceived stress should be screened for at every visit. The AUDIT-C screening questionnaire is a sufficient screening tool; those who test positive should then be asked to complete the full AUDIT questionnaire.

10. **Answer: B.** The most important point of a lifestyle prescription that leads into an action plan is that the patient must be able to perform the agreed upon task. If there is no specific action plan (time allotted to activity, measurement of achievement, or specific amount) the patient will not be able to clearly follow or complete the prescription. Of note, the patient with untreated attention deficit hyperactivity disorder may best be served by using exercise to treat stress, as sitting to perform mindfulness meditation may be more difficult.

SECTION 3 REFERENCES

1. Lianov L., Johnson M. Physician competencies for prescribing lifestyle medicine. *JAMA*. 2010;304(2):202-203.
2. Coleman K. J., Ngor E., Reynolds K., et al. Initial validation of an exercise "vital sign" in electronic medical records. *Med Sci Sports Exerc.* 2012;44(11):2071-2076.
3. Strath S. J., Kaminsky L. A., Ainsworth B. E., et al. Guide to the assessment of physical activity: clinical and research applications: a scientific statement from the American Heart Association. *Circulation*. 2013;128(20):2259-2279.
4. Grant R. W., Schmittdiel J. A., Neugebauer R. S., Uratsu C. S., Sternfeld B. Exercise as a vital sign: a quasi-experimental analysis of a health system intervention to collect patient-reported exercise levels. *J Gen Intern Med.* 2014;29(2):341-348.
5. DeSalvo K. B., Olson R., Casavale K. O. Dietary Guidelines for Americans. *JAMA*. 2016;315(5):457-458. https://doi.org/10.1001/jama.2015.18396.
6. National Institutes of Health. Short dietary assessment instruments. Updated July 24, 2020. https://epi.grants.cancer.gov/diet/screeners.
7. National Institutes of Health. Dietary screener questionnaire in the NHANES 2009-10: background. Updated July 24, 2020. https://epi.grants.cancer.gov/nhanes/dietscreen/.
8. National Institutes of Health. Dietary screener questionnaire in the National Health Interview Survey Cancer Control Supplement 2015. Updated July 24, 2020. https://epi.grants.cancer.gov/nhis/2015-screener/.
9. National Institutes of Health. Dietary screener in the 2009 California Health Interview Survey (CHIS 2009). Updated November 20, 2019. https://epi.grants.cancer.gov/diet/screeners/CHIS2009.pdf
10. US Department of Health and Human Services. National Institutes of Health. National Cancer Institute. National Cancer Institute (NCI) Fruit & Vegetable Intake Screeners from the Eating at America's Table Study: by meal screener. 1998. https://snaped.fns.usda.gov/library/materials/national-cancer-institute-nci-fruit-vegetable-intake-screeners-eating-americas-0.
11. National instititues of Health. Percentage energy from fat screener: overview. Updated July 24, 2020. https://epi.grants.cancer.gov/diet/screeners/fat/.
12. National Instititues of Health. Downloadable dietary assessment screeners, methodological information, and analytic files. Updated July 24, 2020. https://epi.grants.cancer.gov/diet/screeners/files.html.
13. Cherian L., Wang Y., Fakuda K., Leurgans S., Aggarwal N., Morris M. Mediterranean-Dash Intervention for Neurodegenerative Delay (MIND) diet slows cognitive decline after stroke. *J Prev Alzheimers Dis.* 2019;6(4):267-273.
14. Morris M. C., Tangney C. C., Wang Y., et al. MIND diet slows cognitive decline with aging. *Alzheimers Dement.* 2015;11(9):1015-1022. https://pubmed.ncbi.nlm.nih.gov/26086182.
15. Goldhamer A., Myers, T. An Introduction to the whole food plant-based, SOS-free diet. September 18, 2019. https://nutritionstudies.org/an-introduction-to-the-whole-food-plant-based-sos-free-diet/.
16. Cleghorn C., Harrison R., Ransley J., Wilkinson S., Thomas J., Cade J. Can a dietary quality score derived from a short-form FFQ assess dietary quality in UK adult population surveys? *Public Health Nutrition.* 2016;1:1-9.
17. Diet ID. The science behind diet id. https://www.dietid.com/the-science. Accessed February, 2021.
18. Katz D. L., Rhee L. Q., Katz C. S., et al. Dietary assessment can be based on pattern recognition rather than recall. *Med Hypotheses.* 2020;140:109644.
19. Feldman M. D., Christensen, J. F., eds. *Behavioral Medicine in Primary Care: A Practical Guide*. New York, NY: Appleton & Lange; 1997.
20. American Psychological Association. Stress in America key findings: 2010. 2010. https://www.apa.org/news/press/releases/stress/2010/key-findings#:~:text=Nearly%20one%2Dthird%20said%20they,or%20motivation%20(38%20percent).
21. Andreou E., Alexopoulos E. C., Lionis C., et al. Perceived Stress Scale: reliability and validity study in Greece. *Int J Environ Res Public Health*. 2011;8(8):3287-3298.
22. Cohen S., Kamarck T., Mermelstein R. A global measure of perceived stress. *J Health Soc Behav.* 1983;24(4):385-396.
23. Helton William S. Validation of a Short Stress State Questionnaire. *Proceedings of the Human Factors and Ergonomics Society Annual Meeting*. 2004;48(11):1238-1242. https://doi.org/10.1177/154193120404801107.
24. Johns M. W. Sleep propensity varies with behaviour and the situation in which it is measured: the concept of somnificity. *J Sleep Res*. 2002;11(1):61-67.
25. Johns M. About the ESS – Epworth Sleepiness Scale. https://epworthsleepinessscale.com/about-the-ess/.
26. Kobau R., Sniezek J., Zack M. M., Lucas R. E., Burns A.. Well-being assessment: an evaluation of well-being scales for public health and population estimates of well-being among US adults. *Appl Psychol Health Well Being.* 2010;2(3):272-297. https://iaap-journals.onlinelibrary.wiley.com/doi/abs/10.1111/j.1758-0854.2010.01035.x.
27. Global Health Survey Collaborative Group. *Tobacco Questions for Surveys. A Subset of Key Questions from the Global Adult Tobacco Survey (GATS)*. Atlanta, GA: Centers for Disease Control and Prevention; 2011: https://www.who.int/tobacco/surveillance/en_tfi_tqs.pdf.
28. Afshin A., Forouzanfar M. H., Reitsma M. B., et al. Health effects of overweight and obesity in 195 countries over 25 years. *N Engl J Med.* 2017;377(1):13-27.
29. US Department of Veterans Affairs. Personal health inventory. January, 2019. https://www.va.gov/WHOLEHEALTH/docs/10-930_PHI-Short_July2019_508.pdf.
30. US Army. Performance Triad (P3). https://p3.amedd.army.mil/.
31. Mozaffarian D. Mediterranean diet for primary prevention of cardiovascular disease. *N Engl J Med*. 2013;369(7):673-674. http://www.nejm.org/doi/full/10.1056/NEJMc1306659.

32. Ford E. S., Greenlund K. J., Hong Y. Ideal cardiovascular health and mortality from all causes and diseases of the circulatory system among adults in the United States. *Circulation*. 2012;125(8):987-995.
33. American College of Cardiology. ASCVD Risk Estimator Plus. http://tools.acc.org/ASCVD-Risk-Estimator-Plus/#!/calculate/estimate/. Accessed March 9, 2021.
34. McClelland R. L., Jorgensen N. W., Budoff M., et al. 10-year coronary heart disease risk prediction using coronary artery calcium and traditional risk factors: derivation in the MESA (Multi-Ethnic Study of Atherosclerosis) with validation in the HNR (Heinz Nixdorf Recall) Study and the DHS (Dallas Heart Study). *J Am Coll Cardiol*. 2015;66(15):1643-1653.
35. Ridker P. M., Buring J. E., Rifai N., Cook N. R. Development and validation of improved algorithms for the assessment of global cardiovascular risk in women: the Reynolds Risk Score. *JAMA*. 2007;297(6):611-619.
36. World Health Organization. *Waist Circumference and Waist–Hip Ratio: Report of a WHO Expert Consultation, Geneva, December 8-11, 2008*. Geneva, Switzerland: World Health Organization; 2011.
37. Hsu W. C., Araneta M. R. G., Kanaya Alka M., Chiang Jane L., Fujimoto W. BMI cut points to identify at-risk Asian Americans for type 2 diabetes screening. *Diabetes Care*. 2015;38(1):150-158. https://care.diabetesjournals.org/content/diacare/38/1/150.full.pdf.
38. World Health Organization. Regional Office for the Western Pacific. *The Asia-Pacific Perspective: Redefining Obesity and Its Treatment*. Sydney: Health Communications Australia; 2000.
39. World Health Organization. *Obesity: Preventing and Managing the Global Epidemic*. Geneva, Switzerland: World Health Organization; 2011.
40. Ward L. C. Bioelectrical impedance analysis for body composition assessment: reflections on accuracy, clinical utility, and standardisation. *Eur J Clin Nutr*. 2019;73(2):194-199. https://doi.org/10.1038/s41430-018-0335-3.
41. Whelton P. K., Carey R. M., Aronow W. S., et al. 2017 ACC/AHA/AAPA/ABC/ACPM/AGS/APhA/ASH/ASPC/NMA/PCNA guideline for the prevention, detection, evaluation, and management of high blood pressure in adults: a report of the American College of Cardiology/American Heart Association Task Force on Clinical Practice Guidelines. *Hypertension. 2018;71(6):1269-1324.*
42. Whelton P. K., He J., Appel L. J., et al. Primary prevention of hypertension: clinical and public health advisory from The National High Blood Pressure Education Program. *JAMA*. 2002;288(15):1882-1888.
43. Hardy S. T., Loehr L. R., Butler K. R., et al. Reducing the blood pressure-related burden of cardiovascular disease: impact of achievable improvements in blood pressure prevention and control. *J Am Heart Assoc*. 2015;4(10):e002276-e002276. https://www.ncbi.nlm.nih.gov/pmc/articles/PMC4845128/.
44. Brunström M., Carlberg B. Association of blood pressure lowering with mortality and cardiovascular disease across blood pressure levels: a systematic review and meta-analysis. *JAMA Intern Med*. 2018;178(1):28-36. https://doi.org/10.1001/jamainternmed.2017.6015.
45. Ettehad D., Emdin C. A., Kiran A., et al. Blood pressure lowering for prevention of cardiovascular disease and death: a systematic review and meta-analysis. *Lancet*. 2016;387(10022):957-967.
46. Stamler R. Implications of the INTERSALT study. *Hypertension*. 1991;17(1 Suppl):I16-I20.
47. Stamler J. The INTERSALT Study: background, methods, findings, and implications. *Am J Clin Nutr*. 1997;65(2 Suppl):626s-642s.
48. Egger G., Binns A., Rossner S. *Lifestyle Medicine: Managing Diseases of Lifestyle in the 21st Century*. New York, NY: McGraw-Hill; 2010.
49. ATS Committee on Proficiency Standards for Clinical Pulmonary Function Laboratories. ATS statement: guidelines for the six-minute walk test. *Am J Respir Crit Care Med*. 2002;166(1):111-117.
50. Friedewald W. T., Levy R. I., Fredrickson D. S. Estimation of the concentration of low-density lipoprotein cholesterol in plasma, without use of the preparative ultracentrifuge. *Clin Chem*. 1972;18(6):499-502.
51. Jensen M. K., Rimm E. B., Furtado J. D., Sacks F. M. Apolipoprotein C-III as a potential modulator of the association between HDL-cholesterol and incident coronary heart disease. *J Am Heart Assoc*. 2012;1(2):jah3-e000232.
52. Kontush A., Chapman M. J. Functionally defective high-density lipoprotein: a new therapeutic target at the crossroads of dyslipidemia, inflammation, and atherosclerosis. *Pharmacol Rev*. 2006;58(3):342-374.
53. Wallace T. M., Levy J. C., Matthews D. R. Use and abuse of HOMA modeling. *Diabetes Care*. 2004;27(6):1487-1495.
54. Hill N. R., Oliver N. S., Choudhary P., Levy J. C., Hindmarsh P., Matthews D. R. Normal reference range for mean tissue glucose and glycemic variability derived from continuous glucose monitoring for subjects without diabetes in different ethnic groups. *Diabetes Technol Ther*. 2011;13(9):921-928.
55. Hill N. R., Levy J. C., Matthews D. R. Expansion of the homeostasis model assessment of β-cell function and insulin resistance to enable clinical trial outcome modeling through the interactive adjustment of physiology and treatment effects: iHOMA2. *Diabetes Care*. 2013;36(8):2324-2330.
56. National Committee for Quality Assurance. HEDIS measures and technical resources. Updated 2020. https://www.ncqa.org/hedis/measures/.
57. Fields D., Shull J. Systems and practices of clinical care: building upon the foundation of lifestyle medicine. Conducted at: 2019 Asian Society of Lifestyle Medicine Conference; 2019.
58. Krukowski R. A., Lensing S., Love S., et al. Training of lay health educators to implement an evidence-based behavioral weight loss intervention in rural senior centers. *Gerontologist*. 2013;53(1):162-171.
59. Wagner E. H., Austin B. T., Davis C., Hindmarsh M., Schaefer J., Bonomi A. Improving chronic illness care: translating evidence into action. *Health Aff (Millwood)*. 2001;20(6):64-78.
60. Nancarrow S. A., Booth A., Ariss S., Smith T., Enderby P., Roots A. Ten principles of good interdisciplinary team work. *Hum Resour Health*. 2013;11:19.
61. Noffsinger E. B. *Running Group Visits in Your Practice*. New York, NY: Springer-Verlag; 2009.

62. Eisenstat S., Lipps A., et al. *Putting Group Visits into Practice. A Practical Overview to Preparation, Implementation and Maintenance of Group Visits at Massachusetts General Hospital*. Boston, MA:John D Stoeckle Center; 2012.
63. De Vries B., Darling-Fisher C., Thomas A. C., Belanger-Shugart E. B. Implementation and outcomes of group medical appointments in an outpatient specialty care clinic. *J Am Acad Nurse Pract*. 2008;20(3):163-169.
64. Egger G., Binns A., Cole M. A., et al. Shared medical appointments - an adjunct for chronic disease management in Australia? *Aust Fam Physician*. 2014;43(3):151-154.
65. Beck A., Scott J., Williams P., et al. A randomized trial of group outpatient visits for chronically ill older HMO members: the Cooperative Health Care Clinic. *J Am Geriatr Soc.* 1997;45(5):543-549.
66. Scott J. C., Conner D. A., Venohr I., et al. Effectiveness of a group outpatient visit model for chronically ill older health maintenance organization members: a 2-year randomized trial of the cooperative health care clinic. *J Am Geriatr Soc.* 2004;52(9):1463-1470.
67. Trento M., Passera P., Bajardi M., et al. Lifestyle intervention by group care prevents deterioration of Type II diabetes: a 4-year randomized controlled clinical trial. *Diabetologia*. 2002;45(9):1231-1239.
68. Trento M., Passera P., Tomalino M., et al. Group visits improve metabolic control in type 2 diabetes: a 2-year follow-up. *Diabetes Care.* 2001;24(6):995-1000.
69. Trento M., Passera P., Borgo E., et al. A 5-year randomized controlled study of learning, problem solving ability, and quality of life modifications in people with type 2 diabetes managed by group care. *Diabetes Care.* 2004;27(3):670-675.
70. Jordan J. E., Briggs A. M., Brand C. A., Osborne R. H. Enhancing patient engagement in chronic disease self-management support initiatives in Australia: the need for an integrated approach. *Med J Aust.* 2008;189(S10):S9-s13.
71. Flodgren G., Deane K., Dickinson H. O., et al. Interventions to change the behaviour of health professionals and the organisation of care to promote weight reduction in overweight and obese people. *Cochrane Database Syst Rev.* 2010(3):Cd000984.
72. Hetherington S. A., Borodzicz J. A., Shing C. M. Assessing the real world effectiveness of the Healthy Eating Activity and Lifestyle (HEAL) program. *Health Promot J Austr.* 2015;26(2):93-98.
73. Laws R. A., Fanaian M., Jayasinghe U. W., et al. Factors influencing participation in a vascular disease prevention lifestyle program among participants in a cluster randomized trial. *BMC Health Serv Res.* 2013;13:201.
74. Cotton R. T., Andersen R. *Clinical Exercise Specialist Manual: ACE's Source for Training Special Populations.* Philadelphia, PA: Lippincott Williams & Wilkins; 1999.
75. World Health Organization. *Innovative Care for Chronic Conditions: Building Blocks for Action*. Geneva, Switzerland: World Health Oragnization; 2002. http://www.who.int/chp/knowledge/publications/icccreport/en/.
76. US Department of Health and Human Services. Collaborative Care Manager Model. Toolkit for implementing the chronic care model in an academic environment. Updated October, 2014. https://archive.ahrq.gov/prevention/curriculum/chroniccaremodel/index.html
77. Improving Chronic Illness Care. The chronic care model. http://www.improvingchroniccare.org/.
78. Thompson R. S. The prescription for health initiative: some steps on the road to success: what will it take to complete the journey? *Am J Prev Med.* 2008;35(5 Suppl):S431-433.
79. Green L. A., Cifuentes M., Glasgow R. E., Stange K. C. Redesigning primary care practice to incorporate health behavior change: prescription for health round-2 results. *Am J Prev Med.* 2008;35(5 Suppl):S347-349.
80. Agency for Healthcare Research and Quality. Electronic Preventive Services Selector. August, 2013. https://www.ahrq.gov/cpi/about/otherwebsites/epss.ahrq.gov/index.html.
81. Quality Assurance and Performance Improvement. *Five Whys Tool for Root Cause Analysis*. Washington, DC: Centers for Medicare and Medicaid Services; 2017; https://www.cms.gov/Medicare/Provider-Enrollment-and-Certification/QAPI/downloads/FiveWhys.pdf.

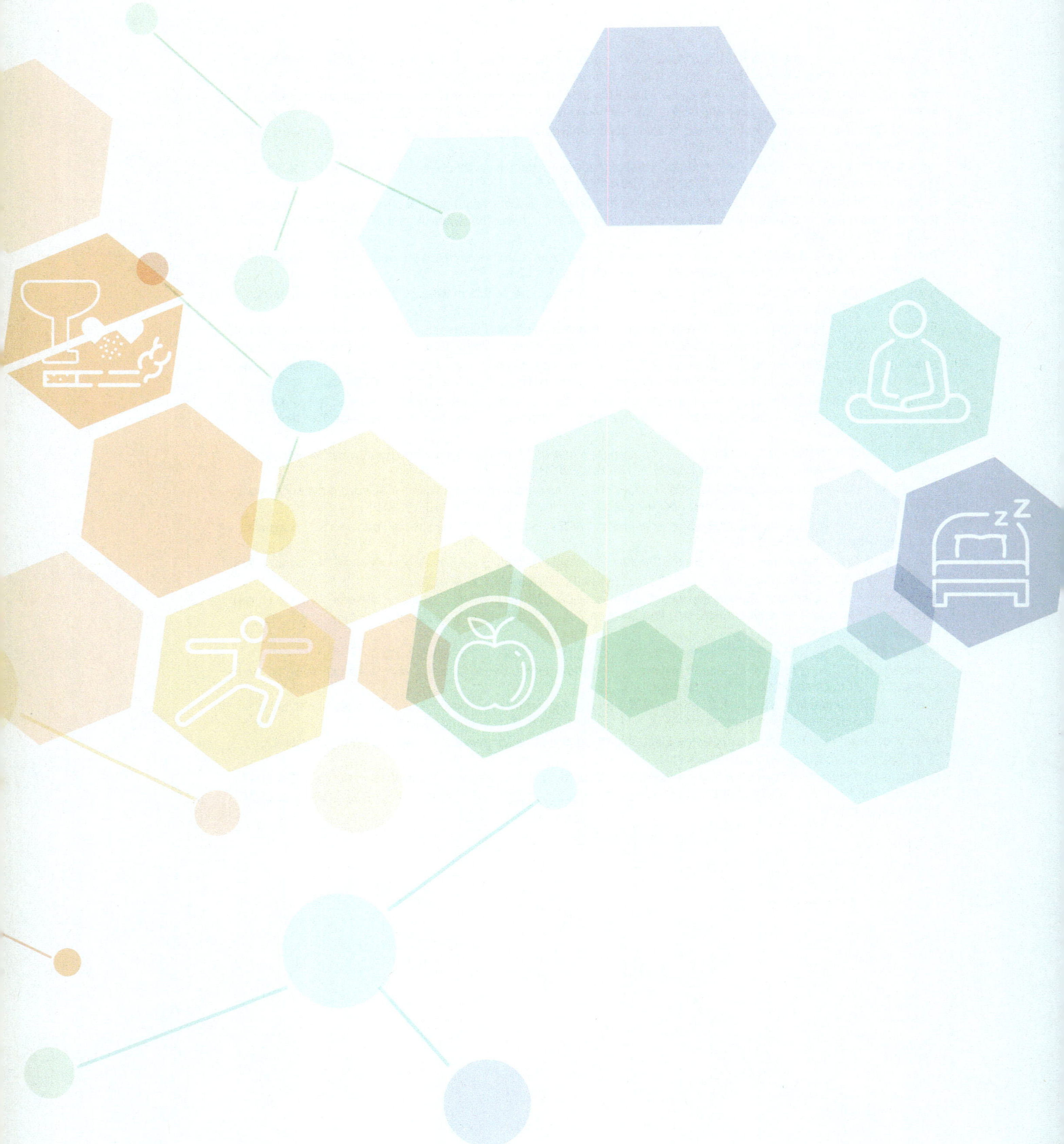

SECTION 4
The Role of Physician Health and the Physician's Personal Health

Objective 1 Cite scientific data supporting that physicians who practice healthy lifestyles are more likely to offer counseling and improve patient outcomes 94

Objective 2 Describe strategies for incorporating a wellness program for providers into a clinic, medical office, or other health care settings (wellness programs for health providers) 95

Objective 3 Conduct personal readiness assessment and develop personal action plan 96

Objective 4 Describe how to conduct effective advocacy on behalf of lifestyle medicine directly with patients and their families, as well as policymakers and decision-makers 97

Section 4 Review Questions 100

Section 4 Review Question Answers and Summaries 101

Section 4 References 102

OBJECTIVE 1

Cite scientific data supporting that physicians who practice healthy lifestyles are more likely to offer counseling and improve patient outcomes

1) Physicians' personal health behaviors

a) Not all physicians are consistently practicing healthy behaviors.

1. In a 2009 survey of Californian physicians, the following health factors were observed (n = 763, 41% response rate)[1]:
   a. Severe to moderate stress: 53%
   b. No or occasional exercise: 35%
   c. 6 or fewer hours of sleep: 34%
   d. Never or occasionally ate breakfast: 27%
   e. Sedative/tranquilizer use: 13%
   f. Depression: 7%
   g. Marijuana use: 4%
2. In a 2012 survey, 53% of primary care physicians (n = 498) were obese.[2]
3. In 2013, 36% of Canadian fourth-year medical students surveyed did not meet physical activity guidelines.[3]
4. In a 2013 article, overweight resident physicians under-acknowledged their overweight status, and their under-acknowledgment increased by training year.[4]

b) Other studies have found physicians are practicing healthy behaviors, therefore, arguing against the "unhealthy doctor."

1. In a 2000 study in men, mortality outcomes suggest that physicians live longer than their same-race professionals and non-professionals in the US population.[5]
2. In 2015, a study found that physicians and medical students engage in more physical activity than the general US adult population.[6]

2) Physicians' personal health and attitudes impact patient care.

a) In *Lifestyle Medicine,* 3rd edition, edited by J. Rippe (pages 1033–1044) and published in 2019, Erica Frank suggests:[7]

1. Providers need to focus on their own health.
2. Healthy doctors are more likely to produce healthy patients.

b) A meta-analysis of 24 studies about health providers' activity habits and their likelihood of counseling patients about physical activity found 19 out of 24 studies showed there was a high correlation between physicians' physical activity habits and counseling frequency, with odds of counseling 1.4–5.7 ($P < 0.05$) times higher among the exercising physicians.[8]

c) A cross-sectional study of 1,349 internists showed physicians' personal health promotion and disease prevention practices were strongly positively associated with more appropriate use of recommended practices for counseling patients ($P < 0.01$).[9]

1. Male internists' personal health practices for smoking, alcohol, seat belt use, and physical activity were positively associated with counseling for each health behavior except alcohol use.
2. Female internists' personal health practices for physical activity were associated positively with counseling patients about exercise and alcohol use.

d) Physicians who exercise (aerobic or strength training) are more likely to counsel patients on exercise than those who do not.[10]

e) Physicians attempting to improve their own poor habits have been found to counsel patients significantly more often than physicians who were not trying to change their own health behaviors.[11]

f) Training primary care physicians in behavioral counseling and providing them with tools and resources helps in their practice of weight-related care.[12]

g) A 2014 study concluded that physicians and medical students who had normal body mass index (BMI) were more likely to feel confident about counseling their patients about physical activity.[13]

h) Non-smoking physicians are more likely to emphasize the risks of smoking.[14,15,16]

i) Physicians were more likely to record a diagnosis of obesity and initiate a conversation if they perceived the patient's weight to be more than their own body weight.[2]

j) Female physicians' personal health practices had a positive correlation with the likelihood they would counsel their patients on health behaviors at least once a year.[14,17]

1. If physicians ate less fat, they counseled more on cholesterol (P = 0.08).
2. If physicians ate five fruits and vegetables per day, they counseled more on nutrition (P = 0.046).
3. Physicians who consumed a vegetarian diet were more likely to counsel on weight loss and nutrition (OR 2.0 and 2.1, respectfully).

k) Poor physician health habits impact the counseling that physicians provide to patients.[18,19,20]

l) The American Medical Association Code of Medical Ethics: "Physician Health and Wellness" states that physicians have a responsibility to maintain their health and wellness for the safety and effectiveness of the medical care they provide.

m) Physicians are at a high risk of burnout.

1. Burnout is defined as a syndrome of high emotional exhaustion, high depersonalization, and a low sense of personal accomplishment from work.[20,21]
2. In a 2019 consensus study report, the National Academy of Medicine (NAM) notes that between 35–45% of US nurses and physicians have substantial symptoms of burnout. Similarly, burnout for medical students is between 45–60%.[10]
3. Suboptimal care for patients may be one of the unintended consequences of physician burnout.
4. NAM suggests a systematic approach to professional well-being to take action against physician burnout. The interventions to prevent and reduce physician burnout need to be both individual-focused and organizationally-focused strategies.[11]

OBJECTIVE 2

Describe strategies for incorporating a wellness program for providers into a clinic, medical office, or other health care settings (wellness programs for health providers)

1) Assure providers have access to physical activity opportunities both inside and outside the providers' office. For example, many local hospitals or health systems may have employee wellness programs, a gym on-site, or local gym discounts.

2) **Implement a culture of wellness in the office with breaks for physical activity and healthy foods.**
   a) Promote healthy meals inside and outside the office (do not serve or provide unhealthy foods at office events).
   b) Install standing workstations or treadmill desks, especially for those who primarily work on the computer.
   c) Consider using technology to assist in tracking activities, such as phone applications or pedometers.
   d) Engage colleagues in health challenges and competitions.
3) **Allow providers time to get involved in local community changes that support healthy living. A well-known event is "Walk with a Doc."[22]**
4) **Supporting and incorporating wellness programs in the office helps promote the practice and sets an example for patients.**

OBJECTIVE 3

Conduct personal readiness assessment and develop personal action plan

1) **Readiness assessment and personal action plans for providers**
   a) Pick a focus area or behavior (e.g., physical activity).
   b) Assess self-readiness to change using the transtheoretical stages of change (see Section 2).
   c) Assess personal confidence in the ability to change and the perceived personal importance of making the change. The scale is 1 through 10; with 1 being the lowest and 10 being the highest.
   d) Develop a specific action plan for behaviors the provider is ready to start or restart.
      1. Use SMART goals.[23] (Also see Section 2)
         a. Specific (identify the exact behavior to be addressed)
         b. Measurable (how one will know she has reached the goal)
         c. Achievable/Attainable (the goal is achievable and can be accomplished)
         d. Relevant (the goal is in alignment with the specific behavior change chosen)
         e. Time (the timeframe for accomplishing that goal or task)
   e) Personalize the plan.
      1. Create a monitoring system like a daily log, checklist, or regular accountability meeting.
      2. Elicit help from a support team, including family, friends, colleagues, structured groups, or online communities.
   f) Follow up at established time intervals.
2) **Reassess progress, confidence, and the importance of making a change.**
3) **Celebrate success, and brainstorm ways to overcome barriers and to help with specific actions.**

OBJECTIVE 4

Describe how to conduct effective advocacy on behalf of lifestyle medicine directly with patients and their families, as well as policymakers and decision-makers

1) **Mobilizing physicians for community-level change[24,25]**
   - **a)** Advocacy
     1. Coordinated efforts to defend, promote, or protect something or someone by influencing public policy debate and interacting with influencers
     2. Occurs at local, state, and federal levels
   - **b)** Community advocacy for public health needs
     1. Identify and target wellness needs and the community's role in addressing them.
     2. Work with community organizations and local partners.
   - **c)** The goals of acquiring advocacy skills
     1. Build one's capacity to advocate and advocate well.
     2. Understand the advocacy process.
     3. Address obstacles to health.
     4. Help make tools and resources accessible to the community and patients.
     5. Develop and implement action plans.
   - **d)** Providers in the advocate role can:
     1. Provide credibility to the change being advocated.
     2. Identify preventive measures and positive solutions.
     3. Personalize an issue with patient stories and frontline experience.
     4. Employ health care change within their clinical care teams.
     5. Extend the impact of work in the clinic by connecting and engaging with the community.
     6. Offer a powerful and credible voice that can help influence policymakers and politicians.
     7. Help create specific responsibilities and expectations for involvement in advocacy.
   - **e)** Ways one can begin to advocate
     1. Be a resource by supplying information and educational materials.
     2. Set an example by being a lifestyle medicine champion in one's social and medical network.
     3. Offer expertise to elected officials, local decision-makers, and community organizations.
     4. Reach out through one's network, both online and in person.
     5. Plan or host an event.
     6. Speak at a community meeting or with the media.
   - **f)** Advocacy checklist
     1. Define the problem and desired solution or policy intervention.
        - a. Consider what the health trends have been for the community recently and in the past and what impact these trends may have on advocacy efforts.
        - b. Reflect on what current issues help address or worsen the problem.
        - c. Problem solve what the solution would be like both in the short and long term.

d. Consider why the community should support this initiative and what goals they could realistically meet.
e. Examples of potential advocacy topics for community health include access to healthy food, walking paths, safe places to be physically active, and neighborhood design.

2. Understand one's audience.
   a. Identify key stakeholders, and work on building connections if possible.
   b. Identify what specific trends and mindsets are present and how they might relate to the advocacy cause.
   c. Identify who could help achieve the goal(s) and who might oppose the issue(s) and the underlying motivations.
   d. Consider the ideal time to approach the audience. For example, legislators are busy in session in the spring, but they would be available to meet in the fall.
3. Determine strategy, tactics, and timeline.
   a. Consider how a change might happen for a particular initiative and what political arenas may need to be addressed.
      (1) Determine who would be best to make this request of the decision-maker(s) and whether it should be done individually or as a group.
      (2) Research whether there are other guidelines (legal or regulatory) to consider.
      (3) Strategize if, how, and when an opportunity for public comment might be best used.
      (4) Develop strategies to achieve the specific goal being advocated for and to overcome resistance from health trends and those who might oppose the change.
4. Evaluate outcomes.
   a. Identify what metrics need to be tracked to determine whether and when the implemented change has worked.
   b. Predetermine what a successful intervention would look like and what goals would be achieved.

2) Examples of lifestyle medicine advocacy:

a) Blue Zones Project

1. This project identifies five geographical locations in the world where people live the longest. These particular communities share nine common characteristics: they move naturally in their day-to-day lives (physical activity); feel a sense of purpose; eat a mainly plant-based diet; stop eating after becoming 80% full; relax; downshift; put family first; find the right tribe to engage with; and belong to something greater than oneself.
2. The Blue Zones Project is a community-led collaboration among community leaders, educators, health providers, public service officials, and the community itself, implemented across North America, along with an international program, to see current cities transform into places of longevity through healthy community systems. https://bluezones.com/services/blue-zones-project/#section-1

b) Robert Wood Johnson Foundation: "Creating a Culture of Health"

1. Communities across the US have showcased their healthy interventions. Community leaders and medical providers often collaborate in these cities to bring about better health for all. https://www.rwjf.org/en/library/features/culture-of-health-prize.html
2. Lessons from the "Creating a Culture of Health" movement: http://www.rwjf.org/en/library/annual-reports/2017-annual-message.html

c) Dean Ornish, MD, has advocated successfully to have a plant-based cardiac rehabilitation program reimbursed by Medicare. https://www.medpagetoday.com/cardiology/prevention/21675

d) Plan4Health initiative by The American Public Health Association and The American Planning Association strives to build local spaces for improving health. http://plan4health.us/

e) Project for Public Spaces is a New York-based non-profit that recently teamed up with Kaiser Permanente to disseminate information supporting the connection between place and health. http://www.pps.org/

f) The Urban Land Institute is a network of real estate and land-use experts engaging in community design and place activation, with a focus on creating opportunities for improving health. https://uli.org/about/

g) Mainstreet America focuses on revitalizing and transforming communities through work in four broad areas, which they call the Four Points: economic vitality, design, promotion, and organization. https://www.mainstreet.org/mainstreetamerica/theapproach

h) Creative Placemaking is an initiative by the National Endowment of the Arts that focuses on creative placemaking, incorporating the arts to transform communities. https://www.arts.gov/artistic-fields/creative-placemaking

i) National Complete Streets Coalition focuses on integrating people and places in the design and construction of streets that are accessible and safe for all members of the community. https://smartgrowthamerica.org/program/national-complete-streets-coalition/

SECTION 4 REVIEW QUESTIONS

1. **Which of the following statements is true?**
   - **A.** Physicians who exercise are more likely to counsel patients on exercise than physicians who do not exercise.
   - **B.** Female physicians who consumed an omnivorous diet were more likely to counsel patients on weight loss and nutrition.
   - **C.** Physicians and medical students who had a normal body mass index (BMI) expressed anxiety and fear about counseling patients regarding their physical activity.
   - **D.** Overweight resident physicians were good at acknowledging their overweight status.

2. **Which of the strategies below represents a collaborative and effective strategy to promote wellness and behavior change in the office setting?**
   - **A.** Stop serving meals at staff meetings and encourage employees to choose their own food.
   - **B.** Encourage employees to order their favorite items for lunch meetings.
   - **C.** Reward employees who have purchased smartwatches with an extra vacation day.
   - **D.** Incorporate 10-minute team "walk breaks" in the office during the workday to encourage physical activity.

3. **Which of the following statements is correct about physicians' healthy behaviors?**
   - **A.** Physicians and medical students engage in the same amount of physical activity when compared to the general US adult population.
   - **B.** Physicians who practice healthy behaviors are more likely to counsel patients to practice healthy behaviors.
   - **C.** Data suggests that provider health is not correlated with patient health outcomes.
   - **D.** Burnout is not a problem with physicians and nurses.

4. **Which of the following is an effective lifestyle medicine advocacy strategy?**
   - **A.** Healthcare providers can extend the impact of work in the clinic by connecting and engaging with the community.
   - **B.** When preparing to give a presentation at a community event, develop a general presentation as you never know who will be in the audience.
   - **C.** Do not engage with media outlets or community groups.
   - **D.** Advocating for short-term solutions is most important.

5 **In preparing a personal readiness assessment for a personal action plan, one should:**
   - **A.** Keep the goals broad and general, not specific.
   - **B.** Assess confidence to change.
   - **C.** Not worry about follow-up meetings, since it is a personal action plan.
   - **D.** Set goals that are difficult to achieve or attain in order to push oneself.

SECTION 4 REVIEW QUESTION ANSWERS AND SUMMARIES

1. **Answer: A.** Physicians who exercise are more likely to counsel patients on exercise than physicians who do not exercise. Female physicians who consumed a vegetarian diet were more likely to counsel on weight loss and nutrition. Physicians and medical students who had a normal BMI were more likely to feel confident about counseling their patients about physical activity. Overweight resident physicians under-acknowledged their overweight status and this increased by training year.

2. **Answer: D.** Incorporate 10-minute team "walk breaks" in the office during the workday to encourage physical activity. Encouraging employees to order their favorite items may backfire if it promotes the consumption of unhealthy foods that harm the employee's health. Mandating food policies, choices, and preferences are touchy subjects in the workplace. Incorporating technology to create health competitions incentivizing movement instead of simply rewarding the purchase of a smartwatch promotes healthier change.

3. **Answer: B.** Physicians who practice healthy behaviors are more likely to counsel patients to practice healthy behaviors. Even physicians attempting to improve their own poor habits have been found to counsel patients significantly more often than physicians who were not trying to change their own health behaviors. Physicians and medical students engage in more physical activity than the general US adult population. Data does suggest that provider health is correlated with patient health outcomes. Between 35–45% of US nurses and physicians have substantial symptoms of burnout.

4. **Answer: A.** Healthcare providers can extend the impact of work in the clinic by connecting and engaging with the community. Advocacy involves coordinated efforts with others and interacting with influencers. When advocating, it is important to know one's audience—identify what specific trends and mindsets are present and how they might relate to the advocacy cause. Ways one can begin to advocate include speaking at a community meeting or with the media. Advocates should problem solve what the solution would be like both in the short and long term.

5. **Answer: B.** Assess confidence to change. Action plans for the goal need to be specific and identify the exact behavior to be addressed. One should pick a specific area or behavior to change, not multiple areas. A specific action plan should be for an attainable goal and should include established time intervals for following up on that goal or task.

SECTION 4 REFERENCES

1. Bazargan M., Makar M., Bazargan-Hejazi S., Ani C., Wolf K. E. Preventive, lifestyle, and personal health behaviors among physicians. *Acad Psychiatry.* 2009;33(4):289-295.
2. Bleich S. N., Bennett W. L., Gudzune K. A., Cooper L.A. Impact of physician BMI on obesity care and beliefs. *Obesity (Silver Spring).* 2012;20(5):999-1005.
3. Holtz K. A., Kokotilo K. J., Fitzgerald B. E., Frank E. Exercise behaviour and attitudes among fourth-year medical students at the University of British Columbia. *Can Fam Physician.* 2013;59(1):e26-32.
4. Leventer-Roberts M., Zonfrillo M. R., Yu S., Dziura J. D., Spiro D.M. Overweight physicians during residency: a cross-sectional and longitudinal study. *J Grad Med Educ.* 2013;5(3):405-411.
5. Frank E., Biola H., Burnett C. A. Mortality rates and causes among U.S. physicians. *Am J Prev Med.* 2000;19(3):155-159.
6. Stanford F. C., Durkin M. W., Stallworth J. R., Blair S. N. Comparison of physical activity levels in physicians and medical students with the general adult population of the United States. *Phys Sportsmed.* 2013;41(4):86-92.
7. Frank E., Holmes D. Physician health practices and lifestyle medicine. In: Rippe J. M., ed. *Lifestyle Medicine Book,* 3rd ed. United Kingdom: CRC Press Taylor & Francis Group; 2019:1033-1044.
8. Lobelo F., de Quevedo I. G. The evidence in support of physicians and health care providers as physical activity role models. *Am J Lifestyle Med.* 2016;10(1):36-52.
9. Lewis C. E., Clancy C., Leake B., Schwartz J. S. The counseling practices of internists. *Ann Intern Med.* 1991;114(1):54-58.
10. Abramson S., Stein J., Schaufele M., Frates E., Rogan S. Personal exercise habits and counseling practices of primary care physicians: a national survey. *Clin J Sport Med.* 2000;10(1):40-48.
11. Fie S., Norman I., While A. The relationship between physicians' and nurses' personal physical activity habits and their health-promotion practice: a systematic review. *Health Educ J.* 2013;72(1):102-119.
12. Steeves J. A., Liu B., Willis G., Lee R., Smith A. W. Physicians' personal beliefs about weight-related care and their associations with care delivery: The U.S. National Survey of Energy Balance Related Care among Primary Care Physicians. *Obes Res Clin Pract.* 2015;9(3):243-255.
13. Stanford F. C., Durkin M. W., Stallworth J. R., Powell C. K., Poston M. B., Blair S.N. Factors that influence physicians' and medical students' confidence in counseling patients about physical activity. *J Prim Prev.* 2014;35(3):193-201.
14. Frank E., Rothenberg R., Lewis C., Belodoff B. F. Correlates of physicians' prevention-related practices. Findings from the Women Physicians' Health Study. *Arch Fam Med.* 2000;9(4):359-367.
15. Frank E., Kunovich-Frieze T. Physicians' prevention counseling behaviors: current status and future directions. *Prev Med.* 1995;24(6):543-545.
16. Meshefedjian G. A., Gervais A., Tremblay M., Villeneuve D., O'Loughlin J. Physician smoking status may influence cessation counseling practices. *Can J Public Health.* 2010;101(4):290-293.
17. Frank E., Wright E. H., Serdula M. K., Elon L. K., Baldwin G. Personal and professional nutrition-related practices of US female physicians. *Am J Clin Nutr.* 2002;75(2):326-332.
18. Frank E., Dresner Y., Shani M., Vinker S.. The association between physicians' and patients' preventive health practices. *CMAJ.* 2013;185(8):649-653.
19. Oberg E., Frank E. Physicians' health practices are better than patients'. *JAMA Intern Med.* 2013;173(12):1155-1156.
20. Elkan A. C., Sjoberg B., Kolsrud B., Ringertz B., Hafstrom I., Frostegard J. Gluten-free vegan diet induces decreased LDL and oxidized LDL levels and raised atheroprotective natural antibodies against phosphorylcholine in patients with rheumatoid arthritis: a randomized study. *Arthritis Res Ther.* 2008;10(2):R34.
21. American Medical Association. Physician health & wellness. https://www.ama-assn.org/delivering-care/ethics/physician-health-wellness. Accessed August 19, 2020.
22. Walk With A Doc. Inspiring communities through movement and conversation. 2020. https://walkwithadoc.org/. Accessed June 17, 2020.
23. White N. D., Bautista V., Lenz T., Cosimano A. Using the SMART-EST goals in lifestyle medicine prescription. *Am J Lifestyle Med.* 2020;14(3):271-273.
24. American Medical Association. Building my public forum participation strategy: A step-by-step outline. September, 2019 https://www.ama-assn.org/system/files/2019-09/public-forum-participation-strategy-outline.pdf.
25. Murphy B. 4 key public speaking tips for physicians. American Medical Association. September 19, 2019. https://www.ama-assn.org/practice-management/career-development/4-key-public-speaking-tips-physicians.

SECTION 5
Nutrition Science, Assessment, and Prescription

Objective 1 Explain the Dietary Guidelines for Americans and why they are important, and the science-base that goes beyond guidelines **105**

Objective 2 Identify the limitations of the Dietary Guidelines for Americans **105**

Objective 3 List the food components most Americans get too much of and the foods in which they're found **106**

Objective 4 List the shortfall (now labeled "underconsumed") nutrients that Americans are failing to sufficiently consume and in which foods they're found . . . **109**

Objective 5 Use these criteria that determine which foods are the healthiest and which are the least health-promoting **111**

Objective 6 Summarize the major (key) nutrition studies and the evidence base for nutrition prescriptions **113**

Objective 7 Evaluate the science behind making nutrition prescriptions **115**

Objective 8 Demonstrate ability to perform a basic nutrition assessment **116**

Objective 9 Prescribe nutrition for basic disease processes including inflammation food patterns / macronutrients, food types / micronutrients, food preparation / oxidation **120**

Objective 10 Describe practical strategies for assisting patients to achieve dietary changes **129**

Objective 11 Summarize nutrition prescriptions for the most common chronic diseases, including hyperlipidemia, diabetes, hypertension, and cancer **131**

Objective 12 Demonstrate ability to make nutrition prescriptions for health maintenance **137**

Objective 13 Describe the role of nutrition in preventing and treating chronic diseases, such as cardiovascular disease **137**

Objective 14 List at least five examples of nutrition interventions for diseases **146**

Objective 15 Describe the role of epigenetics **148**

Objective 16 List at least three key epigenetic influencers................... **150**

Objective 17 Cite the prevalence of diabetes and prediabetes and the associated cost burden **151**

Objective 18 Describe consequences of intensive medication management...... **152**

Objective 19 Describe the pathogenesis of diabetes **152**

Objective 20 Describe the role of nutrition in preventing, treating, and reversing type 2 diabetes **155**

Objective 21 Summarize key dietary research on the impact of diet on diabetes.. **158**

Objective 22 Describe the Diabetes Prevention Program and its applications **160**

Objective 23 List the major physiologic impacts of a plant-based diet in the process of disease reversal.. **161**

Section 5 Review Questions **163**

Section 5 Review Question Answers and Summaries **168**

Section 5 References...**172**

OBJECTIVE 1

Explain the Dietary Guidelines for Americans and why they are important, and the science base that goes beyond guidelines

1) **Dietary Guidelines for Americans (DGA)**[1]
   a) Jointly issued by the US Department of Agriculture (USDA) and the Department of Health and Human Services (HHS).
   b) The guidelines are updated every 5 years.
   c) The guidelines are based on recommendations of the Dietary Guidelines Advisory Committee (DGAC), which is composed of nutrition and medical researchers.[2]
   d) In the US, after experts create the DGAC Scientific Report, the Secretaries of USDA and HHS take public comments and consider both the evidence and public comment in crafting the final DGA.[3] This allows the food industry and other special interests to influence public policy. Therefore, the DGA can include discrepancies between recommendations and scientific evidence.[4]

OBJECTIVE 2

Identify the limitations of the Dietary Guidelines for Americans

1) **Limitation 1: Translation of the Dietary Guidelines for America Committee (DGAC) Report to the DGA is limited by influence from the food industry and other special interests on the DGA writing process. Some experts question the conclusions and methodology of the DGA due to involvement of biased food industries in the creation of the guidelines. In 2017, the National Academies of Sciences, Engineering, and Medicine released a report calling for the overhaul of the DGA process to eliminate bias.**[5]
   a) Dairy is listed as an essential component of MyPlate, which is an eating guide based on the DGA.[6] While "dairy" is shown on MyPlate, this is actually meant to represent calcium-rich foods, including nondairy foods. However, included nondairy foods are not immediately obvious.[6] In the standard American diet, dairy comprises about 10% of calories consumed.[7,8] About half of the dairy is consumed as fluid milk and about half is consumed as cheese.[9]
      1. Dairy has no or only a weak inverse relationship with cardiovascular disease. There is a mild association between dairy and lower stroke risk and with yogurt and lower diabetes risk. Prior studies have shown moderate evidence that dairy consumption is associated with lower risk of high blood pressure and other components of metabolic syndrome,[10] and lowers the risk of diabetes in adults.[11] With substitution analysis, replacing 5% of energy intake from dairy fat with equivalent energy intake from polyunsaturated fat, especially from plant foods, was associated with a 24% decreased risk of cardiovascular disease (CVD).[12] Processed dairy products are typically higher in saturated fat and sodium.
      2. There is evidence of a positive relationship between dairy intake and bone health in children.[13] However, evidence on the effect of dairy intake on fracture risk is mixed.[14] Although fortified dairy products can increase bone mineral density by about 0.7–1.8% over 2 years, this is unlikely to lead to clinically significant reductions in fracture rates.[15]

3. Increasing yogurt consumption may have a protective effect on lowering inflammation (OR = 0.34), but cheese leads to a pro-inflammatory state with higher plasma inflammatory biomarkers.[16]
4. Dairy products do not have an association with all-cause mortality,[17] osteoporosis, hip fracture,[18] or obesity and overweight.[19]

b) Association studies of eggs show mixed results when comparing intake with risk of diabetes and CVD. Some studies show that one or fewer eggs per day is not associated with CVD.[20,21,22,23] Another study looking at the risk of CVD as dietary cholesterol increased did show a significant association.[24] Another meta-analysis found that egg consumption was not associated with the risk of CVD or cardiac mortality, but was associated with an increased incidence of type 2 diabetes in the general population.[25] In a meta-analysis of US, European, and Japanese studies, egg intake was only associated with diabetes in a few US studies, but none of the European or Japanese studies.[26] There was no association of an intake of three or fewer eggs per week with diabetes in any of the studies.[26]

c) While the effects of cholesterol consumption among the general population is a source of active debate, a direct relationship between cholesterol and CVD among individuals with diabetes has been demonstrated.[25]

d) More research is needed on egg consumption in Western countries; very limited research[27] has been conducted that compared zero egg consumption with low levels of egg consumption (most large-scale cohort studies compare lower with higher egg consumption).

1. An egg contains approximately 200 mg of cholesterol,[28] and egg consumption has been found to increase LDL cholesterol with more than one egg per day for less than 12 weeks.[29,30] The 2020–2025 DGA advise eating as little cholesterol as possible, but no limit is given due to inadequate evidence. The prior 2010 guidelines suggested a limit of <300 mg a day.[31]

OBJECTIVE 3

List the food components most Americans get too much of and the foods in which they're found

1) Over-consumed nutrients and their primary food sources

a) Added sugars

1. Added sugars come in many forms and show up on food labels with numerous names, including:
   a. Cane sugar
   b. High fructose corn syrup
   c. Fructose
   d. Sucrose
   e. Dextrose
   f. Lactose
   g. Honey
   h. Brown sugar
   i. Turbinado sugar

j. Beet sugar
k. Raw sugar
l. Malt syrup
m. Maltose
n. Rice syrup
o. Agave
p. Molasses
q. Florida crystals
r. Fruit juice
s. Others

2. Foods and beverages high in added sugars include candies, desserts, sugar-sweetened beverages, condiments, sauces, ketchup, salad dressings, crackers, breakfast cereals, and snack or energy bars.
3. The World Health Organization recommends both adults and children limit their daily consumption of added sugar to less than 10% of total calories (less than 200 calories in a 2000 calories diet; up to 12 teaspoons or 48 grams), with a goal amount of less than 5% of calories (less than 100 calories in a 2000 calories diet; up to 6 teaspoons or 24 grams).[32]
4. The current intake of added sugar among US adults and children >6 yr is approximately 14.1% of total calories.[33]
5. The American Heart Association (AHA) recommends a maximum of 100 calories (6 teaspoons or 24 grams) of added sugar per day for women, children, and teens and no more than 150 calories (9 teaspoons or 36 grams) of sugar per day for men.[34]
6. Some of the top sources of added sugar in the US diet include:[35]
    a. Sugar-sweetened beverages
    b. Breads, rolls, and tortillas
    c. Sweet bakery products
    d. Coffee and tea
    e. Sugars (such as honey, syrups, and jams)
    f. Fats and oils (such as salad dressings and condiments)
    g. Ready-to-eat cereals
    h. Other prepared foods
7. For those in higher deciles of added sugar consumption, liquid calories from sugar-sweetened beverages contribute more sugar calories to the American diet than any other single food or beverage.[35]

b) Cholesterol[36]

1. High cholesterol foods include: eggs, dairy, cheese, organ meats, shellfish; and other meat, including poultry and fish.
    a. Cholesterol is exclusively found in animal foods.
2. Top sources of cholesterol in the US diet[37]
    a. Meat, eggs, grain products, and milk account for 96% of total dietary cholesterol consumption.
    b. Meat: 42% (12% for poultry, 12% for mixed dishes, 8% for red meat, 5% for processed meat, and 5% for seafood)
    c. Eggs: 25%

d. Grain products: 17% (5% for breads, 0% for cooked grains/cereals and ready-to-eat (RTE) cereals, and 12% for other grain products)

e. Milk and milk products: 11%

3. For cardiovascular health, the AHA recommends food-based dietary guidance emphasizing overall dietary patterns that are inherently low in cholesterol (i.e., more plant-based).[38]

c) Saturated fat

1. Saturated fat molecules have no double bonds between carbon molecules because they are saturated with hydrogen molecules and they are usually solid at room temperature, unlike monounsaturated and polyunsaturated fats.
2. The AHA recommends limiting saturated fat intake to no more than 5–6% of total calories.[39]
3. In most foods that contain fat, at least a small proportion of this fat is saturated.[36] However, the following foods have relatively high concentrations of saturated fat:
    a. Higher fat cuts of beef; pork and lamb; salami; sausages and other processed meats (3 ounces); many fast foods (e.g., cheeseburgers); lard; butter; cheese; coconut and coconut oil; palm oil; and palm kernel oil.
4. Whole plant foods mostly contain very low levels of saturated fat, with the exception of tropical oils.[36]
5. While not considered high in saturated fat, the following foods also contain more substantial levels of saturated fat:[28]
    a. Nuts and seeds vary: ≤1–4.3 grams per ounce (most are 1–2 grams per ounce or per 28 grams), with Brazil nuts being the highest
    b. Avocados: 2.1 grams per 100 grams of avocado (about one-half avocado)
    c. Oils: 1–2 grams per tablespoon (15 ml) (except for coconut oil, which is 12 grams per tablespoon (15 ml) and palm oil, which is 7 grams per tablespoon (15 ml)
    d. Eggs: 1.6 grams in one large egg (about 50 grams).
    e. Fish varies: ≤1 to 3 grams per serving.
6. Top five sources of saturated fat in diets of US adults:[40]
    a. Cheese: 16.5%
    b. Beef: 9.1%
    c. Other fats and oils: 8.9%
    d. Milk: 6.7%
    e. Frankfurters, sausages, and luncheon meats: 6.7%

d) Sodium

1. The food groups that are highest in salt are generally those that are commercially prepared. Almost 50% of dietary salt intake comes from mixed dishes defined by the DGA as "burgers, sandwiches, and tacos; rice, pasta, and grain dishes; pizza; meat, poultry, and seafood dishes; and soups."[3]
2. Top sources of sodium in the US diet[41]
    a. Added to food outside the home (70.9%)
    b. Inherent to food (14.2%)
    c. Added in home food preparation (5.6%)
    d. Added at the table (4.9%)
3. Limiting consumption of commercially processed foods is an important strategy to reduce excess sodium intake.[41]

4. Tips for patient counseling around sodium
    a. To help keep sodium in one's diet to 2,000 mg or less, check the nutrition label on packaged foods. Use the rule of thumb developed by registered dietitian Jeff Novick: If the sodium per serving is less than or equal to the calories per serving, someone eating a 2,000 calorie diet total will keep salt intake at approximately no more than 2,000 mg.
    b. If someone is eating mostly whole plant foods, the daily intake of sodium may fall within the low-sodium category (<1,500 mg/day). However, consumption of prepared foods can easily push total sodium intake over this threshold.

e) *Trans* fats

1. The Food and Drug Administration declared *trans*-fatty acids to be unsafe for human consumption and mandated that they be removed from food by 2018.[42,43]
2. *Trans* fats are mostly found in partially hydrogenated plant oils, which historically were used in many processed foods; they also occur naturally in some meat and dairy products.[44]
3. *Trans* fats can be avoided by reducing/eliminating the follow foods from the diet:[44]
    a. Animal foods, especially red and processed meats
    b. Butter
    c. Refined grain products such as doughnuts, cookies, crackers, muffins, pies, and cakes

---

OBJECTIVE 4

List the shortfall (now labeled "underconsumed") nutrients that Americans are failing to sufficiently consume and in which foods they're found

1) An underconsumed nutrient (previously known as "shortfall" nutrient) is a nutrient or food component that is underconsumed by 5% or more of the population or in specific groups relative to the estimated average requirement, adequate intake, or other quantitative authoritative recommendations from the diet alone, as described by the Dietary Guidelines Advisory Committee Report.[2]

2) Underconsumed nutrients include:[1]

a) Calcium*

b) Choline

c) Fiber*

d) Iron

e) Magnesium

f) Potassium*

g) Vitamin A

h) Vitamin C

i) Vitamin D*

j) Vitamin E

* Nutrients of public health concern (low intake is associated with health concerns)

3) **In the food groups listed below, foods considered "high" in a nutrient contain 20% or more of the reference daily intake (RDI) or the daily reference value (DRV) in a serving; foods considered a "good source" of a nutrient have 10–19% of the RDI or DRV per serving.[45,46]**

4) **Selection of underconsumed ("shortfall") nutrients**

   a) Calcium

   1. Foods that are higher in percent daily value (%DV) of calcium[28] include 1/4 cup cheese, 1/4 cup tofu prepared with calcium sulfate, 1/2 cup soybeans, 1 cup enriched cornmeal, 4 oz fortified plant milks, or 1 cup of cooked spinach or collard greens.
   2. Other foods containing calcium include 2 ounces almonds, 1 cup cooked black beans, 1 cup cooked kale or broccoli, 1 cup many fortified cereals, or 1 cup cooked teff.[28]
      a. Some vegetables, including spinach, beet greens, and Swiss chard, are very high in calcium but are also high in oxalates, which limits the absorption of calcium.
      b. Greens, particularly low-oxalate greens such as kale,[47] are reliable sources of calcium.[48,49]

   b) Fiber

   1. Fiber is found exclusively in plant foods,[36] thus, predominantly plant-based diets rich in whole foods make it easy to get plenty of fiber into the diet.[50]
   2. On average, adults in the US consume half the recommended amount of fiber.[51]
   3. Foods that are higher in %DV of fiber include 1/2 cup black beans, 1/2 cup split peas, 1/2 cup lentils, 1/2 avocado, 1/2 cup raspberries, 7 dried figs, 3 tablespoons flaxseeds, 1 cup oatmeal, and 1 cup whole-wheat pasta.
   4. Other foods containing fiber include 1/2 cup blueberries, 1 cup strawberries, 1 cup or 1 piece of most other fruit, 1 cup winter squashes, 1 cup brown rice, a slice of whole-grain bread, 1 cup popcorn, 3/4 cup mushrooms, 1 ounce almonds or peanuts, and 1 ounce sunflower or sesame seeds.[28]

   c) Magnesium

   1. Foods that are higher in %DV of magnesium include 4 Brazil nuts; 1 ounce almonds, cashews, or pine nuts; 2 ounces peanuts; 1 ounce cooked spinach; 1/2 cup amaranth; 3/4 cup edamame; and 2 ounces dark chocolate.[28]
   2. Other foods containing magnesium are 1 slice of whole-grain bread; 4 ounces yogurt; 1/2 cup brown rice; 1 ounce hazelnuts, pecans, pistachios, or walnuts; 1/4 cup tofu; a small potato; 1/2 cup black-eyed peas; and 1/2 cup lima beans.[28]

   d) Potassium

   1. Foods that are higher in %DV of potassium include one small baked potato, 1/2 cup of yams, 1/2 avocado, and beans such as 1/2 cup of either white beans adzuki beans, soybeans, black turtle beans, or lima beans. Other sources include fruits and vegetables (>400 mg/cup equivalent) such as 1 cup mashed banana, 1/2 cup beet greens, 5 dried apricots, or 5 dates.[8,28,52]
   2. Other foods containing potassium are 1 cup yogurt; 3 ounces chicken; 3 ounces tuna; 3 ounces of nuts, such as almonds, hazelnuts or walnuts; and 1/2 cup cooked and green vegetables.[28,36,52]

   e) Vitamin A

   1. Foods that are higher in %DV of vitamin A, retinol include 1/2 cup of cooked sweet potato or spinach, 1/2 cup raw carrots, or 1 cup cantaloupe or butternut squash. Beef liver is very high and 4 ounces exceeds the tolerable upper intake level of 3,000 μg.

2. Other foods containing vitamin A are 1 cup dairy and plant milks, 3 ounces herring, and 1 cup fortified cereals.[28]

f) Vitamin C

1. Foods that are higher in %DV of vitamin C include 1/2 cup bok choy, parsley, daikon radish, broccoli, cantaloupe, Brussels sprouts, pineapple, cabbage, cauliflower, mustard greens, papaya, green peas, kale, tomatoes, strawberries, or turnip greens[28]; 1 orange, guava, kiwi, mango, or red pepper.[28,36]
2. Other foods containing vitamin C are 1/2 cup spinach, most other leafy green vegetables such as collard greens and celery; and fruits including 1 cup cherries, pears, and canned peaches.[36]

g) Vitamin D

1. Foods that are higher in %DV of vitamin D include 1/2 cup salmon, high-fat fish, and 1 cup fortified milks, either dairy or nondairy.[28,31]
2. Other foods containing vitamin D are 1 cup fortified cereals, such as General Mills' Cheerios and Kellogg's Raisin Bran.[28,31]
3. Very few foods contain much vitamin D, so it's added to staple foods. Sunlight is a better source of vitamin D than dietary sources because ultraviolet B (UV-B) radiation will transform a precursor of vitamin D in the skin into vitamin D3. Usually, adequate levels of vitamin D can be synthesized by the body if large body areas, including the face, arms, legs, back, or chest are exposed to direct sunlight between the hours of 10 AM and 3 PM without sunscreen for 5–30 minutes at least 2 days a week. People with darker skin pigmentation require longer amounts of time in the sun. Tanning beds also emit a small amount of UV-B radiation, but they are not recommended due to the increased risk of skin cancer.[53,54]

h) Vitamin E

1. Foods that are higher in %DV of vitamin E include 1 ounce sunflower seeds, almonds, or hazelnuts; 1 tablespoon sunflower or safflower oils; and 1 small fillet trout (113 grams).
2. Other foods containing vitamin E are 2 tablespoons peanut or olive oils, corn oil, or peanut butter.[28]

OBJECTIVE 5

Use these criteria that determine which foods are the healthiest and which are the least health-promoting

1) Nutrient dense foods (ranked by foods that have the most underconsumed nutrients with the least "overconsumed" nutrients per calorie[55])

a) Top food groups to consume based on nutrients per calorie[8,36]

1. Vegetables, including mushrooms
2. Herbs and spices (however, these are eaten in very small quantities)
3. Fruits
4. Legumes
5. Whole-grains
6. Nuts
7. Seeds

b) Plant foods contain phytonutrients, which are antioxidants that protect against environmental toxicants and combat oxidative stress and inflammation in the body.[56]

c) Foods and food groups to avoid/limit based on calorie density and low nutrient density[1]

1. Foods and beverages higher in added sugars, saturated fat, and sodium, such as:
    a. Sugar-sweetened beverages
    b. Desserts and sweet snacks
    c. Sandwiches, especially those with processed meats
    d. Added oils from tropical plants, such as coconut oil, palm kernel oil, and palm oil
    e. Added fats such as butter, shortening, and lard
2. Fried foods
3. Red and processed meats (e.g., hot dogs, sausages, ham, and luncheon meats)
4. Refined grains (white flour, white rice, and white pasta)
5. Alcoholic beverages

2) General principles on foods to consume—patient-facing statements

a) It's important to think beyond a single nutrient and consider the entire "food package" when determining the relative healthfulness of a food. Although some foods are high in a particular nutrient, the rest of the package may not be ideal. Therefore, as a "food package," it may not be a healthy choice.

1. For example, whole fat and 2% milk constitute a top source of calcium but are also one of the top sources of saturated fat.
2. It's important to Ask: "Is there a better source or package to get these nutrients?"

b) Whole foods are unrefined or minimally processed in such a way as to not substantially diminish their nutrient content. Frozen vegetables, for example, are not considered refined foods.

1. Whole foods often do not have an ingredient list because they are single ingredient foods. For example, fresh produce, like an apple or a carrot, has no need for such a list.
2. Another way to decipher what's considered a whole food is that you should be able to visualize everything that has happened to the food before it's consumed. For example, it is easy to imagine what has happened to an apple. It's been picked from a tree, cleaned, shipped, and purchased in a store. It is more difficult to visualize what has happened to an apple when it's incorporated into an apple-flavored hard candy, which would be an example of a processed food.
3. Here's an example of moving an apple from a least-processed whole food to a highly processed food:
    a. Apple → applesauce → apple juice → apple fritter
4. Generally, the more whole the food (or less processed), the more nutritious that food is.

c) Center diet on whole plant foods

1. "Eat food, not too much, mostly plants," is the signature summary guideline of food writer Michael Pollan.[57]
    a. Food: unprocessed, natural foods
    b. Not too much: appropriate portion sizes
    c. Mostly plants: doesn't require vegan or vegetarian, but the diet should consist mostly of plants

    2. Emphasize legumes, vegetables, fruits, whole-grains, nuts, and seeds.

d) Eat a rainbow every day[58,59]
    1. Eating a rainbow refers to eating a variety of plants of different colors. The colors come from different flavonoids and vitamins that are essential to disease prevention and health.
    2. By consuming a wide variety of plant foods every day, most people will be able to meet the daily requirements of macronutrient and micronutrient intake, with possible supplementation needed for vitamins B12 and D.[60]

e) Some institutions that agree with the recommendation that a healthy diet should focus on plants include the United States Department of Agriculture, Dietary Guidelines Advisory Committee, American Institute for Cancer Research, Kaiser Permanente, and the Harvard School of Public Health.[61]

OBJECTIVE 6

Summarize the major (key) nutrition studies and the evidence base for nutrition prescriptions

1) **Major nutrition studies are generally intervention studies or large prospective cohort studies published in high-impact journals.**

2) **The selection of studies that follow include:**
    a) High-impact nutrition studies: large sample sizes and/or published in high-impact journals
    b) Seminal studies for lifestyle medicine: studies demonstrating evidence of disease reversal/remission
    c) Supportive of lifestyle medicine treatment: promising results relevant to disease treatment or cost savings

3) **A dietary portfolio for treatment of hypercholesterolemia[62,63] (high-impact nutrition study)**
    a) Diet: very low saturated fat diet that is high in plant sterols, soy protein, viscous fibers, and almonds.
    b) Patients treated with this dietary portfolio experienced a decrease in low-density lipoprotein (LDL) cholesterol by 28.6%, which was not statistically significantly different from treatment with 20 mg of lovastatin (low-intensity statin treatment), which lowered LDL by 30.9%.

4) **Dietary Approaches to Stop Hypertension (DASH) diet[64,65] (high-impact nutrition study)**
    a) The original study[64] of this diet compared a control diet, a diet rich in vegetables and fruits, and a "combination diet" rich in vegetables, fruits, low-fat dairy products, and reduced in saturated fat, total fat, and dietary cholesterol for their effects on blood pressure. Weight and sodium intake were held constant between the groups. Those in the vegetable and fruit diet reduced their blood pressure compared with the control group, but those assigned to the "combination diet" had the greatest reductions in blood pressure; this was true both for participants with and without hypertension. For those with hypertension (N = 133; defined as systolic blood pressure [SBP] ≥140 or diastolic blood pressure [DBP] ≥90), SBP and DBP were reduced by 11.4 and 5.5 mmHg, respectively, in the combination diet group ($P < 0.001$ for each) compared with the control diet group.

b) A later study[65] of the DASH diet (previously called the "combination diet") compared a control diet to the DASH diet, both with varying levels of sodium (low, intermediate, and high). Those who reduced sodium on either diet reduced their blood pressure. However, the greatest reductions were seen in those assigned to the low-sodium DASH diet as compared with the high-sodium control diet (SBP reduction of 11.5 mmHg for those with hypertension, and 7.1 mmHg for those without hypertension at baseline). Sub-analyses were done by gender and racial background with similar reductions.

5) **The Ornish lifestyle intervention (Lifestyle Heart Trial) for coronary artery disease (CAD)[66,67] (seminal study for lifestyle medicine)**

   a) The intervention in this study included a 10% fat vegetarian diet, moderate aerobic exercise, stress management training, smoking cessation, and group psychological support. Compared with a usual care control group, the intervention group (all of whom had moderate to severe CAD) had reduction in coronary artery stenosis that continued to improve over 5 years, whereas the control group had an increase in coronary artery stenosis over the same time period. During the 5-year follow-up, there were 25 cardiac events in the intervention group (N = 28 patients total) and 45 events in the control group (N = 20 patients total), RR =2 .47 (95% CI, 1.48–4.20) for the control group.

6) **The Ornish lifestyle intervention for prostate cancer[68] (seminal study for lifestyle medicine).**

   a) This was a pilot study of N = 30 participants (all men) with low-risk prostate cancer who declined immediate surgery, hormonal therapy, or radiation in order to participate in the study while undergoing surveillance for tumor progression. After one year, gene expression was altered in the intervention group compared with the control group and this showed that this intensive nutrition and lifestyle intervention may modulate gene expression in the prostate. This was interpreted to favor the intervention group, though a larger trial is needed to confirm the results of this pilot study.

7) **The Lyon Diet Heart Study[69,70] looked at secondary prevention of coronary heart disease with a Mediterranean diet versus the American Heart Association Step 1 diet. (high-impact nutrition study)**

   a) Those assigned to the Mediterranean diet arm had fewer of the composite cardiovascular disease outcomes compared with those in the prudent Western diet arm, demonstrating the protective effects of the Mediterranean dietary pattern. Results were maintained for the extended 4-year study follow-up period after each participant's first myocardial infarction.

8) **The Esselstyn plant-based diet for coronary artery disease[71,72] (seminal study for lifestyle medicine)**

   a) A very low-fat, plant-based diet was shown to reverse and prevent major cardiac events in 177 adherent patients over 3.7 years. Among the 177 adherent patients, cardiac event rates were 0.6%. Among the 21 non-adherent patients, 13 experienced major cardiac events (62%).

9) **The Complete Health Improvement Program (CHIP) program and plant-based dietary interventions with cost savings[73] (supportive of lifestyle medicine treatment)**

   a) The CHIP multifactorial lifestyle intervention was found to be effective in treating type 2 diabetes and to have a positive return on investment within a few months.

10) **Vegan diet for treating diabetes[74] (supportive of lifestyle medicine treatment)**

a) In this 22-week randomized clinical trial of 99 subjects with type 2 diabetes comparing participants assigned to either a vegan diet or the American Diabetes Association (ADA) diet, those assigned to a vegan diet significantly improved their diet quality as measured by the Alternative Healthy Eating index, despite increasing carbohydrate intake. Those assigned to the ADA diet did not improve their diet quality compared with baseline.

11) The above list is not exhaustive. It is beyond the scope of this manual to highlight the many individual foods that have also been shown to improve some diseases.

OBJECTIVE 7

Evaluate the science behind making nutrition prescriptions

1) Nutrition prescriptions are one of the 15 competencies of a lifestyle medicine physician.[75]

2) The US Preventive Services Task Force (USPSTF) recommends intensive behavioral health nutrition counseling and physical activity counseling for overweight people with chronic disease risk factors. This is a grade "B" recommendation. (A "B" rating means to provide service, as there is a high certainty the benefit will be moderate to substantial.)[76,77]

3) The USPSTF recommends that nutrition and physical activity counseling for people with no chronic disease and no risk factors should be based on readiness for change. This is a grade "C" recommendation. (A grade "C" recommendation means that service should be offered in a selective manner to patients based on professional assessment and patient preference.) [76,78]

a) Education and clarity are necessary conditions for successful behavior change.

4) An in-depth guide titled *Primary Care Nutrition: Writing the Nutrition Prescription* details the importance of and process for incorporating nutrition and lifestyle guidance for patients in a primary care setting. Primary care physicians are encouraged to prescribe and endorse plans developed by teams comprised of motivated registered dietitians, nurses, psychologists, physical therapists, and office staff, and tailored for the individual needs of their patients. This guide explains the relationship between nutrition and the immune system, genetics, and numerous chronic disorders and diseases (i.e., gastrointestinal disorders, obesity, heart disease, diabetes, chronic kidney disease, and others). This guide also serves as a practical toolkit by offering clear guidance and recommendations for how to incorporate nutrition and nutrition prescriptions into primary care practices.[79]

a) The Academy of Nutrition and Dietetics provides definitions and guidelines for nutrition screening and assessment.

5) Strong evidence exists for lifestyle prescriptions related to exercise.

a) In 2009, researchers investigated the effectiveness of an exercise prescription given in an outpatient setting. The study was titled, "Effectiveness of Physical Activity Advice and Prescription by Physicians in Routine Primary Care: A Cluster Randomized Trial."[80]

1. For this study, 4,317 physically inactive patients were recruited and divided into two groups: 2,248 in the intervention group and 2,069 in the control group.
2. All patients in the intervention group received physical activity advice, which was given during an office visit. A subgroup of 30% of the intervention patients received an extra intervention that included a tailored physical activity prescription at an additional outpatient appointment.

3. The results at 6 months showed the intervention patients (those who received the physical activity advice, including the subgroup who received a tailored physical activity prescription) increased their exercise by an average of 18 minutes per week (95% CI) compared to the control patients.
4. The intervention patients who received advice showed only a small increase in exercise among older patients (>50 years old) and showed no significant effect among younger patients.
5. Among the exercise prescription subgroup, patients over 50 years old increased activity by 131 minutes per week and doubled their minutes of moderate to vigorous exercise compared to the control group. Patients younger than age 50 increased their activity by 31.5 minutes per week when compared to the control group.

b) Nutrition prescriptions have been used with success among chronic kidney disease patients.[81]

OBJECTIVE 8

Demonstrate ability to perform a basic nutrition assessment

1) Nutrition assessments provide in-depth pictures of the nutrition statuses of patients.

a) They can be performed by a provider with follow up by a registered dietitian (RD) or by a RD in a collaborative team.

b) Information from these assessments helps determine an appropriate nutrition prescription.

c) Nutrition assessments help create a record of a patient's nutrition adequacy and/or needs that can be monitored at future visits.

2) A basic nutrition assessment includes the following elements, referred to by the acronym ABCD.

a) A = Anthropometric data, B = Biochemical data, C = Clinical assessment, D = Dietary assessment

b) A = Anthropometric data includes the following:

1. Weight, height, body mass index (BMI) and waist circumference
    a. Accuracy is important; do not assume height and weight are correct in charts.
2. BMI[82,83] (see box for calculation)
    a. BMI is low cost and easy to calculate based on height and weight measurements
    b. Appropriate uses and limitations:
        (1) High-density muscle and bone mass from extreme physical activity may bias results.
        (2) Calculations in body composition should be adjusted for race when possible.
        (3) BMI is less precise for very short people.

$$\textbf{BMI} = \frac{\textbf{Weight (lbs)}}{[\textbf{Height (in)}]^2} \times 703$$

$$\textbf{BMI} = \frac{\textbf{Weight (kg)}}{[\textbf{Height (m)}]^2}$$

3. Bioelectrical impedance analysis is common, but its accuracy is variable.[82,83]
    a. This analysis uses a small electrical signal to measure the amount of water within a person's body in order to assess body composition. The bioelectrical impedance device is able to calculate body fat percentage based on water measurements because fat tissue and fat-free body mass contain significantly different amounts of water.
    b. This test is more accurate than BMI at measuring percent body fat because body fat is a more accurate assessment of nutrition status.

4. Hydrostatic underwater weighing (hydrodensitometry) is uncommon but accurate.[83]
5. Skinfold measurements with calipers are difficult to perform for adults with overweight or obesity, and results can vary widely by sex and specific techniques used.[82,83] These measurements are not recommended.

c) Biochemical data

1. Lab work
    a. Many common lab tests are linked to nutrition status. While evaluating lab work, keep in mind a patient's medical history and current conditions as well as the effects of hydration status on the lab values.
    b. Commonly ordered labs for general nutrition for general population include sodium, potassium, hemoglobin, hematocrit, glucose, HbA1c, albumin, total cholesterol, low-density lipoprotein (LDL) cholesterol, high-density lipoprotein (HDL) cholesterol, triglycerides, calcium, vitamin D, vitamin B12, iron, and ferritin.

d) Clinical assessment

1. Age
2. Gender
3. Medical and surgical history
4. Activity level
5. Nutrition history
    a. Weight history (e.g., highs, lows, changes, the weight a patient feels/felt best at, etc.)
    b. Any history of nutrition deficiencies, gastrointestinal diseases, or other states contributing to malabsorption (e.g., history of bariatric surgery, celiac disease, etc.)
6. Vital signs (see Section 3)
7. Physical exam (see Section 3)

e) Dietary assessment

1. The dietary assessment looks at components of the patient's current diet and behavioral drivers for food choices, including food insecurity/food access, abilities/tools for meal preparation, and more. The assessment may be completed using a variety of questionnaires or tools. Some examples are:
    a. Daily intake of solids and liquids
    b. 24-hour recall
        (1) Recall asks the patient what they ate during the last 24 hours.
        (2) The recall is often done in an office visit as a verbal interview, and it may be easier to work backwards, asking the patient what they most recently ate.
        (3) An example that can be viewed online is the National Cancer Institute's Automated Self-Administered 24-Hour Dietary Assessment Tool (ASA24).[84]
        (4) To increase accuracy, clarify:
            (a) How was the food prepared (broiled, baked, grilled, etc.)?
            (b) How big was the portion?

> **Note**
>
> The provider may wish to have this variety of questionnaires completed by a registered dietitian; these assessments can be time consuming, and dietitians are trained to do them and have the appropriate tools (food models, measuring utensils, etc.).

(c) How often is that food or drink consumed?
(d) Did you eat any food, snacks, or beverages between meals?
(e) Did you have drinks during or after meals?
(f) Were there any desserts or sweets?
(g) Was this day typical?
(h) If not, how did it differ from a typical day?
(i) Does intake change on the weekends?
(j) If so, how?
(k) Do you use any nutrition supplements (bars, shakes, pills, etc.)?
(l) If so, how much and how often?

c. 3-day food record
   (1) 3-day food intake[85]
      (a) It's best if the patient is able to catch a range of eating behaviors, for example eating habits during 2 work days and 1 day off, or eating habits on a "good" day, "bad" day, and an "average" day.
      (b) Be sure to be specific about portion sizes, type of foods, brand name of prepared food, preparation methods, anything added to the food (salt, ketchup, brown sugar, etc.), and whether the food was homemade.
   (2) The 3-day food record is often given as an assignment to bring to the next appointment.

Practical Tip

It may help to have food models, as many people are not skilled at estimating portions.

d. Mini Nutritional Assessment (MNA) for the elderly[86]
   (1) This is a validated nutrition screening and assessment tool that can identify patients 65 years of age and above who are malnourished or at risk for malnourishment.
e. Online and/or interactive individual dietary assessment tools include the following, which may be helpful in prompting conversation during an appointment:[87]
   (1) In-depth assessment by a dietitian
   (2) Block Dietary Fat Screener (online version at NutritionQuest)[88]
      a) Tracks one's fat intake and compares it to the average American fat intake
   (3) Fruit/vegetable/fiber screener from NutritionQuest[89]
      a) Compares current fruit and vegetable intake to what is needed to reduce disease risk.
   (4) Healthy Body Calculator from Ask the Dietitian[90]
   (5) Calculates recommended amounts of nutrients and physical activity based upon one's body frame size, BMI, and waist-to-hip ratio.
   (6) Nutrition calculators and counters made available by the Centers for Disease Control and Prevention include:[91]
      (a) Interactive Dietary Reference Intake (DRI) Calculator for Healthcare Professionals
      (b) Basal Energy Expenditure: Harris-Benedict Equation calculator
      (c) BMI Percentile Calculator

f. Mobile apps for dietary self-assessment (while not endorsing any specific platforms, some examples include: MyPlate Calorie Counter, Calorie King, LoseIt, Healthwatch 360, My Fitness Pal, Cronometer, and others)

2. Ask about the patient's meal schedule, including timing, duration, place, and activities during eating.
3. Ask about patient's social history, including family structure, psychosocial factors, and cultural considerations. All are important elements of a thorough dietary assessment.
   a. Readiness to change
   b. Self-efficacy
   c. Nutrition knowledge
   d. Motivation
   e. Social support from family/friends
   f. Cultural or religious restrictions or preferences (certain foods may be prohibited such as pork or shellfish)
   g. Financial resources or food budget
   h. Functional ability (ability to chew, intolerances to gluten, etc.)
   i. Special dietary needs (history of kidney failure, constipation, etc.)
4. Assess emotions at times of eating.
5. Assess for food groups or nutrients being under consumed.
6. Assess for food groups or nutrients being over consumed.

f) Highlights of a collaborative nutrition assessment completed by an interdisciplinary team

1. The general approach to collaborative nutrition assessments includes:
   a. A physical exam and basic nutrition assessment completed by a physician or advanced practice provider
   b. Possible referral and follow-up scheduled with a RD
      (1) Patients with food-related disease or complex chronic diseases should be referred to a RD for comprehensive assessment in addition to the provider's basic assessment.
         (a) Patients may have conditions that include prediabetes, diabetes, renal disease, cardiovascular disease, weight related disorders, history of bariatric surgery, cancer, a compromised immune system (HIV), liver disease, gastrointestinal disorders (celiac, Crohn's), and patients taking weight-promoting medications if they cannot be changed or discontinued.
2. Role of the physician or medical provider in nutrition assessments
   a. Obtain a baseline history and physical examination.
   b. Determine patient risk factors for chronic conditions and current diagnoses.
   c. Create a framework for treatment.
      (1) For most chronic conditions, nutrition should be emphasized as a key part of treatment.
      (2) Explain importance of nutrition specifically in terms of patient's current medical treatment and goals for disease prevention or remission/reversal.
   d. Lead a multidisciplinary care team.
   e. Help patients set short- and long-term dietary and other lifestyle goals.
   f. Oversee recommendations made by the RD.

3. Role of the RD
    a. Assess and monitor nutrition status.
    b. Determine macronutrient and/or micronutrient needs/deficiencies.
    c. Develop individualized dietary recommendations.
    d. Coach patients toward personal goals with consideration of medical history.
    e. Track progress, such as the impact of dietary measures on biomarkers (in conjunction with the physician).
    f. Provide ongoing support and education.
    g. Provide medical nutrition therapy.

OBJECTIVE 9

Prescribe nutrition for basic disease processes including inflammation: food patterns / macronutrients, food types / micronutrients, food preparation / oxidation

1) Macronutrients

a) All macronutrients (fat, protein, and carbohydrate) are present in all whole foods, just in varying proportions.

b) No single food is equivalent to a single macronutrient.

c) Table 5.1 shows macronutrients, primary functions, and Recommended Dietary Allowance (RDA) or Adequate Intake (AI) below:[92]

Table 5.1 Macronutrients, Primary Functions, and RDA or AI

Macronutrient	Function	RDA or AI*
Carbohydrate	Primary energy source for the brain (RDA); calories needed to maintain body weight	130 g/day
Fiber	Improves laxation, increases satiety, lowers risk of coronary heart disease, helps to maintain normal blood glucose levels	Men 38 g/day* Women 25 g/day* (based on 14 g per 1,000 calories energy consumed)
Protein	Serves as the major structural component of all cells in the body and functions as enzymes, in membranes, as transport carriers, and as some hormones	0.8 g/kg Or, approximately: 46 g for women 56 g for men
Fat (n6 fatty acids)	Essential component of structural membrane lipids, involved with cell signaling, and precursor of eicosanoids; required for normal skin function	Men 17 g* Women 12 g*
Fats (n3 fatty acids)	Involved with neurological development and growth; precursor of eicosanoids	Men 1.6 g/day* Women 1.1 g/day*

Recommended Dietary Allowance (RDA)—The average daily dietary intake level that is sufficient to meet the nutrient requirements of nearly all (97.5%) healthy individuals in a particular life stage and gender group.

Adequate Intake (AI)—The recommended average daily intake level of a nutrient based on observed or experimentally determined approximations or estimates of intakes that are assumed to be adequate for a group (or groups) of apparently healthy people; used when the RDA cannot be determined.

d) Protein

1. In the US, protein is typically associated with animal proteins (e.g., meat, poultry, and eggs) and protein powder, but all essential amino acids (which are the building blocks of protein) originally come from plants and microbes.[93]
2. Labeling animal foods as "protein" is a misnomer; the majority of calories for most animal foods (though not necessarily all, including low-fat dairy or egg whites) are from fat (saturated fat), not protein.
   a. "Complete" vs "Incomplete" proteins
      (1) Historically, a "complete protein" has been defined as one that contains all of the essential amino acids in the approximate amounts needed by humans, while an "incomplete" protein contains only some of the essential amino acids.[94] Essential amino acids are those that the human body cannot manufacture.

   b. Both animal and plant proteins contain all nine essential amino acids, though most plant proteins are limited in either lysine or sulfur containing amino acids, (methionine is the only essential sulfur-containing amino acid). (Soybean is the only plant source of "complete" protein.)

   c. Because amino acids in various plant foods tend to complement each other, it is nearly impossible to become deficient in any one essential amino acid.[95,96]

   d. All proteins, both plant and animal, entering the stomach are digested similarly. They are broken down into their amino acid building blocks by hydrochloric acid and protease enzymes, absorbed by cells, and built into proteins in the body as needed.[94]

   e. Examples of the protein content of plant and animal foods are in Tables 5.1 and 5.2.
      (1) While the RDA for protein is calculated based on body weight, not as a percentage of calories, there is utility in understanding the percentage of calories from protein from different foods.
      (2) The 0.8 g/kg of body weight translates to a recommended intake of roughly 10–11% calories from protein.
      (3) Overall, the protein content of plant foods is more than adequate to meet human needs if a variety of foods is consumed, and it is actually easy to consume more than 10–11% (even more so if any emphasis is given to greens, legumes, and whole-grains).
      (4) Example
         (a) 150 lb (68.2 kg) person eating 2,000 calories per day
         (b) 0.8 g × 68.2 = 55 g protein required per day
         (c) Protein is 4 calories per gram, so →
         (d) 55 g × 4 calories = 220 calories from protein
         (e) 220 calories ÷ 2,000 calories = 11% energy from protein

Table 5.2 Plant Protein Content as % Energy[28]

Foods	US Nutrient Database #	Energy (kcal) / 100g	Protein (g)	Protein (% Energy)
Spinach	11457	23	2.86	50%
Soybeans	16109	172	18.21	42%
Lettuce	11257	16	1.33	33%
Brussels Sprouts	11099	36	2.55	28%
Broccoli	11091	35	2.38	27%
Seaweed (wakame)	11669	45	3.03	27%
Peas	11305	84	5.36	26%
Chickpeas	16057	164	8.86	22%
Tomatoes	11529	18	0.88	20%
Oats	20038	389	16.89	17%
Green Pepper	11333	20	0.86	17%
Quinoa	20137	120	4.4	15%
Baked Potatoes	11356	290	7.86	11%
Corn	20014	365	9.42	10%
Walnuts	12155	765	17.82	9%
Banana	09040	89	1.09	5%
Apples	09003	52	0.26	2%

Table 5.3 Animal Protein Content as % Energy[28]

Foods	US Nutrient Database #	Energy (kcal) / 100g	Protein (g)	Protein (% Energy)
Chicken Breast	1098452	175	26.37	60%
Tuna Fillet	1145081	174	25.29	58%
Lean Pork Chops	1098246	211	27.69	52%
Beef (Skirt Steak)	171787	220	26.13	48%
Eggs	748967	143	12.4	35%
Low-Fat Yogurt	170886	63	5.25	33%
Milk, Skim or 1%	1097520	43	3.38	31%
Cheddar Cheese	1098007	408	23.3	23%
Ice Cream, Vanilla	1097924	207	3.5	7%

f. One concern for which some evidence exists is that of "diet-derived metabolic acidosis," in that the consumption of animal protein causes an acidic condition in the body which needs neutralizing.[97] Calcium can be extracted from the bones to generate more of a buffering substrate. Some evidence exists that supports extracting calcium from the bones may contribute to poor bone health,[97] but more research is needed.[98]

g. A healthy, totally plant-based diet can still provide a complete amino acid profile, provided the diet is based on whole foods and a variety of foods are generally consumed. It is not necessary to combine specific protein foods within the same meal or the same day, but rather to consume a variety of food over time.[99]

3. Protein needs are adequately met when following a varied, whole food plant-based diet.
    a. Evidence supports some increased need for protein above general population needs for the following populations: the elderly, children, pregnant women, and athletes.[100]
4. Example SMART goal prescription for protein-rich foods: I will prepare and eat 1 cup of beans in lunch or dinner every day for 3 months.
    a. Type of food: legumes (i.e., beans, peas, and lentils)
    b. Amount of food: 1 cup cooked (198 grams; or two servings, approximately 200 calories)
    c. Frequency: once daily for 3 months

e) Fat

1. As stated above, almost all whole foods contain some amount of fat. Most foods that contain fat have a variety of types.
2. Dietary patterns and food packages are far more important in the reduction of cardiovascular disease (CVD), diabetes, and other chronic diseases than total fat consumed. Foods containing predominantly monounsaturated and polyunsaturated fats (e.g., healthy plant, fish, and seafood sources) should replace those containing predominantly saturated fats (e.g., processed foods, meat, dairy, and tropical plant oils). *Trans* fats should be avoided whenever possible.[101,102]
3. Different types of fats
    a. Polyunsaturated
        (1) Omega 3s (usually considered anti-inflammatory)
        (2) Omega 6s (usually considered pro-inflammatory)
            (a) **Author's note:** This breakdown is oversimplified. The inflammatory effect occurs with arachidonic acid, which is one type of omega-6 fatty acid. However, dihomo-γ-linolenic acid is also an omega-6 fatty acid, but it's generally considered to be anti-inflammatory. Several studies have shown higher linolenic acid, which is also an omega-6 fatty acid, intake does not increase inflammation. The relationship between omega-3 and omega-6 fatty acids and inflammation is complex and still not well understood.[103,104,105,106,107]
    b. Monounsaturated[39]
        (1) Fats that contain a substantial proportion of monounsaturated fats are generally liquids at room temperature (e.g., olive, canola, peanut, safflower, and sesame oils).
        (2) If monounsaturated fatty acids are used in place of *trans* fats or saturated fats, they may help lower LDL cholesterol and reduce a known risk factor for CVD, lower risk of cardiovascular events, and reduce all-cause mortality.[39]
    c. Saturated
        (1) Sources of saturated fat in Western or US diets[108]
            (a) Lauric acid (found in coconuts)
                1. Increases total cholesterol, HDL, and LDL[109]
                    a. HDL may not lower heart disease risk, and increasing LDL is known to increase the risk of heart disease.[110,111,112]
            (b) Stearic acid has harmful health effects (found in cheese, meat, poultry, and dairy)

1. Though it doesn't appear to raise cholesterol as much as other long-chain saturated fatty acids (SFAs), all SFAs are strongly correlated with coronary heart disease (CHD). Replacing stearic acid with an equivalent number of calories from polyunsaturated fats, whole-grain carbohydrates, or plant proteins would lead to a 6-8% reduction in the risk of CHD.[113,114]
2. Associated with increased endothelial damage and cell death[115] and decreased function of endothelial progenitor cells essential to vascular repair[116]
3. Associated with increased risk of colorectal cancer[117]

(c) Palmitic acid, which is harmful[117,118]

1. Found in palm oil, butter, cheese, milk, and meat[36]
2. Most common saturated fat
3. May lead to increased heart disease risk and associated with insulin resistance[118]

(d) Myristic acid, which is harmful[119] and is found in dairy products (i.e., cheese, butter, and milk) and tropical oils (i.e., coconut, palm, and palm kernel oils).

1. Is hypercholesterolemic[120]
2. Associated with CVD,[119] risk of all-cause mortality, and type 2 diabetes[121]

d. Trans fat

(1) Found in partially hydrogenated vegetable oils

(a) Associated with an increased risk of CHD[43]

(2) The FDA mandated that the food industry must remove *trans* fat from foods by 2018.[122]

(3) *Trans* fats are found in:

(a) Partially hydrogenated oils (shortenings, margarines)

(b) Fried foods (French fries, doughnuts)

(c) Commercially baked goods and snack foods (crackers, cookies, microwave popcorn)

(d) Coffee creamers

(e) Refrigerated doughs

(f) Naturally found in meat and dairy products

e. Lower-fat foods prescription

(1) Instructions to reduce fat are most commonly prescribed as a "negative" prescription, meaning patients are advised to limit intake, particularly of saturated fats.[101]

(2) It's less helpful to count fat grams, and it's more helpful to limit specific kinds of foods. Suggesting specific replacements is more helpful than just prohibiting foods.

(3) Prescriptions should be tailored to patient's dietary preferences (i.e., no need to limit foods they are already not consuming).

(4) Example SMART goal prescription: I will find a salad dressing to replace my oil-based dressings for 1 week of salads at dinner. I will start by trying a balsamic vinaigrette.

(a) Type of food: limit oil-based salad dressing and replace with balsamic vinaigrette

(b) Amount of food: 1/4 cup (32 grams)

(c) Frequency: every day for 1 week

f) Carbohydrates

1. Carbohydrate quality is important; complex and unrefined carbohydrates from legumes, vegetables, whole-grains, and fruits differ in their health effects from refined carbohydrates.[123]
2. They must be addressed in the context of whole foods versus processed foods.[124,125]
    a. Whole-food carbohydrates are the healthiest carbohydrate-rich food options (e.g. vegetables, fruits, legumes, and whole-grains). Foods and dietary patterns rich in highly processed carbohydrates (e.g., added sugars, white flours, etc.) are associated with negative health outcomes (e.g., overweight, obesity, metabolic disorders,[126] heart disease,[127] and type 2 diabetes[128]) and should be limited or avoided.[123]
3. Components of carbohydrates
    a. Fiber
        (1) Essential to gut health and immune function, often overlooked as it has almost no nutrients or calories.[129] Higher intake is associated with lower risk of coronary artery disease,[74] insulin resistence,[130] and colonic diseases.[131,132]
        (2) Found intact in whole foods; often removed in the processing of carbohydrates.
        (3) Physiology
            (a) Insoluble fiber is not absorbed from the gut and therefore increases stool bulk.
            (b) Fiber increases stool viscosity and holds extra water.[133]
            (c) Though indigestible to humans, intestinal bacteria feed on insoluble fiber to produce short-chain fatty acids for energy and support a healthy colony of protective bacteria for immune function and to control pathogens.[134]
            (d) Fiber heals and protects the intestinal barrier, keeping it intact, avoiding "leaky gut," and providing immune defense.[135]
            (e) Soluble fiber is absorbed into the blood stream and slows digestion, increases insulin sensitivity,[136] and carries out cholesterol.[137]
        (4) Increasing fiber in the diet can improve a variety of conditions.
            (a) Improves stool consistency and decreases constipation
            (b) Lowers cholesterol[63]
            (c) Stabilizes blood glucose [137,138]
            (d) Increases satiety and decreases cravings[139]
            (e) Decreases risk of diabetes[130]
            (f) Decreases risk of colon cancer[140]
        (5) Daily fiber recommendations: Dietary Reference Intakes for total fiber is based on 14 g per 1000 calories per day.[141]
            (a) Women: 25 grams per day, greater benefits if >40 grams per day
            (b) Men: 38 grams per day, greater benefits if >45 grams per day
        (6) Best sources of fiber
            (a) Legumes, whole-grains, vegetables, fruits, nuts, and seeds.
            (b) There is no fiber in animal products (e.g., meat, poultry, fish, seafood, dairy, and eggs).
    b. Added sugars
        (1) Note: The naturally occurring sugars contained in whole foods are healthy and are not associated with adverse effects. They have been found to be consistently protective against chronic disease.

c. Starch is a healthy complex carbohydrate.

d. Foods that contain starch can be healthy or unhealthy, driven by the degree to which food is intact or refined.

   (1) Examples of intact, healthy, starch-containing foods include potatoes, corn, legumes, and whole-grains.

   (2) Examples of refined, unhealthy starch-containing foods include potato chips, corn chips (which both have added fat and salt), textured vegetable protein (which is a refined protein), and white flour pasta (refined grains).

2) Micronutrients

a) Micronutrients are chemical elements or substances that are essential in small or minute amounts for growth and health. Micronutrients are vitamins and minerals.

b) Beneficial non-nutrients are valuable to health but are not proven to be essential for life. They include antioxidants, anti-inflammatory molecules, phytochemicals, polyphenols, phytosterols, glucosinolates, and carotenoids.

c) In the US, it's a common misperception that supplements are needed to achieve micronutrient balance.

1. Multiple studies indicate a variety of whole foods helps achieve micronutrient balance better than taking supplements.[142,143,144,145,146]
2. It's important to note that the body is trying to maintain homeostasis (remain in a stable state), and harm can occur with overdosing of micronutrients, which can occur with supplementation.
3. However, it is also important to recognize that supplements may be warranted. For example, those who are on a plant-only diet should take a vitamin B12 supplement.

d) Types of foods

1. Micronutrients can be prescribed as "food families."
   a. Note that food prescriptions usually need to be more specific than a food family. A specific micronutrient is generally not prescribed.

e) Micronutrient value

1. High in antioxidants
   a. Decrease oxidation thereby decrease inflammation and a variety of disease states
2. Increase cell health[147]
   a. Increases strength of immune system to detect and fight disease
   b. Inflammation is considered the mechanism of most chronic disease.
3. Antioxidant foods are anti-inflammatory foods.
   a. Cruciferous vegetables:
      1) Contain sulforaphane and indole-3-carbinols
      2) Broccoli, cauliflower, Brussels sprouts, bok choy, kale, and Chinese cabbage
      3) Example of a positive prescription: 1 cup (91 grams) fresh or 1/2 cup (92 grams) cooked daily
   b. Dark berries and fruits
      (1) Contain polyphenols such as ellagic acid, anthocyanidins, and anthocyanins
      (2) Blueberries, raspberries, strawberries, cranberries, and pomegranates
      (3) Example of a positive prescription: 1/2 cup (170 grams) daily

c. Allium vegetables
    1) Rich in organosulfurs
    2) Garlic, onions, and leeks
    3) Example of a positive prescription: one garlic clove daily

d. Orange, yellow, and dark green vegetables and fruits
    1) Contain carotenoids that stimulate natural killer cells, which fight foreign inflammation
    2) Carrots, yams, and mango
    3) Example of a positive prescription: one medium carrot daily

e. Dark green leafy vegetables
    1) High in potassium, calcium, and magnesium
    2) Spinach, collards, Swiss chard, dark lettuces, mustard, and turnip greens
    3) Example of a positive prescription: 1 cup fresh or 1/2 cup (170 grams) cooked spinach daily

3) Foods that increase inflammation

a) Processed grains (flour) and sugar

1. Have a high glycemic index and increase insulin production
2. Are found in a high percentage of packaged foods
3. Example of negative prescription: no more than one serving of refined carbohydrates per day (e.g., sugar or white bread)

b) Processed meat and red meat[148]

1. Processed meats include sausage, bacon, lunch meat, cured meats, jerky, ham, and hot dogs. Includes any meats that have been salted, smoked, fermented, cured, or processed in another way.
    a. Known Group 1 carcinogen (see Box) for colon cancer, stomach cancer, pancreatic cancer and prostate cancer
2. Red meats include beef, pork, lamb, goat, and horse.
    a. Probable carcinogen associated with colorectal cancer

Group 1: Carcinogenic to Humans

aflatoxin, alcoholic beverages, benzene, coal-tar, formaldehyde, hepatitis B virus, hepatitis C virus, processed meat, tobacco (smokeless and smoking), and X and gamma radiation.

Note: *For a more complete list, see American Cancer Society's "Known and Probable Human Carcinogens"*[152]

c) Harmful fats[39,149,150,151]

1. *Trans* fats (which are mainly in highly processed oils)
2. Oxidized fats (products of oxidation formed by heat or rancidity)
3. Solid fats (from lard, butter, meat, dairy, and tropical oils)

4) Food preparation can also affect nutrient value through oxidation

a) AGEs (advanced glycation end products)

1. Are a family of oxidative stress inducers
2. Have known pathologic mechanisms

a. AGEs affect the same systems that are damaged in type 2 diabetes and may be a partial cause of this disease.

b) AGE biochemistry

1. AGEs are products formed by a spontaneous chemical reaction between an amino acid (protein) and a monosaccharide (simple sugar such as glucose).
    a. Research has found AGEs are associated with oxidative stress and inflammation, which may lead to the development of chronic diseases.
    b. A small amount of AGEs will be produced in the body daily. However, most AGEs are from tobacco products or consumed foods.
    c. AGEs in food occur more:
        (1) In protein rich foods than fatty foods, and lastly, carbohydrate rich foods
        (2) When temperatures are higher
        (3) When heat is applied for a longer amount of time
        (4) When food is dry; moisture lowers AGE formation
        (5) When the pH of the food is more acidic or basic
        (6) In the presence of higher amounts of trace minerals
    d. Cooking methods can affect amount of AGEs in food. AGEs increase with grilling, broiling, roasting, searing, and frying.[153]
2. AGEs increase over time
    a. AGEs accumulate at higher amounts with increasing age in the proteins of the lens of the human eye and the skin collagen.[154]
3. The body can detoxify some AGEs, but it processes them slowly.
4. AGEs can build up when too many are present.
5. AGE build up can lead to cell damage, especially in cells that have a long life (nerve and brain cells, collagen proteins in kidney, blood vessels, and eye cells).
6. Increased AGEs have been directly related to:[155]
    a. Diabetes, type 1 and type 2
    b. Atherosclerosis
    c. Kidney disease
    d. Slow wound healing

c) AGEs in food[153]

1. A 6-year study at Mt. Sinai Medical Center tested for AGEs in foods that were regularly eaten and found.
    a. Whole foods (AGE kU/serving): 10 (carrots) to 799 (dried fig)
    b. Processed foods (AGE kU/serving): 17 (Snickers) to 1,522 (fast food french fries)
    c. Animal products (AGE kU/serving): 515 (smoked salmon) to 11,905 (bacon fried for 5 minutes)
    d. Dairy products (AGE kU/serving): 1 (fat-free milk) to 325 (heavy, ultra-pasteurized cream)
    e. Nuts and seeds (AGE kU/serving): 753 (raw sunflower seeds) to 3,363 (roasted pine nuts)

d) Summary for food preparation

1. Increase consumption of unprocessed whole foods such as vegetables, fruits, legumes, and whole-grains.
2. Decrease consumption of fatty meats, solid fats, full dairy products and highly processed foods.

3. Prepare foods less often by dry heat cooking, such as grilling, baking, and frying.
    a. AGEs form at temperatures in excess of 248 °F (120 °C).
4. Prepare foods more by moist heat cooking, such as boiling, stewing and broiling.
    a. Moisture and lower heat produce fewer AGEs.

OBJECTIVE 10

Describe practical strategies for assisting patients to achieve dietary changes

1) Nutrition prescription format

- **a)** Use SMART goals format (see below).
- **b)** Include the patient's name, the date, and the provider's signature.
- **c)** Core prescription components (pneumonic TAF—opposite of FAT)
    1. Type of food (be specific)
    2. Amount of food to be eaten (be exact)
    3. Frequency food should be eaten
        a. May be time limited (e.g., once a day for 2 weeks, or three times a week for 2 months)
- **d)** Positive prescriptions
    1. Eat more of one type of food (e.g., whole-grains, legumes, or leafy greens), or swap (e.g., brown rice for white).
    2. Generally, this is more accepted by patients.
- **e)** Negative prescriptions
    1. Consume less of a type of food (e.g., processed meats, milk products, or sweets)
    2. Suggesting replacements and swaps of foods is easier (suggestions below)

2) Use SMART goals as basic guideline for nutrition prescription.

- **a)** Consider these when talking about nutrition prescriptions.
- **b)** SMART goals can be used in many instances, except in deficiency states.
- **c)** SMART goals should be determined largely by the patient, with coaching and engagement from the provider
- **d)** SMART stands for:
    1. Specific
        a. What are you prescribing?
            (1) Describe exactly what that new habit will be: not "eat more vegetables," but "eat 1/2 cup cooked spinach or broccoli each dinner."
            (2) Involve patient in identifying where their diet could benefit from change.
            (3) Engage them in the process to determine specific changes they would like to work on.
            (4) Help them align their targets with healthy dietary behavior changes.
            (5) Avoid generic statements such as, "my goal is to eat healthier."
    2. Measurable
        a. How much? How many (e.g., one medium [apple], 1/2 cup (125 ml), 1 cup (250 ml), etc.)?

3. Achievable/Attainable/Action-oriented
    a. Describe how the goal will be attained. For example, think about who will do the food shopping, prepare the food, and more.
4. Realistic/Relevant: Improvement is the goal, not perfection.
    a. This refers to making sure the SMART goal is something the patient can accomplish, as well as directly related to bigger goals.
        1) Often patients will set very high goals, like wanting to go from six sodas a day to zero sodas starting the following morning or wanting to lose 20 pounds in 5 weeks. The health provider needs to help oversee goals to make sure they are realistic (and safe/healthy) for the patient to achieve.
5. Time-connected/Time-limited
    a. How frequent (e.g., daily, each meal, weekly)?
    b. How long (e.g. 3 months)?
    c. Time limits may encourage compliance versus open-ended amounts of time, which can be overwhelming, especially if the change is going to be difficult for the patient.

e) More examples of SMART dietary changes

1. Instead of white rice for dinner, my goal is to eat 1 cup brown rice instead of white rice.
2. My evening snack will be a sliced apple and 6 almonds, instead of __________.
3. I will eat 1/2 cup of spinach or green vegetable at every dinner.

f) Examples in practice

1. The patient has a practical discussion with his provider about the role of nutrition in treating his current conditions and preventing additional conditions.
2. Provider should approach discussion with patient with sensitivity to the Stages of Change[156] and tailor suggestions or prompts to the patient's readiness to change.
3. When the patient is ready for action, develop a specific written nutrition plan (nutrition prescription) and/or refer to a registered dietitian, health coach, or other appropriate provider for additional support.
    a. Focus on the positive by beginning with what to add to the diet.
    b. Be realistic: If the patient is drinking 2 liters of soda each day, they may not be ready to cut it all out. The initial step may be exchanging one glass of soda for soda water with a splash of pomegranate juice or pure blueberry juice—just enough juice to flavor it.
    c. Be specific: Help the patient see where they can add things in (e.g., antioxidant- and fiber-rich berries plus omega-3 rich ground flaxseeds on morning cereal).
    d. Base goals on the patient's readiness to change; self-efficacy and confidence (see Section 2); medical and weight history; schedule; and food preferences.
    e. Base goals on the 24-hour recall results and current habits.
    f. Set measurable goals.
        (1) It may be helpful to have a list of healthy behaviors pre-written and allow patients to choose which items they would like to work on (example list below)
            (a) Eat two more pieces of fruits daily.
            (b) Take a 15-minute walk on your lunch break.
            (c) Add one more vegetable to lunch and dinner.
            (d) Cook dinner at home two more times per week.
            (e) Start eating breakfast based on whole foods such as oatmeal, fruit, and nuts.

g. Help patients adopt healthy habits by encouraging them to:
    (1) Maintain a healthy eating pattern.
    (2) Choose a variety of foods.
    (3) Remember balance and moderation.
    (4) Increase their awareness by:
        (a) Keeping a food and exercise journal
        (b) Developing a consistent meal schedule
        (c) Increasing self-awareness of eating cues, including hunger, satiety, stress and environmental cues
    (5) Develop healthy eating behaviors, such as mindful eating.
        (a) Slow down, chew well, and pay attention to hunger and satiety cues.
        (b) Avoid eating in the car or on the run, which may cause people to eat too quickly and to overeat.
    (6) Encourage cognitive behavior therapy techniques: self-monitoring, structured eating patterns, rewards and reinforcements, social support, cognitive restructuring and stress management (see Section 2).
h. Remember that nutritional counseling is complex.
    (1) A team approach and collaboration are important and helpful, due to time constrains, training, and skills.
    (2) Frequent and long-term follow up are paramount.
    (3) A collaborative approach is essential, and a paternalistic approach is not as effective. Health professionals are educators, and it is their responsibility to provide accurate, comprehensive information about the evidence for the need to make therapeutic lifestyle change. However, for change to occur, the patient must be engaged and choose to change.

4. Provide each patient online, digital, and community resources to support their ongoing healthy dietary practices.
5. Offer resources to patients, such as:
    a. Patient-facing materials that are available through American College of Lifestyle Medicine's website and Resources & Tools webpage
    b. Email newsletters
    c. Patient potlucks and meetups
    d. Shared medical appointments[157]

OBJECTIVE 11

Summarize nutrition prescriptions for the most common chronic diseases, including hyperlipidemia, diabetes, hypertension, and cancer

1) Nutrition prescriptions can be written for prevention and treatment.

- **a)** The same prescriptions often help multiple diseases (e.g., diabetes, arthritis, and heart disease).
- **b)** Patients with more advanced disease states typically need more focused and intense nutritional treatments.
- **c)** Appropriate dosing is essential.[158]

2) **Foundation diet for nutrition prescriptions:**

   a) A whole food, plant-predominant diet composed of:
      1. Vegetables (greens, red and yellow, and starchy)
      2. Fruits
      3. Legumes
      4. Whole-grains and pseudo grains
      5. Nuts and seeds

   b) High in fiber, antioxidants

   c) Low in total added fat, saturated fat, added sugar, added salt

3) **Table 5.4 includes some, but not all, of the conditions which have demonstrated a response to more plant-based dietary patterns.**

Table 5.4

Condition	Diet Component
Hyperlipidemia	Decreased meat; more plant foods; replace *trans* and saturated fats with unsaturated fats; increased nuts; and omega-3 fat intake
Hypertension	Increased proportion of plant foods; reduced sodium; limited alcohol consumption
Type 2 Diabetes	Increased high-fiber foods; reduced overall fat and simple/refined carbohydrates
Cancer	Antioxidant rich; high-fiber diet; lower total protein; lower animal protein

   a) Hyperlipidemia is a condition in which there are high levels of blood lipids. Examples of lipids include cholesterol and triglycerides.
      1. Reduce intake of certain fats, including:
         a. *Trans* fats[122]
         b. Saturated fats which are found naturally in dairy (especially full-fat products) and meat (especially high-fat cuts and processed meat).
         c. Because food manufactures were to eliminate *trans* fats by 2018, they're using more saturated fats, such as coconut oil, palm oil, and lard.
         d. Omega-6 fatty acids, which are not as harmful as *trans* or saturated fats, however they should still be limited.
      2. Eat a diet that lowers hyperlipidemia.
         a. Hyperlipidemia is less common in vegans than in non-vegetarians (<5% vs 15%). Vegan diets are traditionally associated with lower fat intake and higher intake of whole foods.[159,160]
         b. Replacing saturated and trans fats with unsaturated fats, especially polyunsaturated fats, and eating high-quality complex carbohydrates can lower risk of heart and vascular disease.[161]
         c. Countries with high intake of processed foods and animal products have higher amounts of hyperlipidemia.[162]
            (1) Hyperlipidemia increases in direct proportion to the amount of meat consumed.[160]
         d. Increase intake of fiber to at least 40–45 grams (1.4–1.6 ounces) per day. Some plant-based diets provide closer to 70 grams (2.5 ounces) per day.
            (1) Foods that are high in fiber include:

(a) Legumes (beans, lentils, garbanzos, etc.)

(b) Vegetables (eggplant, okra, sweet potatoes, etc.)

(c) Fruits (figs, pears, raspberries, etc.)

(d) Whole-grains (barley, rye, wheat, oats, etc.)

e. Increase nut intake to a handful each day (almonds, walnuts, and pecans).

f. Increase omega-3 fatty acid intake (flax seeds, chia seeds, walnuts, fish, etc.).

g. Increase intake of plant sterols and stanols (soybeans, green peas, legumes, nuts and seeds, sprouts, avocado, wheat germ, and Brussels sprouts). Vegetable oils (corn, sesame, canola, and olive oil) also contain plant sterols and stanols, but they are highly processed and are high source of calories, so they should be limited.

h. In the study, "Effects of a Dietary Portfolio of Cholesterol-Lowering Foods Versus Lovastatin on Serum Lipids and C-Reactive Protein," by Jenkins, et al., the researchers surmised that feeding patients a portfolio diet (that is, a group of cholesterol-lowering foods) could be as effective as placing patients on a low-dose, cholesterol-lowering medication called lovastatin.[62]

(1) There were three groups involved in the study (Figure 5.1) the portfolio diet group, the lovastatin group, and the control group.

Figure 5.1 Change From Baseline in LDL-C, LDL-C–HDL-C Ratio

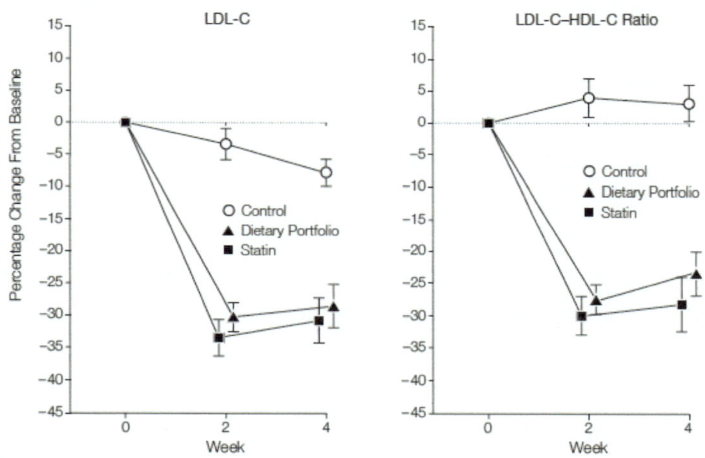

LDL-C indicates low-density lipoprotein cholesterol; HDL-C, high-density lipoprotein cholesterol. Values are expressed as mean (SE) because, with the number of participants involved, approximately twice the SE represents a significant difference.

(a) The portfolio diet intervention group was fed a diet high in cholesterol-lowering foods that contained plant sterols and viscous fibers (oatmeal, soybeans, almonds, eggplant, and okra) and foods that were low in saturated fat.

(b) The medication intervention group was started on lovastatin 20 mg, and they were also fed a low saturated-fat diet.

(c) The control group was advised to eat a low saturated fat diet, but they didn't start medications, and they didn't receive counseling about specific cholesterol-lowering foods.

(2) In 2 weeks, both the portfolio diet group and the 20 mg lovastatin group lowered the percentage of low-density lipoprotein (LDL) cholesterol by 28.6% and 30.9% respectively. Those in the control group lowered LDL cholesterol by only 8.0%.

b) Hypertension

1. Hypertension is uncommon in people who eat plant-based diets.[160]
   a. 7% of vegans have hypertension, but 23% of non-vegetarians have hypertension (risk ratio >3.0).
   b. There is a positive association between intake of animal products and risk of hypertension.
2. To improve hypertension, reduce:
   a. Sodium
      (1) Reduced sodium intake is broadly effective to lower blood pressure and control hypertension in older individuals, with similar reductions seen among African-Americans and the elderly as with the general population.[163]
      (2) The tolerable upper limit for daily intake for adults is 2,300 mg per day.[1,164]
      (3) American Heart Association ideal limit is <1,500 mg per day.[165]
      (4) The largest sources of sodium in the US are:
         (a) Processed foods
            1. Processed foods account for 75% of American dietary sodium intake.
            2. Pizza, breads, rolls, crackers, luncheon meats, cold cuts and processed meats, among others.
         (b) Canned foods, such as soups and vegetables
   b. Saturated fat (cheese, high-fat dairy, processed foods, and animal fats)
   c. Alcohol
      (1) Men should limit intake to ≤2 drinks per day, and women should limit intake to ≤1 drink per day.
      (2) There is a J-curve response between alcohol consumption and high blood pressure.[166,167]
         (a) Those with excessive alcohol intake have much higher blood pressure.
         (b) Those without any alcohol intake have slightly higher blood pressure.
   d. Caffeine, excess weight, tobacco, stress, and physical inactivity
3. Improve hypertension by increasing intake of:
   a. Potassium, which is found in:
      (1) Potatoes and sweet potatoes
      (2) Fruits (cantaloupe, bananas, and peaches)
      (3) Vegetables (squash, broccoli, and spinach)
      (4) Legumes (white beans, lentils, soy, and lima)
   b. Calcium, which is found in:
      (1) Greens (choose low-oxalate greens such as collards, kale, turnip greens, mustard greens, and bok choy). Essentially all greens are good sources of calcium except for beet greens, chard and spinach, because these are high in oxalates, which reduces the absorption of calcium that is present in the greens.
      (2) Beans (white beans, black-eyed peas, etc.)
      (3) Fortified nondairy milks
      (4) Low-fat dairy is recommended in the DASH diet, which has been shown to reduce systolic blood pressure by approximately 11 mmHg over 8 weeks. However, recent studies show dairy has no or only a weak inverse relationship with cardiovascular disease prevention. It appears replacing dairy fat with plant-based or polyunsaturated fat may produce a significantly lower risk of heart disease.[7,168]

c. Magnesium, which is found in:
   (1) Nuts (almonds, cashews, and peanuts)
   (2) Beans (black, soy, and kidney)
   (3) Amaranth, quinoa, avocados, and potatoes
d. Garlic which can lower systolic blood pressure.[169]
   (1) Systolic blood pressure (SBP) of 5.1 ± 2.2 mmHg ($P < 0.001$)
   (2) Diastolic blood pressure (DBP) of 2.5 ± 1.6 mmHg ($P < 0.002$)

4. Water-only fasting has been found to lower blood pressure.[170]
   a. Fasting was done under medical supervision and took place over 18–21 days, including fast and refeeding.
   b. Potential mechanisms may include the substantial down-regulation of diurnal insulin secretion associated with fasting and the accompanying loss of body fat,[171,172] although weight loss was not controlled for in the final analysis of the intervention.[170]

c) Type 2 diabetes

1. Diabetes is less prevalent among people who eat high amounts of fiber and more of a plant-based diet.
   a. The prevalence of diabetes among vegans is less than 2.9%, compared to a prevalence of 7% among people who eat meat.[173,174]
   b. Fiber is associated with a lower risk of diabetes ($r = 0.16$, $P < 0.03$).[175]
2. Diabetes risk is related to intake of dietary fat and processed simple sugars.[158]
   a. Diabetes prevalence and macronutrient intake[175]
      (1) Risk increases with dietary fat intake ($r = 0.84$, $P < 0.001$) and corn syrup ($r = 0.83$, $P < 0.001$)
   b. Diabetes is correlated with fat just as strongly as it is with sugar
3. Dietary changes to help reduce the risk of diabetes
   a. Reduce intake of simple carbohydrates, including:
      (1) Processed sugars
         (a) Common names include sugar, syrup, malt, fruit concentrate, and anything ending with "-ose" (glucose, sucrose, fructose).
         (b) Artificial sweeteners have been associated with dysbiosis and can adversely affect weight control. They are generally best avoided.[176]
         (c) Dysbiosis in the gut microbiota is associated with type 2 diabetes and may be improved with increased dietary fiber.[177]
      (2) Processed grains
         (a) White flour, unbleached white flour, rice flour, and others, and products made from these flours (wheat bread, crackers, and baked goods)
         (b) Puffed (puffed rice or rice cakes) or flaked cereals (cornflakes)
         (c) White rice
         (d) Ground, flaked, and puffed whole-grains
   b. Reduce intake of high glycemic index foods (these have a similar effect to ingesting glucose).
   c. Reduce intake of saturated and *trans* fats.
   d. Reduce total caloric intake, because excess calories will raise serum triglycerides and lead to weight gain.

e. Increase dietary fiber and low glycemic index foods.

4. Aggressive therapeutic lifestyle changes can decrease or reverse type 2 diabetes in most individuals.

   a. Multiple books document plant-based eating and diabetes reversal.

      (1) *Goodbye Diabetes*, by Wes Youngberg

      (2) *Defeating Diabetes*, by Brenda Davis and Tom Barnard

      (3) *The End of Diabetes*, by Joel Fuhrman

      (4) *Dr. Neal Barnard's Program for Reversing Diabetes*, by Neal Barnard

      (5) *The 30-Day Diabetes Miracle*, by Franklin House, Stuart Seale and Ian Blake Newman

d) Cancer

1. Factors that reduce risk for cancer include:

   a. Lifestyle choices that minimize both gene mutation (cancer initiation)[178,179] and development of tumors (cancer progression)[180,181]

   b. A healthy immune system with natural killer cells, which are tumor-fighting immune cells

   c. Low inflammatory processes in the body, for example:

      (1) Lung cancer is related to bronchial inflammation from cigarette smoking.

      (2) Cervical cancer is related to cervical inflammation from the human papilloma virus.

   d. Lower total protein at younger ages[182]

   e. Increased proportion of protein from plant foods instead of animal foods[183]

2. To help lower the risk of cancer through dietary practices, people should aim to support the immune system and decrease inflammation. This can be done by making healthy food choices (whole food plant-based diet) and choosing healthy food preparation methods (avoiding increased advanced glycogen end products from thermal processing).

   a. Reduce pro-inflammatory foods that are associated with an increased risk of breast and colon cancer.

      (1) These include foods with saturated fat, processed sugar, processed meat, red meat and highly processed foods.

   b. Increase antioxidant-rich foods[36]

      (1) Beta-carotene (carrots, sweet potatoes, spinach, kale, etc.)

      (2) Lycopene (tomatoes, watermelon, guava, pink grapefruit, etc.)

      (3) Resveratrol (red grapes, blueberries, peanuts, soy, etc.)

      (4) Selenium (Brazil nuts, sunflower seeds, fish, mushrooms, etc.)

      (5) Vitamin C (cantaloupe, citrus fruits, kiwi, mango, berries, etc.)

      (6) Vitamin E (almonds, peanuts, green leafy veggies, etc.)

      (7) Note: Antioxidant supplements do not seem to help reduce cancer risk, whereas whole foods do.[184]

   c. Increase fiber in diet to at least 30–35 grams (1.1–1.2 ounces) per day.[185,186]

3. Nuances for specific cancers

   a. Breast cancer: Obesity (BMI ≥30) and increased meat intake both increase the risk for developing breast cancer. Eating more soy, fruits, and vegetables decreases the risk.[48,187]

   b. Prostate cancer: Eating more foods high in lycopene and selenium lower the risk of prostate cancer. Whole food soy (but not processed soy) may also provide a protective benefit.[187]

c. Colon cancer: Eating more red meat and processed meats increases the risk of cancer occurrence. A diet high in fiber, calcium, and folate lowers the risk.[187]

d. Gastric cancer: Eating more processed meats increases the risk for developing gastric cancer. Eating more fruits and vegetables decreases the risk.[187]

e. Other cancers: There's no clear evidence yet for nutrition associations with pancreatic, ovarian, endometrial, or other types of cancers.[187]

OBJECTIVE 12

Demonstrate ability to make nutrition prescriptions for health maintenance

1) **Identify patients for whom a dietary lifestyle approach may yield benefits.**
2) **Implement strategies for supporting patients in Objective 10 of this section, "Describe practical strategies for assisting patients to achieve dietary changes."**
3) **Apply motivational interviewing techniques.**
4) **Support patients in self-determination of goals.**
5) **Provide support using SMART goals format.**
6) **When possible, provide follow-up resources to encourage adherence to prescription.**

OBJECTIVE 13

Describe the role of nutrition in preventing and treating chronic diseases, such as cardiovascular disease

1) **Predominantly plant-based diets play a role in reducing risk and treat a variety of conditions.**
2) **Western-style diets, with high consumption of animal foods, refined foods, added sugar, fat, and salt overall increase chronic disease risk.**
3) **Historical development of ideas connecting Western lifestyles with disease:**
   - **a)** In 1972, the *Canadian Journal of Family Medicine* published the article, "The Etiological Significance of Related Diseases," by Dr. Dennis Burkitt. This article highlighted the patterns of emergence of several diseases seen in Western civilizations. The lack of dietary fiber was proposed to be a common cause for these related diseases.[188]
   - **b)** The related diseases discussed in the 1972 paper continue to be common problems in the Western world. Diseases as described in the article:
     1. Ischemic heart disease: most common cause of death
     2. Gallbladder surgery: most common cause for abdominal surgery
     3. Appendicitis: most common cause for emergency abdominal surgery
     4. Diverticular disease: most common disease of the intestine
     5. Cancer of the colon or rectum: second most common cause of cancer death after lung cancer

6. Hemorrhoids: estimated to be present in almost half of people over age 50
7. Varicose veins: affect approximately 20% of the population
8. Hiatus hernia: detectable in nearly one of five upper gastrointestinal tract radiological examinations
9. Obesity: the most common nutritional problem

4) In 1982, Dr. Dennis Burkitt wrote a follow-up landmark article titled, "Western Diseases and Their Emergence Related to Diet."[189]

a) He concluded the most significant public health finding of our time is that diseases of the 21st century are lifestyle related, and, in particular, diet-related and therefore preventable. He proposed dietary changes to prevent and treat these diseases.

5) In 1987, Dr. Trowell and Dr. Burkitt published an article, "The Development of the Concept of Dietary Fiber." This piece described how, during the industrial revolution, fiber was taken out of flour due to the belief that dietary fiber was a gastrointestinal irritant. In place of the starchy and high-fiber foods, people began increasing their intake of animal products, salt, and sugar.[190]

6) Thinking on dietary risk factors for disease and mortality continue to evolve.

a) Poor dietary practices are now recognized as a major cause of non-communicable disease, according to the Global Burden of Disease report in 2017.[55]

b) Poor diet is responsible for more deaths globally than tobacco, high blood pressure, or any other health risk.

c) Dietary habits account for one in every five deaths globally.

d) Figure 5.2 shows the top dietary factors:[55]

Figure 5.2 Dietary Risk Factors

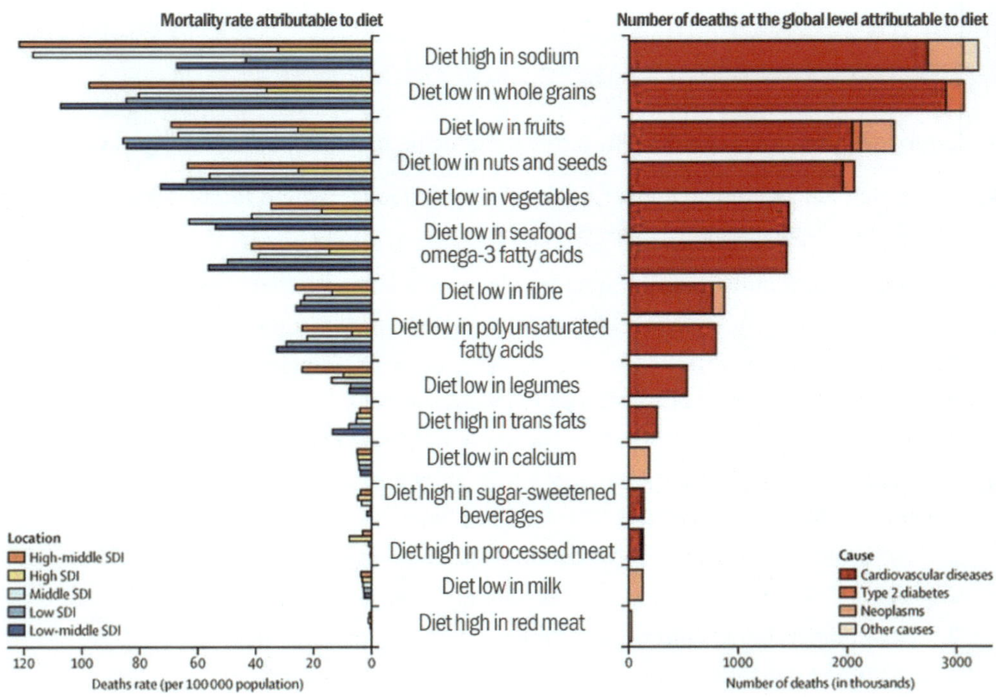

7) **The role of nutrition in cancer**

a) There was a 2-year follow-up for the Prostate Cancer Lifestyle Trial, a clinical trial comparing a lifestyle intervention (low-fat, plant-based diet, exercise, stress management, and group support) to usual care among patients with early-stage prostate cancer who were initially undergoing active surveillance.[191]

1. Results
    a. In the intervention group, only 2 of 43 patients eventually required prostate cancer treatment. Prostate cancer cell growth measured in the serum was suppressed by 70%.
    b. In the control group, 13 of 49 patients underwent prostate cancer treatment. Prostate cancer cell growth in the serum was only suppressed by 9% in the control group.
2. Conclusion: Patients with early-stage prostate cancer who choose active surveillance may be able to delay treatment by making lifestyle changes.

b) A study on the effects of a low-fat, high-fiber diet on breast cancer cell growth followed 12 women who served as both a control and an experimental subject. The women had 2 weeks off and then 2 weeks on the intervention.[192]

1. Breast cancer cell growth after 2 weeks of eating a plant-based diet and walking was significantly reduced, with a concurrent increase in cancer cell apoptosis.
2. Cancer promoting growth hormone IGF-1 (insulin-like growth factor1) dropped. At the same time, levels of IGF-1 binding protein, which removes excess IGF-1 from blood stream, had increased.
3. Both diet and exercise appeared to play a role in inhibiting cancer cell growth.

c) The 2007 prospective study discussed in, "Greater Survival After Breast Cancer in Physically Active Women with High Vegetable-Fruit Intake Regardless of Obesity," followed 1,490 women through diagnosis and treatment of breast cancer.[193]

1. Women who ate five servings of fruits and vegetables per day and who did 180 minutes of moderate intensity exercise each week showed almost a 50% reduction in mortality.
2. Implementing the lifestyle factors above produced almost the same risk reduction for those who were overweight and obese as those who were normal weight.

8) **The role of nutrition in type 2 diabetes**

a) The potential to prevent diabetes is considered one of the greatest recent discoveries in the field of nutrition.[194]

b) Vegetarian diets and incidence of diabetes[195]

1. Among those who ate more plants, there was a step-wise drop in rates of diabetes.
2. Diet Group diabetes prevalence
    a. Non-vegetarian 1.00
    b. Semi-vegetarian 0.72
    c. Pesco-vegetarian 0.49
    d. Lacto-ovo-vegetarian 0.39
    e. Vegan 0.22
3. The same results occurred regarding BMI; the more plants people consumed, the closer their BMI was to a healthy body weight.
4. The incidence of diabetes was significantly lower even after controlling for BMI, indicating vegetarian diets are helpful even beyond controlling weight.

c) Anderson, in a small study of 20 men with type 2 diabetes, tested the theory that a plant-based diet improved diabetes because it was lower in calories, which led to weight loss. Patients in the study were placed on a high-fiber (65 grams/day), plant-based diet with sufficient nutrition so that they did not lose weight. The following was observed:[196,197]

   1. Insulin use was discontinued in 11 patients and reduced in the remaining patients within 16 days.
   2. A high-fiber, plant-based diet helped to reverse diabetes despite no weight loss occurring, implying the types of foods consumed impact blood glucose regulation.

d) In a small retrospective study, 13 patients who had an average HbA1c of 8.2% dropped their HbA1c average to 5.8% after 7 months of eating a high nutrient density diet (meaning a diet high in phytochemicals and antioxidants from greens, fruits, nuts/seeds, and beans/legumes).[198]

   1. Most of their prior diabetes medications had been stopped, and patients on an average of four medications went down to an average of one.

9) A randomized control trial showed a low-fat vegan diet is superior to the American Diabetes Association diet.[199]

10) The role of nutrition in hypertension

a) There is a dose-dependent drop in blood pressure and an improvement in diabetes as diets become more plant-based.[200]

   1. Vegans more so than vegetarians had lower systolic and diastolic blood pressures and less diagnosis of hypertensive. Omnivores had the highest rates of elevated blood pressure and antihypertension medications.

b) Blood pressure can significantly improve within 2 weeks while on a whole food plant-based diet even while hypertensive medications are being tapered down or off.[201]

11) The role of nutrition in cataracts

a) People who eat the most plant-based diets have the lowest risk of cataracts.[202]

12) The role of nutrition in chronic obstructive pulmonary disease

a) Increasing fruit intake by 100 grams was associated with a 24% lower chronic obstructive pulmonary disease mortality.[203]

b) Fruit and vegetable intake led to an improvement of lung function.[204]

13) The role of nutrition in kidney disease

a) There are three dietary risk factors for kidney function decline and resultant albuminuria[205]

   1. Animal protein
   2. Animal fat
   3. Cholesterol

14) Nutrition and immune function[206]

a) Those with higher intake of fruits and vegetables showed an increase in immune response to the pneumonia vaccine without over-stimulating the immune system.

15) Nutrition and Crohn's disease[207]

a) A semi-vegetarian diet produced remission rates of 80% in people with Crohn's.

16) **Nutrition and multiple sclerosis**[208]

a) People who restricted their saturated fat were without progression of disease at 34 years from diagnosis.

17) **The more behavioral change providers ask for, the more changes patients end up making. It's not necessary to prescribe smaller changes that may not create an effect. Dramatic change is often more acceptable to patients than we think.**[209]

a) **Author's Note:** This point is very important to emphasize as lifestyle medicine prescribers—we must prescribe lifestyle medicine treatment at the optimal therapeutic dosing.

18) **A closer look at cardiovascular disease (CVD)**

a) Epidemiology of CVD

1. Leading cause of death for men, women, and people of most racial and ethnic groups in the United States[210]
2. Number one cause of death globally, taking an estimated 17.9 million lives each year[211]
3. Death rates higher in upper-income countries but rates in affluent countries now peaking and rates in lower-income countries are increasing[212]
4. Established risk factors include diet, obesity, smoking, high blood pressure, hypercholesterolemia, family histories of CVD, chronic kidney disease, and type 2 diabetes[213,214]
5. Costs the US $219 billion each year (2014), which includes health care services, medication, and lost productivity due to death[215]
6. Dietary risk factors are:[162,216,217,218,219]
    a. Saturated fat
    b. Animal foods
    c. Dietary cholesterol
7. Whole food plant-based diets show promising results for treatment, and achieving reversal of atherosclerosis.[66,72,216,220]
8. Mechanisms
    a. Plant-based diets contribute to improvements in artery function, blood flow, angina, and ultimately the reversal of CVD by allowing plaque to dissolve, which opens up arteries.
    b. Plant-based diets reduce inflammation.[58] Macronutrient ratios of the plant-based foods may result in lower blood cholesterol[221] and reduced inflammation due to increased antioxidants.
    c. Antioxidants reduce reactive nitrogen species, which are identified in the pathophysiology of atherosclerosis and consequential CVD development.[222]
    d. Examples of promising research: The following studies contain results with encouraging outcomes for lifestyle medicine treatment in the scope of research on serum-cholesterol, diet, and coronary artery disease (CAD).[223]
        (1) In Uganda, coronary heart disease is almost non-existent.
            (a) Diet is comprised of vegetables and whole-grains, and protein is mainly derived from plants.
            (b) Average total cholesterol at age 40 was 145 mg/dL (3.75 mmol/L). This is similar to the levels seen among vegans, who average approximately 141 mg/dL (3.64 mmol/L).[224]

(2) Dr. Caldwell Esselstyn Jr., a leading researcher in lifestyle medicine, described how cardiac disease is an illness acquired from food in his article, "Is the Present Therapy for Coronary Artery Disease the Radical Mastectomy of the Twenty-First Century?"[213]
(3) In Western civilizations where diets are high in fat, CVD is common.
(4) In cultures where diets are plant-based and low in fat, CAD is almost non-existent including:
    (a) The Tarahumara Indians of northern Mexico, who have a diet of beans and corn[225]
    (b) The Papua highlanders of New Guinea, who have a diet of sweet potatoes[226]
    (c) The inhabitants of rural China, who have a diet of rice and vegetables[162]
    (d) The inhabitants of rural Africa, who have a diet of green plantains, sweet potatoes, pumpkins, tomatoes, and green leafy vegetables[223]
(5) An article written by T. Colin Campbell called "Diet, Lifestyle and Etiology of Coronary Artery Disease," described the differences between the diet among those living in rural China and those in the United States and the differences in the incidence of CVD.[162]
    (a) The diet in rural China compared to the diet in the United States had about half the fat, one-tenth of the meat intake, and three times the fiber intake.
    (b) Mean total cholesterol was 127 mg/dL (3.28 mmol/L) in rural China versus 203 mg/dL (5.25mmol/L) in the US.
    (c) There's a 16.7-fold greater CAD mortality in US men and a 5.6-fold greater CAD mortality in US women compared to their Chinese counterparts.
    (d) There were no recorded coronary heart disease events in a 3-year period among 246,000 males ≤64 years of age from five counties and 130 villages in rural mainland China.
(6) CAD affects less than 1% of people in South African Bantu.[227]
    (a) One study looked at 1,328 consecutive autopsies over a period of 5 years. Among those, there were only seven cases of coronary thrombosis (a blood clot in a heart vessel that restricts blood flow to the heart) or myocardial infarction.
(7) Another study compared the incidence of myocardial infarction in 632 Ugandans and Americans by age and gender matched autopsies.
    (a) Among black Ugandans, there was one myocardial infarction (0.2%).
    (b) Among Caucasian Americans, there were 136 myocardial infarctions (22%).
    (c) The study above was expanded in Uganda, East Africa. There was only one healed myocardial infarction among 1,427 Ugandan patients who were older than 40.
    (d) All autopsies were performed at missionary hospitals with US trained surgeons.

e. Heart disease facts and principles, learned from the 2013 Baylor University Conference[228]
    (1) The main risk factor for heart disease is cholesterol.

(2) According to Dr. W.C. Roberts, Baylor Cardiovascular Institute, "If the serum total cholesterol is 90–140 mg/dL (2.327–3.620 mmol/L), there is no evidence that cigarette smoking, systemic hypertension, diabetes mellitus, inactivity, or obesity produces atherosclerotic plaques. Hypercholesterolemia is the only direct atherosclerotic risk factor; the others are indirect."

(3) America's "normal" cholesterol level may be too high to be protective.

(a) 75% of heart attack patients had LDL cholesterols that fell into recommended target range.[229]

(4) What is the optimal LDL?

(a) Optimal LDL is 50–70 mg/dL (1.293–1.810 mmol/L).[230]

(b) Lower is better, and physiologically normal LDL is 50–70 mg/dL (1.293–1.810 mmol/L).

1. This is the threshold for development of atherosclerotic disease.

(c) Healthy neonates and wild primates have LDLs between 40–80 mg/dL (1.034–2.069 mmol/L).

1. Only adult humans have a mean LDL over 80 (2.069 mmol/L) and total cholesterol over 160 mg/dL (4.138 mmol/L).

(5) Regression suggests atherosclerosis does not progress when LDL is ≤70 mg/dL (1.810 mmol/L).

(a) Reaching the ideal LDL levels of 50–70mg/dL (1.293–1.810 mmol/L)

(b) In the article, "Introduction: More Than Coronary Artery Disease," Dr. Caldwell Esselstyn Jr., discussed how past cholesterol guidelines were not as strict as they needed to be simply because advocating for an LDL level between 50–70 (1.293–1.810 mmol/L) might frustrate the general public and they may, in turn, make no change.[220]

f. The 2017 American Heart Association and American College of Cardiology guidelines on lifestyle management to reduce cardiovascular disease recommend a dietary pattern that achieves no more that 5–6% of calories from saturated fat. This is difficult to achieve on a non-vegetarian diet. A whole food plant-based diet is much more likely to produce the goal of 50–70mg/mL (1.293–1.810mmol/L) of LDL cholesterol.[231]

g. Any intake of *trans* fat, saturated fat, or cholesterol above 0% energy may increase LDL cholesterol.[232]

h. A prospective study of intake of *trans*-fatty acids found that it appears *trans* fats are associated with increased cardiovascular risk, whether the *trans* fats occur naturally or are processed.[71]

i. Preventing and arresting coronary atherosclerosis[233]

j. Plaque progression ceases when total serum cholesterol is less than 150 mg/dL (3.879mmol/L).

k. Although the average cholesterol of a vegetarian is less than 150 mg/dL (3.879 mmol/L), lipid-lowering medications are often used to get cholesterol levels to this level or below since many people will not adhere to a vegetarian lifestyle.

l. Average serum LDL cholesterol[224]

1) Omnivores: 123.43 ± 42.67 mg/dL (3.192 ± 1.103 mmol/L)

2) Lacto-ovo-vegetarians: 101.47 ± 28.07 mg/dL (2.624 ± 0.726 mmol/L)

3) Lacto-vegetarians: 87.71 ± 41.67 mg/dL (2.268 ± 1.077 mmol/L)

4) Vegans: 69.28 ± 29.53 mg/dL (1.792 ± 0.764 mmol/L)

m. Effects of plant-based diets on plasma lipids[234]

(1) A decrease in HDL may occur as people transition to a plant-based diet, but the ratio of the drop of LDL compared to that of HDL still provides a benefit.

n. The pathophysiology of CAD[235]

o. The best way to manage CAD is to lower LDL cholesterol and triglycerides. This can be achieved through:

(1) A vegetarian diet, which works best, has an excellent side effect profile, and through which patients report feeling better.

(2) Diet and drug therapy, which may or may not have drug-related side effects.

p. A study on the effects of a very-high-fiber diet with vegetable, fruit, and nut consumption on serum lipids and colonic function showed:[132]

(1) The very-high-fiber vegetable, fruit, and nut diet resulted in a reduction of cholesterol that was equivalent to a therapeutic dose of a statin medication.

(2) The above results were achieved in 2 weeks.

(3) The greater the dietary changes, the greater the cholesterol reduction.

(4) The high-fiber diet out-performed both low-fat and starch-based diets.

q. Findings from the Lifestyle Heart Trial, by Dr. Dean Ornish showed a 10% fat, whole food vegetarian diet along with aerobic exercise, stress management training, smoking cessation, and group psychosocial support produce regression of plaque stenosis and a reduction in cholesterol.[67]

(1) The 5-year follow-up study, "Intensive Lifestyle Changes for Reversal of Coronary Heart Disease,"[67] showed continued regression of plaque stenosis in the intervention group. At 1 year, the average percent diameter stenosis at baseline had decreased 1.75%, and at 5 years it had decreased by 3.1%. The control group worsened. At 1 year, the control group's average percent diameter stenosis at baseline had increased by 2.3%, and at 5 years it had increased by 11.8%.

r. "The Effects of Stress Management Training and Dietary Changes in Treating Ischemic Heart Disease," a randomized control trial of 24 intervention and 24 control patients, resulted in:[236]

(1) A 91% reduction in frequency of angina (pain or discomfort in the chest, caused by insufficient blood flow to the heart) episodes and a 44% mean increase in exercise duration in intervention patients compared to controls in 24 days.

s. The "Angina Pectoris and Atherosclerotic Risk Factors in the Multisite Cardiac Lifestyle Intervention Program" was a large multi-site study of 757 men and 395 women with mild to limiting angina. The study assessed how changing to a 10% fat plant-based diet, achieving moderate exercise 3 hours a week, and practicing stress management 1 hour per day affected angina symptoms (which are a frequent medical indication to undergo a revascularization procedure).[216]

(1) The intervention group experienced significant improvements in angina in 12 weeks:

(a) 74% were angina free.

(b) 9% changed from the "limiting" angina to the "mild" angina category.

(c) The observed decreases were similar to those reported in the studies of coronary artery bypass graft or percutaneous coronary intervention, meaning that making intensive lifestyle changes could reduce the need for revascularization procedures.

t. "Updating a 12-year Experience With Arrest and Reversal Therapy for Coronary Heart Disease (an Overdue Requiem for Palliative Cardiology)" is an article about the effect of dietary changes on severe CVD. The article was based on the experiences of an original cohort of 24 patients with severe cardiovascular disease, and it was written by Dr. Caldwell Esselstyn, Jr.[237]

(1) The intervention was to eat a whole food plant-based diet, eliminate oil, eliminate meat products and dairy (except skim milk and nonfat yogurt) and increase fruits, vegetables, whole-grains, beans, and legumes.

(2) After 12 years, adherent patients experienced no extension of clinical disease, no coronary events, and no cardiac interventions.

(3) Prior to the dietary intervention, the 18 compliant patients had experienced 49 coronary events in the preceding 8 years. Of the six patients who were not compliant and were released in the first 12–18 months of the study, there were 13 new cardiac events.

(4) Note: Dr. Esselstyn refers to the current treatment of CAD as "palliative cardiology" because current cardiovascular treatments and interventions may help alleviate symptoms without addressing the disease itself, whereas lifestyle interventions actually treat and reverse the cause of the disease.[220]

u. More recent results from Dr. Esselstyn's patients[72]

(1) The intervention: eat a whole food plant-based diet, eliminate oil, eliminate meat products, and increase fruits, vegetables, whole-grains, beans, and legumes (no dairy)

(2) 2014 case series of 198 consecutive patients found a recurrence rate of 0.6% for major cardiac events among adherent patients (n = 177) and 62% among nonadherent participants

v. Despite the powerful and consistent results, widespread implementation of nutrition with a whole food plant-based diet for CVD has not yet occurred. One driving factor for this may be the lack of reimbursement for lifestyle treatments. However, in 2010, Centers for Medicare and Medicaid did approve the Ornish and Pritikin programs for reimbursement.[238]

OBJECTIVE 14

List at least five examples of nutrition interventions for diseases

1) Omnivorous diets well-studied in research

a) Mediterranean diet

1. Typically defined as a diet including some variation of the following components:[1,239]

   a. High monounsaturated-to-saturated fat ratio (often using olive oil as main cooking oil)

   b. High fruit and vegetable intake

   c. High consumption of legumes

d. High grain and cereal intake
e. Moderate red wine consumption
f. Moderate consumption of dairy products
g. Low consumption of meat and meat products with increased intake of fish

2. May contribute to cardiovascular health, including improvements in blood pressure, serum triglycerides, and cholesterol.[240]
3. There is limited evidence to support reduced incidence of cardiovascular events, breast cancer, and type 2 diabetes when this diet is practiced with no restriction on fat intake.[239]

b) Vegetarian diet

1. Mainly a plant-based diet where animal flesh foods are avoided and the following foods are included:[1,241]
   a. Beans, peas, and lentils
      (1) Includes soy products, especially tofu and other processed soy products
   b. Nuts and seeds
   c. Grains and grain products
   d. Fruits and fruit juices
   e. Vegetables and vegetable juices
   f. May include some dairy, eggs, and fish/seafood
2. Variations of this diet include the following:
   a. Semivegetarian (flexitarian) diet: minimizes but does not completely eliminate animal flesh foods
   b. Pesco-vegetarian (pescatarian) diet—includes some fish/seafood but no other animal flesh foods (i.e., no meat or poultry)
   c. Lacto-ovo-vegetarian diet: includes some eggs and dairy but no animal flesh foods (i.e., no meat, poultry, or fish)
   d. Strict vegetarian (vegan) diet: restricts all animal flesh foods (i.e., no meat, poultry or fish) and foods produced by animals (i.e. no eggs or dairy) or insects (i.e., honey)
3. Lacto-ovo-vegetarian and vegan diets are associated with favorable cardiometabolic risk factor profiles (lower values for BMI total and LDL cholesterol, triglycerides, and blood glucose).[241]
4. These dietary patterns are also associated with lower risk of chronic diseases such as obesity, type 2 diabetes, ischemic heart disease, and cancer.[241]

c) Dietary Approaches to Stop Hypertension (DASH) diet

1. This diet is focused on foods that meet these criteria:[242]
   a. Low in saturated and *trans* fats
   b. Rich in potassium, calcium, magnesium, fiber, and protein
   c. Lower in sodium (1,500–2,300 mg/day sodium)
2. Recommendations include the following:[242]
   a. Eat vegetables, fruits, and whole-grains.
   b. Include fat-free or low-fat dairy products, fish, poultry, beans, nuts, and vegetable oils
   c. Limit foods high in saturated fat (i.e., fatty meats, full-fat dairy products, and tropical oils, such as coconut, palm kernel, and palm oils).
   d. Limit sugar-sweetened beverages and sweets.

3. Associated with lower incidence of cardiovascular disease[243] and related health outcomes (i.e., coronary heart disease, stroke, and heart failure)[244] and improvements in blood pressure[243,245]
4. May help with weight management and, for people with overweight and obesity, weight reduction[246]

2) Intervention diets more commonly utilized in lifestyle medicine

a) Whole food plant-based diet[60]

1. Defined as a diet comprised of plant-based foods (i.e., no meat, poultry, fish, eggs, dairy, or honey) that are minimally processed (e.g., no refined oils).
    a. Whole-grains (preferably intact) or minimally processed grains and grain products
    b. Beans, legumes, and whole soy or minimally processed soy and soy products
    c. Vegetables
    d. Fruits (typically may limit high-fat fruits like avocado, coconut, palm fruit, and olives)
    e. Nuts and seeds (typically encouraged in limited quantities)
2. Low-fat whole food plant-based diets are associated with favorable health outcomes, including weight loss or maintenance, improved BMI, reduced total cholesterol, lower risk of cardiovascular events (and improved cardiovascular risk factors[247]), and fewer medications.[248]
3. Associated with favorable quality of life outcomes (i.e., general self-efficacy, nutritional self-efficacy, self-esteem, average daily exercise, food enjoyment, and food costs).[248]
4. Some examples of specific programs:
    a. Ornish Program for Reversing Heart Disease[238,249]
        (1) Also known as the Multisite Cardiac Lifestyle Intervention Program, Multicenter Cardiac Lifestyle Intervention Program, and the Lifestyle Heart Trial program
        (2) Based on comprehensive lifestyle modifications, including:
            (a) Exercise
            (b) A low-fat diet
            (c) Smoking cessation
            (d) Stress-management training
            (e) Group support sessions
    b. Pritikin Program[238,250]
        (1) Also known as the Pritikin Longevity Program
            (a) Provided in physician's office and incorporates the following:
                1. Specific diet (10–15% of calories from fat, 15–20% from protein, and 65–75% from complex carbohydrates)
                2. Exercise
                3. Counseling lasting 21–26 days
                4. Option for residential component
    c. Dr. Esselstyn's Prevent & Reverse Heart Disease Program[251,252]
        (1) A low-fat, whole food plant-based diet with the following criteria:
            (a) Avoid all animal products
            (b) Avoid all oils
            (c) Reduce or avoid soybeans, nuts, and avocados

d. Complete Health Improvement Program (CHIP)[253]
   (1) Intensive lifestyle intervention program focused on the following six pillars:
      (a) Activity
      (b) Nutrition: A whole plant food diet focused on "food as grown"
         1. Increase consumption of:
            a. Whole-grains
            b. Legumes
            c. Fruits
            d. Vegetables
            e. Water
            f. Wholesome breakfasts
         2. Decrease consumption of:
            a. Fats and oils
            b. Sugars
            c. Foods containing cholesterol
            d. Salt
            e. Alcohol and caffeine
      (c) Sleep
      (d) Risky substances
      (e) Social connection
      (f) Stress management

OBJECTIVE 15

Describe the role of epigenetics

1) Key take-home message for patients: Your genes are not your destiny, but your lifestyle is your destiny. The changes you make today will change your lifestyle, and ultimately change your future.

2) Epigenetics (Figure 5.3)[254]

   a) Epi: near, upon, at

   b) Genetics: hereditary material

   c) Epigenetics is the study of the non-DNA sequence components of genetic inheritance

      1. These non-DNA sequence components act like gene-switches that modify and control gene expression through:
         a. DNA-methylation
         b. Micro-RNA
         c. Histone acetylation
         d. Growing number of other molecular changes

Figure 5.3 Epigenetics

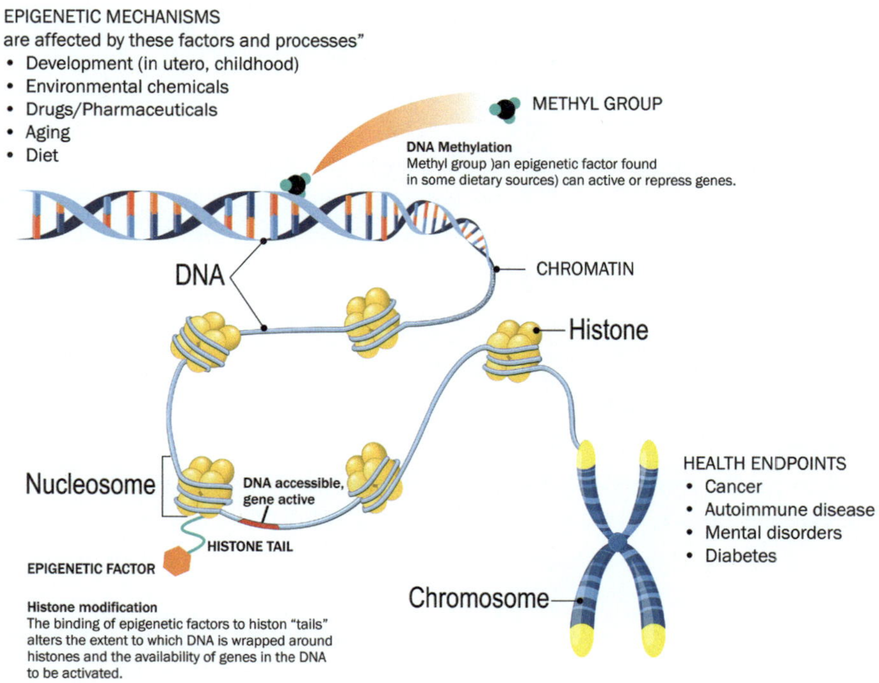

3) **Epigenetic sequences are passed on from parents to child as "set switches."**

   a) Dutch Hunger Winter was a famine that occurred during the winter of 1944–1945.[255]

      1. Scientists have since studied the unfortunate consequences of an extreme dietary change (<1,000 calories per day) during pregnancy.

         a. Children born to mothers who were pregnant during the famine had increased rates of obesity, diabetes, schizophrenia, fingerprint alterations, and decreased fertility.

         b. Continued studies have revealed that the subsequent three generations have all been affected.

   b) Agouti mice research[256]

      1. Genetic expression of obesity, heart disease, and diabetes could be turned on and off by lifestyle changes in genetically identical mice.

   c) Maternal diet influences the methylation status of a promoter region (RXRA) that is strongly correlated with adiposity and metabolic syndromes in her children.[257,258]

      1. If mothers are eating a diet low in plants, they are lacking in methylation capability.

         a. Methyl groups come through plant foods and B vitamins.

4) **Although epigenetic sequences are inherited with certain predispositions, unlike the genes themselves, those sequences can and are changed and modified by numerous environmental and genetic factors. Lifestyle—and especially diet—have a major influence.**

   a) Ornish and colleagues in a study on prostate cancer, found that intensive nutrition and lifestyle changes altered the expression of more than 500 genes, down-regulated 453 genes and up-regulated 48 genes. Each of these genes had critical roles in tumorigenesis of prostate cancer.[68]

b) Key epigenetic aspects of diet and exercise
   1. Variants, such as minor alleles like PGC-1α, are associated with an increase susceptibility to forming type 2 diabetes among individuals who are Chinese, Japanese, Korean, Italian, and some European, such as those who are Danish. [257,259,260]
   2. Exercise-induced expression of GLUT4 in skeletal muscle regulates glucose uptake. With increased exercise and GLUT4 activity, glycemic control can be improved. However, studies show glycemic control for even 3–5 years may not reduce the risk of macrovascular complications. That is likely because of the epigenetic effect caused by the proinflammatory state of hyperglycemia, which may take longer than 5 years to correct.[260,261]

c) Sleep deprivation is found to alter expression of >700 genes in adults.[262]

d) Dietary and environmental factors can predispose to worsen diabetes.[257]

e) If altered DNA-methylation or histone micro-RNA changes occur, gene expression can be changed, leading to altered insulin sensitivity. Altered insulin sensitivity is an example of subclinical phenotype changes.[263]

f) When insulin sensitivity is altered, the risk of acquiring type 2 diabetes is increased. When type 2 diabetes occurs, this is an example of clinical phenotype changes.

g) Type 2 diabetes is associated with altered DNA methylation and further changes in histone micro-RNA.

h) Hyperglycemia induces epigenetic changes by increasing production of inflammatory proteins by acting on the NF-kß p65 promoter unit. Inflammatory proteins can lead to endothelial cell damage of the blood vessels which can result in vascular injury and disease.

i) When glycemic control was improved for 3–5 years with medication, it did not reduce macrovascular complications due to epigenetic changes. Genome-wide studies have shown that cell-type specific changes in histone methylation patterns under diabetic conditions persist for 5 years. This likely helps explain how macrovascular complications are not improved with glycemic control.[260,264]

OBJECTIVE 16

List at least three key epigenetic influencers

1) **Key influencers of epigenetic expression during pregnancy/early childhood[265]**
   a) Maternal nutrition during pregnancy
   b) Presence or absence of breastfeeding
   c) Early child nutrition
   d) Gut microbiota
   e) Chemical food contaminants

2) **Key lifestyle influencers[266]**
   a) Diet
   b) Physical activity
   c) Smoking and alcohol consumption
   d) Sleep habits
   e) Chronic stress

f) Conditions such as obesity, infections, and exposure to environmental chemical contaminants

3) **Examples of epigenetic influence**[267,268,269]

a) Diet: Among rat fetus models, high-fat diets alter gene expression in the developing rat fetuses and result in anatomic changes in their brains.[270]

b) Exercise: Physical activity alters gene expression of the GLUT4 receptor and improves glucose uptake.[271]

c) Sleep: Sleep deprivation alters gene expression.[272]

d) Obesity: Obesity alters gene expression.[273]

OBJECTIVE 17

Cite the prevalence of diabetes and prediabetes and the associated cost burden

1) **The prevalence of diabetes in the US, based on 2017 data published in 2020**[274]

a) 34.2 million people have diabetes.
   1. 26.9 millionpeople are diagnosed, 7.3 million are undiagnosed.[274]
   2. 5.2% (1.4 million) people have type 1 diabetes.[275]
   3. The prevalence of prediabetes in the US based on 2018 data, published in 2020[275]
      a. 88 million adults have prediabetes in the US (approximately 34.5% of the adult US population).
      b. 46.6% of adults 65 years of age or older have prediabetes.

b) The prevalence of diabetes in adults over 18 years of age by race/ethnicity is below. Note the overall prevalence of diabetes is 10.5% of the US population.[275]
   1. 14.7% of American Indian/Alaska Native
   2. 11.4% of black, non-Hispanic
   3. 12.5% of Hispanic
   4. 10.0% of Asian, non-Hispanic
   5. 7.5% of white

c) It's estimated that 60.6 million people will have diabetes in 2060 (approximately two in five of the US population).[276,277]

d) Prevalence will increase in all race-sex groups, with black women and men continuing to have the highest diabetes percent prevalence.[277]

2) **Diabetes in the worldwide population**[278]

a) Global prevalence in 2019 was 9.3% (463 million).

b) One in two people living with diabetes do not know they have it (50.1%).

c) Global prevalence of impaired glucose tolerance in 2019 was 7.5% (373.9 million).

d) Projected increases globally are 9.2% by 2030 and 9.6% by 2045.

3) **Diabetes cost estimates from 2017 in the US**[279]

a) $327 billion is spent annually on direct and indirect costs. This is a 26% increase from 2012 estimates of $245 billion.

1. $237 billion in direct medical costs
2. $90 billion in indirect costs from absenteeism, reduced productivity, disability, and premature death

b) Medical costs are 2.3 times higher for those with diabetes compared to those without diabetes.[279]

1. People with diagnosed diabetes incur average medical expenditures of $16,750 per year, of which $9,600 is attributed to diabetes.

OBJECTIVE 18

Describe consequences of intensive medication management

1) Conventional progression relies on medication management.

a) Current "disease management" approach for patients with type 2 diabetes is primarily aimed at delaying progression of the disease[280] (not remission)[158]

b) Causes for concern in increasing medication include the development of end-stage organ damage, such as retinopathy, nephropathy, end-stage renal disease, nonalcoholic fatty liver disease, and CVD[280,281]

2) An intensive medication intervention trial, called the ACCORD (Action to Control Cardiovascular Risk in Diabetes) study was completed in 2008. The study aimed to aggressively lower blood glucose into tightly controlled levels with medications to help lower CVD risk.[282]

a) Results: Intensively reducing blood glucose below guidelines with medications produced harm in high-risk patients with type 2 diabetics.

3) Increased insulin dosing is associated with increased risk of cancer, CVD and weight gain.[283]

OBJECTIVE 19

Describe the pathogenesis of diabetes

1) Pathogenesis of type 2 diabetes[284]

a) Eating excess calories leads to an increase in adipose tissue, fatty infiltrate in muscle and liver cells, and leptin production. All of this leads to weight gain and an increase in inflammatory mediators. The Western diet and other factors, such as antibiotics, disrupt the microbiome. This disruption promotes dysbiosis and decreases the production of short-chain fatty acids, such as butyrate, that assist in blood glucose management.[130]

b) Fatty deposits in the liver lead to increased blood glucose levels due to the failure of the liver to suppress gluconeogenesis (production of glucose, which generally occurs only in fasting states) and increase triacylglycerols. (Triacylglycerols are fatty acids that are stored in muscle cells and adipocytes).

c) Insulin resistance begins to occur as inflammatory mediators cause damage to liver and beta cells and as muscle and adipocyte cells begin resisting further fat storage. Intramyocellular fat accumulation disrupts insulin receptors via production of lipotoxic mediators, which increases insulin resistance.

- **d)** To overcome insulin resistance, the pancreas begins increasing the amount of insulin produced and excreted into the blood stream. Therefore, a rise in insulin is often seen before a rise in blood glucose levels.
- **e)** Insulin increases appetite, leading to further excess calorie consumption, which repeats the process above (points a through d) and further increases fatty deposits in liver.
- **f)** The beta cells in the pancreas that produce insulin are damaged by fatty acids (triacylglycerols). This damage suppresses insulin secretion that is in response to glucose in the blood stream. Eventually, the beta cells are unable to produce sufficient insulin to push glucose into cells, and blood glucose begins to rise.
- **g)** When blood glucose is elevated above normal, this can be captured on fasting lab work, a hemoglobin A1c, or with an oral glucose tolerance test. Based on well-defined criteria, the diagnosis of prediabetes, diabetes types 1 or 2, or gestational diabetes can be made.
- **h)** When the pancreas stops producing insulin due to an autoimmune cause (type 1 diabetes) or due to damage from inflammation and overuse (type 2 diabetes), a patient becomes insulin dependent.

2) Time sequence of pathogenesis of type 2 diabetes[285]

- **a)** Muscle insulin resistance determines the rate of fatty liver progression.
- **b)** Fatty liver progression and the deposit of fatty acids in the pancreas are responsible for the rate of hepatic insulin resistance (failure to appropriately respond to blood glucose levels) and beta cell dysfunction.

3) Whether insulin resistance occurs is dependent upon epigenetic, dietary, and lifestyle factors.[286]

4) Insulin resistance cascade[261,287]

- **a)** Adipocytes (fat cells) are key factors in the development of insulin resistance.
    1. As weight gain occurs, adipocytes undergo hyperplasia and hypertrophy (that is, they grow in number and in size) and begin accumulating in ectopic tissues, such as the liver and muscle cells.
        - a. Intracellular lipid accumulation in ectopic tissues leads to impaired insulin signaling within the cells.
        - b. Adipocyte growth increases inflammation and lipolysis (fat break down), which leads to increased production of inflammatory mediators and macrophage recruitment.
            - (1) Inflammatory mediators and cytokines include TNF-alpha, MCP-1, IL-6, c-reactive protein, PAI-1 and increased plasma FFA.
            - (2) An increase in inflammation and FFA leads to a decrease in adiponectin.
                - (a) Adiponectin is protective. It clears triglycerides, reduces TNF-alpha, and protects endothelium. It's important for hippocampal growth and for decreasing depression.
                - (b) When TNF-alpha is increased, it leads to further inflammation.
            - (3) Lipolysis and lipotoxicity
                - (a) Lead to production of DAG = diacylglycerol, TAG = triacylglycerol; associated with insulin resistance (see cited articles for more details)
                - (b) Lead to Ceramide (CER) and Sphingosine (Sph); also associated with increased insulin resistance
        - c. Adipocytes produce:
            - (1) Leptin, a hormone and marker related to obesity and inflammation.

(a) A resistance to excess leptin can occur in the body. When it does, leptin resistance results in the inability to detect satiety signals, which further drives the sensation of hunger and a person to consume even more calories.[288]

(b) Leptin is proangiogenic, meaning it triggers new blood vessel growth (angiogenesis) to adipocytes. Increased angiogenesis can heighten the risk of cancer cell growth, provide more opportunities for metastasis, and increase cytokine production, leading to further inflammation.

(2) Epithelium-derived factor desensitizes cell further to insulin.

(3) Retinol-binding protein prevents activation of glucose carrying proteins.

2. If activated, the inflammatory cascades can cause endothelial cell damage via physical stress and oxidative damage.

a. NF-kß pathway

(1) The NF-kß pathway is initiated through inflammation and free radicals, which can come from radiation, food, and toxins.

(a) When NF-kß is produced and activated inside the cell, it can impact 400 genes, causing worsening inflammation.

(b) NF-kß can activate telomerase, cytokines, adhesion molecules, VEGF, and TNF.

(c) It's associated with atherosclerosis, cancer, diabetes, asthma, allergies, aging, colitis, gastrointestinal diseases, autoimmune diseases, Alzheimer's disease, and arthritis.[289]

(2) Diet modifies and regulates NF-kß through phytonutrients and antioxidants.

(a) Down-regulates NF-kß production and gene modulation that occurs from NF-kß

(b) NOTE: The ability to down-regulate has not yet been successfully achieved with pharmaceuticals.

3. Macrophages are part of the immune system and can be recruited when inflammatory pathways are activated.

a. Inflammatory pathways that lead to macrophage recruitment include:

(1) Cytokine pathway activation (IL-6, IL-1Beta, and TNF-alpha)

(2) NF-kß and JNK inflammatory cytokine pathways

b. Macrophages, if recruited near beta cells, can lead to beta cell death.

b) Of note: Heme iron and diets high in red and processed meat are associated with an increased risk of type 2 diabetes and insulin resistance.[290,291]

c) Heme iron stores are pro-oxidants.[292]

1. A reduction in heme iron could reduce insulin resistance by reducing inflammation.

5) Beta cells in the pancreas are responsible for producing insulin.

a) Over time, with exposure to poor diet and lifestyle factors, beta cells experience progressive injury. If injury is severe enough, beta cells can cease to function or die, causing insulin deficiency and hyperglycemia.

b) Beta cell healing and regeneration may be possible. However, it takes time to repair the injury (like paying off a credit card debt), and sometimes drastic change is required to halt or reverse the disease.

6) Beta cell death can occur due to multiple genetic, environmental, and lifestyle factors.

a) Dyslipidemia: very low-density lipoprotein and low-density lipoprotein are pro-apoptotic and can lead to beta cell death.[293,294]

1. Dyslipidemia risk is increased with obesity and a high-fat diet, especially *trans* fat and saturated fat.

b) Glucotoxicity triggering IL-1Beta leading to beta cell apoptosis

c) Cytokines (NF-kß and JNK pathways)

d) Leptin can stimulate cytokine pathways, inducing apoptosis.[295]

e) Oxidative stress can cause endothelial cell injury from hyperglycemia and free fatty acids via NF-kß and JNK pathways.

OBJECTIVE 20

Describe the role of nutrition in preventing, treating, and reversing type 2 diabetes

1) Lifestyle is the primary cause and the cure of type 2 diabetes.[158]

a) The increase in type 2 diabetes in the last half century is directly related to changes in lifestyle.[296]

b) Lifestyle-related risk factors include:[296]

1. Overweight or obese[297]
2. High blood pressure
3. Low level of high-density lipoprotein or "good" cholesterol, or a high level of triglycerides[293,294]
4. Not physically active[298,299]

c) Dietary risk factors include consumption of:[296]

1. Higher total fat
2. Higher cholesterol
3. Red meat[291]
4. Added sugars
5. Overnutrition/overconsumption of total energy

d) Type 2 diabetes is preventable with lifestyle.[297,298,299,300]

e) Type 2 diabetes improvements occur with structured intervention programs that produce significant weight loss.[300,301]

f) Targeted lifestyle interventions are found to be clinically effective and cost effective for diabetes prevention and treatment.[73,302]

2) The United States Department of Agriculture Economic Research Service in 2009, plus research from the *American Journal of Clinical Nutrition* looked at current US food consumption as a percentage of calories:[303,304]

a) 63% of American diet is processed food.

1. Added fats, oils, sugars, and refined grains

b) 25% is from animal foods.

1. Meat, dairy, eggs, fish, and seafood

c) 12% is from plant foods.

1. 6% processed plant foods (almonds in candy, apples in apple pie, etc.)
2. 6% unprocessed vegetables, fruits, legumes, whole-grains, and nuts and seeds

3) **The US diet has changed from 100 years ago to the present.**[305,306]

   a) Per person, per year

      1. Sugar intake (Figure 5.4) has increased from <10 lbs to >140 lbs (<4.5 kg to >63.5 kg)

Figure 5.4 Sugar Intake and Obesity Prevalence

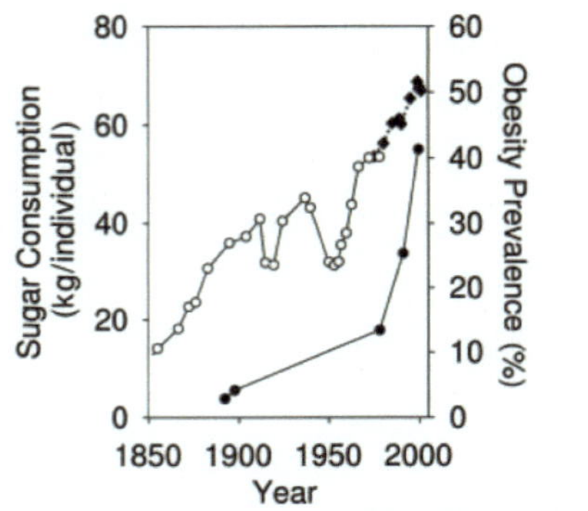

Sugar intake per capita in the United Kingdom (○) and in the United States (◆) compared with obesity rates in the United States in non-Hispanic white men aged 60–69 y (●).

      2. Oil intake has increased from 4 lbs to 70 lbs (1.8 kg to 41.7 g).
      3. Cheese has increased by 25 lbs (11.3 kg).
      4. Television has increased from 0–4 hours per day.

4) **Definitions (Table 5.5):**

   a) American College of Lifestyle Medicine defines "reversal" of type 2 diabetes as the normalization of blood glucose and HbA1c and the discontinuation of all diabetes medications (oral and injectable).

   b) According to Buse et al., published in Diabetes Care: remission requires HbA1c <5.7 for at least one year with no active pharmacology or procedures.[307]

Table 5.5

Measure	Partial Remission	Complete Remission	Prolonged Remission
HbA1c %	<6.5	<5.7	<5.7
FBG mg/dl (mmol/L)	100–125 (5.6-6.9)	<100 (<5.6)	<100 (<5.6)
Time	≥1 year	≥1 year	≥5 years
Therapy	No active pharmacology or procedures		

5) **Dietary interventions**[158]

   a) Whole food plant-based nutrition is a diet that maximizes the intake of whole plant foods and minimizes the intake of processed and animal-derived foods.

      1. Maximized: Vegetables, fruits, whole-grains, beans, peas (chickpeas and split peas), lentils, mushrooms, herbs, spices, seeds, and nuts.
      2. Minimized: Industrial sugars, animal products, refined grains, and oils.

6) **Pathway of healing from type 2 diabetes**

   a) Diet is the cornerstone of type 2 diabetes control, treatment, and reversal. It outweighs all other lifestyle changes, and it can undo almost all medical treatments.

   b) Exercise can help. It acutely lowers blood glucose; improves weight control; helps with insulin resistance; and lowers the percentage of fat in muscles and liver.

c) Stress management can help lower blood glucose by decreasing the amount of exposure to cortisol (a stress hormone that raises blood glucose levels).

7) **Type 2 diabetes is reversible with lifestyle.**

a) Normalization of beta cell function can occur in association with decreased pancreas and liver triacylglycerol levels.[308]

b) Blood glucose and HbA1c levels can normalize to nondiabetic ranges with intentional weight loss in a home setting by motivated individuals.[309]

c) High rates of type 2 diabetes reversal occurred in newly diagnosed Asian Indian young adults with intensive lifestyle therapy.[310]

d) Youth who adhered to a very-low-energy diet reversed type 2 diabetes.[311]

e) Though in a murine model, a fasting-mimicking diet can promote beta-cell regeneration, which may have future implications for the role of reversing insulin-dependent type 2 diabetes.[312]

8) **Diabetes interventions for weight loss and resulting diabetes benefits**

9) **Almost any diet that reduces weight will effectively reduce markers of inflammation and increase insulin sensitivity.**

10) **Gastric bypass in patients with type 2 diabetes**[313]

a) Despite being a high-risk surgery, when weight loss was achieved there was a reduction in HbA1c levels, all-cause mortality, and medication requirement by 8.7%–31.8%.

b) At 18 to 24 months, remission rates with bariatric surgery vary from 39% to 93%. Longer term remission outcomes are lower but still significant. Remission rates at 5 years with the STAMPEDE (Surgical Treatment and Medications Potentially Eradicate Diabetes Efficiently) trial were 29%, and 30% at 15 years in Swedish Obese Subjects study follow up.[314,315,316]

11) **High-protein, low-carbohydrate diets in patients with type 2 diabetes**[317]

a) These can achieve weight loss, reduced insulin requirements, and reduced HbA1c levels.

b) Health Professionals Follow Up Study (HPFS) showed a 37% increased risk of diabetes on a low-carbohydrate diet.

c) Note: High dietary protein levels may put the kidneys of someone with diabetes at risk for injury or worsening disease.

12) **Mediterranean diet in patients with type 2 diabetes**

a) Shown to reduce HbA1c levels, reduce incidence of diabetes, and improve insulin sensitivity[318]

b) Improved HbA1c 0.30–0.47% and insulin sensitivity (inverse relationship)

c) Patients experienced a 20–30% reduced risk of developing type 2 diabetes

13) **Very-low-calorie diets**

14) **Whole food plant-based diets (low-fat)**

OBJECTIVE 21

Summarize key dietary research on the impact of diet on diabetes

1) **A vegan diet intervention improved hemoglobin HbA1c levels more than the traditional American Diabetes Association (ADA) diet in a 22-week randomized trial.**[74]

a) Among 49 participants in the vegan diet group, 48% reduced diabetes medications, and the average drop of HbA1c was 1.23% in those who did not change medications. This was compared to the 50 participants in the ADA diet group, where 23% reduced medications and HbA1c levels improved 0.38% in those who did not change medications.

2) **A low-fat vegan diet was associated with weight loss and reductions in fasting glucose in patients with non-insulin dependent diabetes without changes in exercise.**[319]

3) **The 8-year follow up of the Nurses' Health Study followed 91,246 women.**[320]

   a) Consumption of processed meat five or more times per week was associated with an increased risk of diabetes.

      1. Suggested pathology:

         a. Nitrite exposure

         b. Inflammation

         c. Heme iron stores

4) **The 16-year follow up Nurses' Health Study**[321]

   a) This was a retrospective analysis of a prospective study in 84,941 diabetes-free female nurses.

   b) Relative Risk = 0.09 of type 2 diabetes for a low-risk group of 3,300 cases during the 16-year follow-up.

      1. Body mass index (BMI) <25
      2. Diets high in cereal fiber and polyunsaturated fat and low in *trans* fat and glycemic load
      3. Moderate-to-vigorous exercise 30 or more minutes per day
      4. Nonsmoking
      5. Average one half serving of alcohol per day

   c) 91% of type 2 diabetes cases attributed to exceptions to these five factors.

5) **Adventist Health Study**[322]

   a) This was a cross-sectional study.

   b) Regular meat consumption nearly doubled the risk of having diabetes. Diabetes occurred at 40% higher prevalence in meat-consuming women and 80% higher prevalence in meat-consuming men.

   c) Adventists who ate meat compared to those who did not eat meat (age adjusted) had a 97% increased risk of diabetes for men, and a 93% increased risk of diabetes for women.

6) **EPIC study, which followed 38,094 participants**[323]

   a) Every 5% of calories from animal protein resulted in a 30% increased risk of diabetes.

   b) Vegetable protein was not associated with an increased risk of diabetes.

7) **Dietary research on eggs**[26]

   a) Nurses' Health Study and Health Professionals Follow Up Study (HPFS)

      1. People with diabetes who consume more than one egg a day doubled their risk of cardiovascular disease compared to those who ate less than one egg a week.
      2. Eating more than five eggs per week was associated with an increased risk of developing diabetes.
      3. The carnitine and choline found in meat and eggs produced inflammation that may contribute to diabetes.

8) **A National Institutes of Health (NIH) funded study looked at 49 participants on a plant-based diet versus 50 participants on the ADA diet (2002 recommendations).[74]**

   a) HbA1c dropped three times as much on plant-based diet (1.23% vs 0.38%).

   b) LDL dropped twice as much (21.2% vs 9.3%).

   c) Weight dropped more than two times (14.3 lbs vs 6.8 lbs) (6.5 kg vs 3 kg).

   d) Medication requirements dropped about two times (43% vs 26%).

9) **Vegetarian versus ADA diet[324]**

   a) This was a 24-week randomized parallel design with 74 subjects with type 2 diabetes.

   b) The experimental group ate a vegetarian diet, while the controls ate a conventional diabetes diet.

   c) The vegetarian group had:

      1. More reduction in medications and weight and an improvement in insulin sensitivity compared to the diabetes diet group
      2. Increased adiponectin, vitamin C, and superoxide dismutase
      3. Decreased leptin

10) **Meat consumption and type 2 diabetes risk (Figure 5.5)[325]**

   a) The relative risk (95% CI) for acquiring type 2 diabetes by consuming 100 grams of unprocessed red meat per day and for 50 grams of processed red meat per day, were 1.19 (1.04, 1.37) and 1.51 (1.25, 1.83), respectively.

   b) The risk of forming diabetes is estimated to be 16–35% lower if one serving of red meat per day is substituted with one serving of nuts, low-fat dairy, or whole-grains.

Figure 5.5 Diabetes Associated with Replacement of Other Food Groups for Red Meat Intake

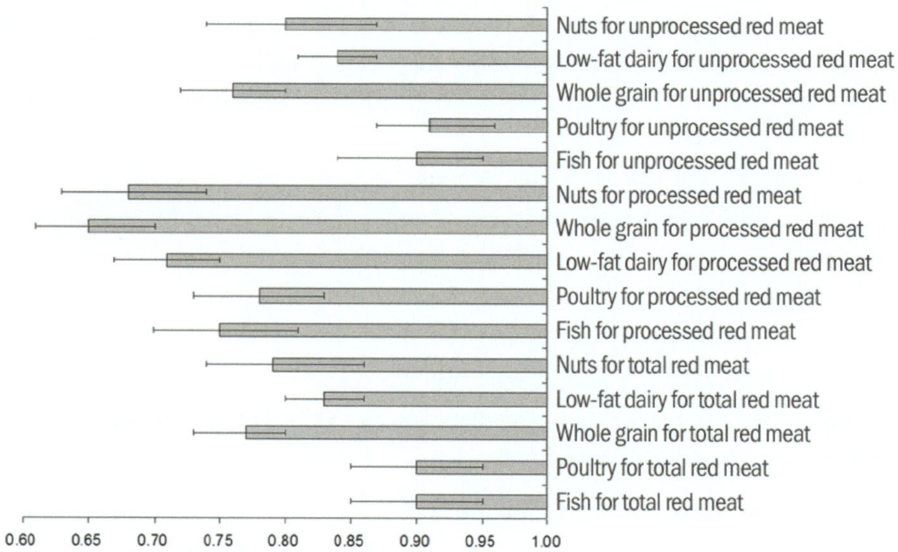

HRs and 95% CI for diabetes associated with replacement of other food groups for red meat intake. Adjusted for age (continuous), BMI category (kg/m^2; <23, 23–24.9, 25–29.9, 30–34.9, or ≥35), alcohol consumption (0, 0.1–4.9, 5.0–14.9, or ≥15 g/d), physical activity level (<3, 3–8.9, 9–17.9, 18–26.9, or ≥27 metabolic task hours/week), smoking status (never; past; current: 1–14, 15–24, or >24 cigarettes/d), race (white or nonwhite), menopausal status and hormone use in women (premenopausal, postmenopausal never hormone users, postmenopausal past hormone users, or postmenopausal current hormone users), family history of diabetes, history of hypertension and hypercholesterolemia, and quintile of total energy intake.) Change in type 2 diabetes risk from substituting miscellaneous foods for red meat.

11) Plant-based foods and risk of type 2 diabetes in three large cohorts[326]

- **a)** Data from three large cohorts (Nurses' Health Study 1984–2012, Nurses' Health Study 1991–2011, and HPFS 1986–2010)
  1. >200,000 US male and female health professionals were followed for 20+ years.
  2. There were regular data collections on diet, lifestyle, medical history, and new diagnoses.
- **b)** Results showed diets emphasizing plant foods and low in animal foods had ~20% lower risk of diabetes.
  1. Plant-based diets that specifically emphasized healthy plant-based foods had ~34% lower risk.
  2. Plant-based diets that were high in less healthy plant foods (such as processed foods) had 16% increased diabetes risk.

OBJECTIVE 22

Describe the Diabetes Prevention Program and its applications

1) The Diabetes Prevention Program (DPP)[327] (see article 1 In Appendix)

- **a)** The Centers for Disease Control and Prevention led an intensive lifestyle intervention program designed to help reduce the progression of prediabetes and at-risk groups. The intervention program included advice on healthy eating and physical activity, as well as assistance with problem solving and coping skills.
- **b)** Program
  1. 12-month program
     - a. Meetings were weekly with a research team for 6 months, then monthly for 6 months.
     - b. Instructions were to meet physical activity guidelines of 150 minutes of moderate intensity exercise per week via walking or body weight resistance.
     - c. The program focused on sustainable lifestyle change without gym memberships or intensive physical activity.
  2. Dietary change was less fat, fewer calories.
     - a. Dietary advice followed "MyPlate" recommendations for healthier choices.
  3. Support was virtual or live.
- **c)** DPP conclusions:
  1. Lifestyle habits can prevent diabetes.
  2. The DPP offers effective clinical applications.
  3. Lifestyle is preferable for managing diabetes, as it doesn't have the negative effects of intensive medication management.

2) Clinical application of lessons learned from the DPP

- **a)** Begin talking with patients about prediabetes and the need to treat it.
- **b)** Screen with lab work and questionnaires.
- **c)** Discuss the long-term implications.
- **d)** Include honest conversations about medical and lifestyle interventions.
  1. Discussing all treatments, including lifestyle treatment, is part of informed consent for treatment of chronic disease. Discuss opportunities for change, challenges, and sustainability.

e) Focus on the positive aspect of lifestyle.
   1. Lifestyle is cost effective (cost of treating disease over lifetime).
   2. There is co-morbid risk reduction.
   3. General well-being and daily health are improved.
   4. Provide success stories.
   5. End with encouragement to support healthier choices and minimize fear of follow-up.

OBJECTIVE 23

List the major physiologic impacts of a plant-based diet in the process of disease reversal

1) **A whole food plant-based diet:**
   a) Changes epigenetics and overall lowers risk of chronic disease, treats chronic disease, and may even reverse disease
   b) Normalizes angiogenesis reducing comorbid disease (cancer and heart disease)
      1. Especially leafy greens, cruciferous vegetables, onions, and mushrooms
   c) Lowers total caloric intake and reduces feelings of hunger that result from weight loss, improved HbA1c, and normalization and sensitization of leptin and adiponectin levels.
   d) Improves insulin sensitivity independent of weight loss
   e) Works to lower inflammation through the addition of antioxidant foods and the reduction of pro-inflammatory foods
   f) Lowers overall endothelial cell injury, oxidative stress, and the NF-kß and JNK inflammatory cascades
   g) Protects beta cells by:
      1. Normalizing the lipid profile
      2. Normalizing the leptin/adiponectin pathway
      3. Down-regulating inflammatory cascades
      4. Normalizing glucose levels, which protects against apoptosis
      5. Stabilizing immune system via multitude of pathways
   h) Improves glycemic control and optimizes the microbiome via production of short-chain fatty acids from intake of fiber[328]
      1. Short-chain fatty acids are produced by the microbiome
         a. Digestion produces butyrate
         b. Butyrate:
            (1) Enhances insulin sensitivity
            (2) Enhances mineral absorption
            (3) Decreases cholesterol and triglycerides
            (4) Decreases glycolysis in the liver
            (5) Improves satiety
   i) Reduces pain associated with peripheral neuropathy[329]

1. After changing to a whole food plant-based diet, 81% of participants reported significant improvement in symptoms, including improvement in numbness within 4–16 days, which is faster than what would have been expected for nerve regrowth.

j) Assists with overcoming food addictions and dependency by helping to reprogram taste buds and break eating patterns.

   1. Also, phytochemicals from plants may help to normalize the dopamine reward system in brain.

k) Reduces total costs by lowering the need for medical treatments and interventions

l) Is sustainable, as it's a message of abundance and not caloric restriction, whereas diets with caloric restriction have a success rate of 3% over 5 years

   1. Ornish Lifestyle Heart Trial showed 71% adherence at 5 years.[66,67]
   2. In the peripheral neuropathy study mentioned above, 17 participants from the original 21 patients were followed for 1–4 years. Of those, 71% remained on the diet and exercise program, and all but one continued to have relief from peripheral neuropathy pain.[329]

m) Reversal of diabetic retinopathy[330]

n) Take-home messages for patients

   1. Focus on a whole food plant-based diet.
      a. Aim for mix of raw and cooked foods.
      b. Encourage the addition of beans and lentils.
   2. Focus dietary advice around improving glycemic load over the glycemic index.
      a. Short-term fluctuations are not as important as long-term trends.
   3. Provide education on true and false hunger signals.[331]
      a. Food addictions and withdrawal symptoms are not true hunger.
      b. Encourage patients to endure withdrawal symptoms, as they will eventually normalize.

SECTION 5 REVIEW QUESTIONS

1. **A 34-year-old male presents for a routine physical. On brief review of his diet, you find he eats fast food for breakfast and lunch, but typically chicken or fish for dinner with a vegetable or salad. He consumes processed or red meat 1–2 times a day and drinks four cans of soda. Which nutrient is he most likely over consuming in his diet?**
   - **A.** Fiber
   - **B.** Vitamin E
   - **C.** Vitamin C
   - **D.** Saturated fats
2. **A patient asks how to lower his intake of saturated fat. You suggest replacing it with foods higher in polyunsaturated fat. Which of the following would be the best source?**
   - **A.** Sharp cheddar cheese
   - **B.** Coconut oil
   - **C.** Chicken
   - **D.** Walnuts
3. **Which statement best describes the clinical findings in the study, "Effects of a Dietary Portfolio of Cholesterol-Lowering Foods Versus Lovastatin on Serum Lipids and Hypercholesterolemia," by Jenkins, et al., in the *American Journal of Clinical Nutrition*, 2006:**
   - **A.** Diets that focus on low saturated fat and increased viscous fiber, plant sterols, vegetable protein and nuts do not statistically reduce low-density lipoprotein (LDL) cholesterol levels.
   - **B.** Study participants were able to lower their LDL cholesterol more than 20%, which was almost equal (not significantly different) to the response of the group placed on 20 mg of lovastatin, a first-generation statin medication.
   - **C.** The US Food and Drug Administration now permits health claims that foods that deliver adequate amounts of plant sterols reduce the risk for coronary heart disease (CHD).
   - **D.** The portfolio diet group showed a reduction in the LDL cholesterol but not the cardiovascular inflammatory marker c-reactive protein.
4. **A 55-year-old male patient presents for follow up of coronary artery disease (CAD) status post balloon angioplasty 1 year prior and hypertension. He is highly motivated to change his diet in order to reverse his CAD and reduce future risk of any further heart disease. Which dietary plan would be best to prescribe?**
   - **A.** DASH Diet
   - **B.** Ornish Diet
   - **C.** Mediterranean diet
   - **D.** Ketogenic diet

5. **Of the following, which is the strongest support for including nutrition counseling into clinical care for patients who are overweight or obese?**
   - **A.** The US Preventative Services Task Force recommends that nutrition and physical activity counseling for people who are overweight and have chronic disease is intensive and focused on specific behavioral interventions.
   - **B.** Patients receiving physical activity prescriptions and advice from their health care provider increased their exercise by 18 minutes per week.
   - **C.** Nutrition prescriptions are believed to be helpful in changing patients' behavior toward food.
   - **D.** Nutrition prescriptions can be written for prevention and treatment for multiple chronic diseases, such as diabetes and heart disease.

6. **A nutrition prescription should follow the SMART goal format. Which of the following is the best example of this?**
   - **A.** Eat 1/2 cup of broccoli or spinach every weekday for 4 weeks. Vegetables will be purchased every Sunday.
   - **B.** Increase vegetable intake by purchasing vegetables in season for next 3 months.
   - **C.** Begin eating seven servings of vegetables a day for next 6 months.
   - **D.** Eat more vegetables. Purchase in-season vegetables on Sundays. Follow up with provider when goal is completed.

7. **Advanced glycation end products (AGEs) are a family of oxidative stressors found in proteins and glucose that cause inflammation and cell damage. Certain types of food preparation can increase AGEs. The best way to prepare food in order to decrease the amount of AGEs produced is:**
   - **A.** Roasting
   - **B.** Frying
   - **C.** Boiling
   - **D.** Grilling

8. **Reducing the intake of what micronutrient will decrease the risk of hypertension?**
   - **A.** Calcium
   - **B.** Sodium
   - **C.** Potassium
   - **D.** Vitamin C

9. **A 45-year-old male presents for a preventive exam with a BMI of 32 and reports eating red meat or processed meats 1–2 times a day, exercising 150 minutes per week, taking a multi-vitamin daily, and only drinking two cans of soda per day. You counsel him on his personal risk factors for cancer. Which information would be most important to share?**
   - **A.** Foods high in saturated fats, foods high in sugar, and processed and red meat increase the risk of colon and breast cancer.
   - **B.** Obesity increases the risk of breast cancer.
   - **C.** Prostate cancer risk is decreased with the consumption of red and processed meats.
   - **D.** Antioxidant-rich foods, such as carrots, berries, nuts, and green leafy vegetables decrease the risk of cancer.

10. Which one of the following statements best describes a situation with zero risk of developing heart disease from hypercholesterolemia?

- **A.** Trans-fatty acid consumption is associated with an increased risk of heart disease.
- **B.** A whole food plant-based diet, as demonstrated in the Lifestyle Heart Trial, produces regression of plaque stenosis and reduction in cholesterol.
- **C.** A decrease in high-density lipoprotein (HDL) cholesterol may occur with a plant-based diet, but the ratio of the drop of LDL compared to HDL still provides a benefit.
- **D.** If the serum total cholesterol is 90–140 mg/dl (2.327–3.620 mmol/L), and the LDL is less than 70 mg/dL (1.810mmol/L), there is no evidence of atherosclerotic plaque formation or risk of heart disease.

11. The Diabetes Prevention Program (DPP) trial was the first major study to compare lifestyle intervention to medications to prevent diabetes. During this trial, striking findings were revealed. The lifestyle intervention showed a 58% reduction in the incidence of diabetes compared to controls whereas the metformin group had only a 31% reduction. The two major goals of the lifestyle intervention were to achieve 7% weight loss and 150 minutes weekly of physical activity similar to brisk walking. Based on the study, what kind of weight-loss counsel did the lifestyle intervention group receive that made it so effective?

- **A.** Participants were encouraged to gradually achieve the fat and calorie levels through better choices of meals and snack items; healthier food preparation techniques; and careful selection of restaurants, including fast food and the items offered.
- **B.** The initial focus of the dietary intervention was on caloric restriction to 1,200 calories per day for all participants.
- **C.** The dietary advice was based on meeting an extremely low intake of dietary fat at 10% of calories from fat per day.
- **D.** Participants who began with the highest starting weights (>250 lbs) were advised to have a lower caloric intake than those who began with a lower initial weight of (120–170 lbs).

12. The pathogenesis of diabetes is best described as:

- **A.** Insulin resistance in muscle facilitates the development of fatty liver. Increased fatty acids produced by the liver damage pancreatic beta cells, suppressing glucose-mediated insulin secretion, and leading to hyperglycemia.
- **B.** Muscle insulin resistance determines the rate at which fatter liver digresses.
- **C.** Eventually the pancreas is unable to produce sufficient amounts of leptin to push glucose into the cells, so serum glucose levels rise.
- **D.** Loss of sensitivity to insulin causes a decrease in adipose tissue and leptin levels.

13. Ornish and colleagues found that intensive nutrition and lifestyle changes down-regulated 453 genes and up-regulated 48 genes. Each of these genes had critical roles in the tumorigenesis of which of the following:

- **A.** Colon cancer
- **B.** Cardiovascular disease
- **C.** Prostate cancer
- **D.** Chronic kidney disease

14. The outcome of the 8-year follow-up of the Nurses' Health Study showed:

- **A.** Meat-eating Adventists compared to non-meat-eating Adventists showed a 97% increased risk for diabetes in men and a 93% increased risk in women.
- **B.** Every 5% increase in calories from animal protein resulted in a 30% increase in risk of diabetes.
- **C.** HbA1c dropped more than three times for participants on a plant-based diet compared to participants on the American Diabetes Association diet.
- **D.** Consuming processed meat more than five times per week was associated with an increased risk of type 2 diabetes.

15. The theory that a plant-based diet improved diabetes because it was lower in calories, which led to weight loss, was challenged by Anderson in a small study of 20 men with type 2 diabetes. Patients in the study were placed on a high-fiber (65 grams/day), plant-based diet with sufficient calories to prevent weight loss. Insulin use was discontinued in 11 patients and decreased in the other nine men. How quickly did insulin discontinuation or reduction occur and in what relation to weight loss?

- **A.** Weeks, independent of weight loss.
- **B.** Months, independent of weight loss.
- **C.** Weeks, but only if weight was lost.
- **D.** Months, but only if weight was lost.

16. In results from the Adventist Health Study-2 among white subjects, a dose-dependent drop in blood pressure was noted as diets became more plant-based. Which of the following is true regarding this dose-dependent effect?

- **A.** Blood pressure-lowering effects occurred in those with a BMI of >25 for systolic blood pressure only.
- **B.** After adjusting for age and gender, vegans and lacto-ovo-vegetarians had significantly lower blood pressure compared to omnivores.
- **C.** Blood pressure-lowering effects were different for individuals consuming alcohol.
- **D.** Adjustment for BMI resulted in reversal of the dose-response blood pressure-lowering effect for vegans, lacto-ovo-vegetarians and partial vegetarians.

17. A study by Pierce, et al. "Greater Survival After Breast Cancer in Physically Active Women with High Vegetable-Fruit Intake Regardless of Obesity," assessed whether fruit and vegetable intake and physical activity in obese women affected breast cancer survival. This study demonstrated that:

- **A.** Within all fruit and vegetable intake and physical activity level categories, women who were obese had apparent increased mortality compared with those who were not obese.
- **B.** Compared to non-obese sedentary women with low fruit and vegetable intake, obese women in the same category had greater chances of survival.
- **C.** Mortality of physically active obese women consuming high amounts of fruits and vegetables was similar to that of non-obese, physically active women consuming high amounts of fruits and vegetables.
- **D.** Mortality rates were highest for obese and non-obese physically active women consuming low amounts of fruits and vegetables.

18. Which component would be most damaging in terms of causing a rise in total blood cholesterol?

- **A.** Dietary cholesterol
- **B.** Saturated fats
- **C.** *Trans* fats
- **D.** Insoluble fiber

19. **The leading source of saturated fat in the American diet is:**
   - **A.** Beef
   - **B.** Eggs
   - **C.** Cheese
   - **D.** Olive oil

20. **Which of the following statements are true?**
   - **A.** Insoluble fiber is mostly found in legumes, fruits, and oats.
   - **B.** Plant foods contain more than 100,000 phytochemicals associated with protection against major chronic diseases. Animal products contain no phytochemicals.
   - **C.** The best way to lose weight is to outline a daily 60-minute exercise program and do it with a partner.
   - **D.** It's difficult to find atherosclerosis or CHD in societies with total blood cholesterol levels below 200 mg/dL (3.879 mmol/L).

21. **Which of the following is a proven clinical outcome of the DASH Diet?**
   - **A.** As effective in lowering LDL cholesterol as statins
   - **B.** Regression of CAD and atherosclerosis
   - **C.** Telomere length increase
   - **D.** Reduced hypertension

22. **Which of the following is proven clinical outcome of the Esselstyn diet?**
   - **A.** Equally effective in lowering LDL cholesterol as statins
   - **B.** Inhibition of prostate cancer cells
   - **C.** Telomere length increase
   - **D.** Regression of CAD and atherosclerosis; coronary event rate was 100 times higher over 4 years in those who did not adhere versus those who did

23. **Which of the following is a proven clinical outcome of the Ornish Diet and lifestyle intervention?**
   - **A.** Equally effective in lowering LDL cholesterol as statins
   - **B.** Regression of CAD and atherosclerosis and inhibition of prostate cancer cells
   - **C.** Telomere length decrease and inhibition of prostate cancer cells
   - **D.** Coronary event rate was 100 times higher over 4 years in those who did not adhere versus those who did

24. **Which of the following is a proven clinical outcome of the portfolio diet?**
   - **A.** As effective in lowering LDL cholesterol as statins
   - **B.** Regression of CAD and atherosclerosis
   - **C.** Telomere length increase
   - **D.** Inhibition of prostate cancer cells

25. **Which of the following statements is true?**
   - **A.** The World Health Organization declared red meat a group 1 human carcinogen.
   - **B.** Coconut oil has been shown to reduce Alzheimer's disease.
   - **C.** Ground up flax seed is an excellent source of omega-3 fatty acid.
   - **D.** A more optimal daily dietary fiber content would be 28 grams (almost twice the recommended amount).

SECTION 5 REVIEW QUESTION ANSWERS AND SUMMARIES

1. **Answer: D.** This patient is eating a high amount of processed foods, animal proteins, and sugary drinks. He is likely overconsuming saturated fat along with added sugars, processed grains, cholesterol, sodium, and *trans* fats. Answers A through C listed, fiber, vitamin C, and vitamin E, are common shortfall nutrients in the standard American diet as they are predominately found in nutrient-dense, whole, plant-based foods.

2. **Answer: D.** Walnuts are high in polyunsaturated fats and low in saturated fats. Cheddar cheese would be high in saturated fat. Coconut oil is also very high in saturated fat, but does contain small amounts of monounsaturated and polyunsaturated fats. Chicken is low in polyunsaturated fat and saturated fat. https://www.nal.usda.gov/sites/www.nal.usda.gov/files/polyunsat_fat.pdf https://fdc.nal.usda.gov/fdc-app.html#/food-details/1103857/nutrients

3. **Answer: B.** Participants who ate the dietary portfolio of cholesterol-lowering foods (plant sterols, soy protein, nuts and viscous fiber) were able to lower LDL cholesterol concentrations >20%. This was statistically significant compared to the control group (on a low saturated fat diet, not a high fat diet) and almost equal (no significant difference found) to the response to lovastatin 20 mg, a first-generation statin medication. The US Food and Drug Administration now permits health claims that foods that deliver adequate amounts of plant sterols reduce the risk for coronary heart disease (CHD) but this does not best describe the study. Both LDL-cholesterol and the cardiovascular inflammatory marker c-reactive protein were reduced.

4. **Answer: B.** The Ornish diet would be best to prescribe for coronary artery disease (CAD). It is a low-fat, plant-based diet capable of reversing CAD stenosis in one year and maintained reversal at the 5-year follow-up, according to the Lifestyle Heart Trial. The DASH Diet for hypertension (a combination of vegetables, low salt and low-fat dairy) has been found to be adequate first-line treatment for essential hypertension. The Mediterranean diet for secondary prevention but not reversal of CAD, as it was found to be superior to a prudent Western diet in preventing recurrence of CAD events. Ketogenic diets have shown to reduce weight, help improve blood sugar, increase HDL cholesterol and lower triglycerides. However, there have been several studies linking low-carbohydrate diets to increased mortality, cardiovascular disease, and LDL cholesterol; but the evidence is mixed. https://www.ncbi.nlm.nih.gov/pmc/articles/PMC6124862/. https://www.ncbi.nlm.nih.gov/books/NBK537084/

5. **Answer: A.** It is a Grade B recommendation from the US Preventive Services Task Force to offer intensive behavioral health nutrition counseling and physical activity counseling for overweight people with chronic disease risk factors. The B rating means to provide service, as there is a high certainty of a moderate to substantial benefit.

6. **Answer: A.** The SMART acronym for nutrition prescriptions stands for specific, measurable, achievable/attainable, realistic, and time. Specific type of foods. Measurable, meaning how much of the food. Achievable/attainable goals for who will be doing the cooking and the shopping. Realistic goals for what food is available, the budget, time commitment, and what will the patient actually do. Time connected, meaning what is the frequency for eating the food, and for what duration of time is the prescription written.

7. **Answer: C.** Foods that are fried, smoked, grilled, baked, or roasted have higher advanced glycation end products (AGEs). Foods that are prepared with moist heat cooking, such as boiling, stewing, and broiling, have fewer AGEs.

8. **Answer: B.** Sodium restriction typically reduces blood pressure by 2.5–7 mmHg. According to the American Heart Association, the ideal limit of sodium should be less than 1.5 grams daily, with the upper limit being 2,300 mg daily. The largest sources of sodium in the US are processed foods and canned foods.

9. **Answer: A.** The risk of breast, colon, and prostate cancer are increased with the consumption of red meat, processed meat, highly processed grains, added sugars, high saturated fats, and *trans* fats. Processed meat was categorized as a Group 1 carcinogen to humans and red meat has been classified as a Group 2a carcinogen, meaning it's probably carcinogenic to humans. It would be most important to have the patient reduce consumption of processed and red meats to reduce his risk of colon cancer; they are not known to increase the risk of prostate cancer. Long term, encouraging antioxidant rich foods could help reduce his overall risk of cancer.

10. **Answer: D.** Facts learned from 2013 Baylor University Conference: If the serum total cholesterol is 90–140 mg/dL (2.327–3.620 mmol/L), there is no evidence that cigarette smoking, systemic hypertension, diabetes, inactivity, or obesity produces atherosclerotic plaques. Hypercholesterolemia is the only direct atherosclerotic risk factor; the others are all indirect. Optimal LDL is 50–70 mg/dL (1.293–1.810mmol/L). Plaque progression ceases with total cholesterol <150 mg/dL (3.879 mmol/L).

11. **Answer: A.** Participants were encouraged to gradually achieve set fat and calorie levels through better choices of meals and snack items; healthier food preparation techniques; and careful selection of restaurants, including fast food and the items offered. The initial focus of the dietary intervention was on reducing total fat rather than calories. This allowed participants to accomplish a reduction in caloric intake while at the same time emphasizing overall healthy eating. It also streamlined the self-monitoring requirements, which was important given the diversity of educational and literacy levels among participants. After several weeks, the concept of calorie balance and the need to restrict calories as well as fat was introduced. The calorie goals were calculated by estimating the daily calories needed to maintain the participant's starting weight and subtracting 500–1,000 calories per day (depending on initial body weight) to achieve 1–2 pounds of weight loss per week. The fat goals, given in grams of fat per day, were based on 25% of calories from fat. Four standard calorie levels were used: 1,200 calories per day (33 grams fat) for participants with an initial weight of 120–170 lbs; 1,500 calories per day (42 grams fat) for participants with a weight of 175 to 215 lbs; 1,800 calories per day (50 grams fat) for participants with a weight of 220–245 lbs; and 2,000 calories per day (55 grams fat) for participants weighing >250 lbs. The fat and calorie goals were used as a means to achieve the weight loss goal rather than as a goal in and of itself. Therefore, if a participant reported consuming more than the calorie or fat goal but was losing weight as planned, the coach did not emphasize greater calorie or fat reduction.

12. **Answer: A.** Insulin resistance begins to occur as inflammatory mediators cause damage to liver and beta cells and as muscle and adipocyte cells begin resisting further fat storage. Adipocytes are key factors in the development of insulin resistance. As weight gain occurs, adipocytes undergo hyperplasia and hypertrophy (that is, they grow in number and in size) and begin accumulating in ectopic tissues, such as the liver and muscle cells. Intramyocellular fat accumulation disrupts insulin receptors via production of lipotoxic mediators, causing insulin resistance. Muscle insulin resistance determines the rate of fatty liver progression. Fatty liver progression and the deposit of fatty acids in the pancreas are responsible for the rate of hepatic insulin resistance (failure to appropriately respond to blood glucose levels) and beta cell dysfunction.

13. **Answer: C.** Ornish and colleagues, in a study on prostate cancer, found that intensive nutrition and lifestyle changes altered the expression of more than 500 genes, down-regulated 453 genes, and up- regulated 48 genes. Each of these genes had critical roles in tumorigenesis of prostate cancer.

14. **Answer: D.** The eight-year follow-up to the Nurses' Health Study showed that the consumption of processed meat greater than five times weekly increased the risk of diabetes. The Adventist Health Study showed regular meat consumption was associated with two times greater risk of diabetes. Among meat eating Adventists compared to non-meat eaters, there was a 97% increased risk of diabetes in men and 93% increased risk in women. The EPIC study showed that for every 5% of calories consumed from animal protein, there was a 30% increase in diabetes. The National Institutes of Health study compared a plant-based diet to the American Diabetes Association diet. It found that participants following the plant-based diet dropped their HbA1c three times more, decreased their LDL cholesterol twice as much, lost more weight, and had greater reductions in medications. Data from three large cohorts (Nurses' Health Study 1984–2012, Nurses' Health Study 1991–2011, Health Professionals Follow-Up Study 1986-2010) found the type of plant-based diet is important in diabetes risk. A plant-based diet that specifically emphasized healthy plant-based foods had ~34% lower risk of diabetes. Whereas, plant-based diets that were high in less healthy plant foods (such as processed foods) had a 16% increased risk of diabetes.

15. **Answer: A.** Researchers tested the effect of a low-fat, high-carbohydrate (9% of energy from fat, 70% from carbohydrate) near-vegetarian diet containing 65 grams of fiber and 65 grams of cholesterol per day. Participants were 20 normal-weight men with insulin-treated type 2 diabetes, and it was a 16-day trial. No significant weight changes occurred for any of the participants. By the end of the study period, insulin use was discontinued in 11 participants. In the rest of the participants, it was reduced from a mean of 26 to 11 units per day ($P < 0.001$). Despite this reduction in medication use and no meaningful weight loss, mean fasting plasma glucose concentration still decreased from an average of 164 mg/dL to 152 mg/dL (amount decreased was not significant).[196]

16. **Answer: B.** For BMI of <18 to >32, there is a linear association with blood pressure, from lowest to highest for both systolic and diastolic. Adjusted for age and gender, significantly lower blood pressure was found in non-treated vegans and lacto-ovo-vegetarians compared to omnivores. Adding alcohol intake to the models studied did not identify an alcohol effect, however alcohol intake was infrequent and small. For vegans, lacto-ovo-vegetarians, and partial vegetarians, effects were reduced (but not reversed) after adjustment for BMI.

17. **Answer: C.** The study found women who were obese but had high levels of physical activity (≥540 metabolic equivalent minutes per week) and ate high amounts of fruits and vegetables daily (>5 servings per day) had the same mortality rates as women who were not obese but also had high physical activity and high fruit and vegetable intake.[193]

18. **Answer: C.** *Trans* fats are the most damaging fats and are formed by adding hydrogen to liquid vegetable oils to make them solid. *Trans* fats also occur naturally in meat and dairy products. They are known to increase LDL cholesterol and lower HDL cholesterol, increasing risk for heart disease. Saturated fats come mainly from meat and dairy products. Plant foods that contain saturated fats include coconut, coconut oil, palm oil, and cocoa butter. The American Heart Association recommends keeping the amount of saturated fat in the diet to less than 5–6% of total daily calories. The 2015 Dietary Guidelines for Americans[332] no longer include a recommendation to limit dietary cholesterol to less than 300 mg a day. But the guidelines acknowledge this does not mean dietary cholesterol should not be limited, as diets lower in dietary cholesterol are associated with lower risk of heart disease and obesity. Of note, foods high in dietary cholesterol are mainly higher in saturated fats, except those egg yolks and shell fish that are high in cholesterol but low in saturated fat. Polyunsaturated fats may help improve blood cholesterol levels, especially if they are used to replace saturated and *trans* fats. Insoluble fiber is a carbohydrate, and that may help lower cholesterol levels by not allowing it to be reabsorbed in the colon.

19. **Answer: C.** Foods that are high in saturated fat (more than 8 grams of saturated fat per serving) include higher fat cuts of beef, pork, and lamb; salami, sausages and other processed meats; many fast foods (e.g., cheeseburgers); and coconut and coconut oil. Cheese is moderately high in saturated fat with 4–7 grams per serving, but it's consumed in high quantities, making it the number one source of saturated fat in the US according to the NHANES 2003-2006 study. https://www.ncbi.nlm.nih.gov/pmc/articles/PMC3546624/table/nutrients-04-02097-t005/?report=objectonly. https://www.ncbi.nlm.nih.gov/pmc/articles/PMC3546624/

20. **Answer: B.** Insoluble fiber is mainly found in vegetables, wheat, wheat bran, nuts, and seeds. Legumes, fruits, and oats are high in soluble fiber. Phytochemicals are only produced by plants. Exercise is great for maintenance of weight loss, but caloric restriction must be included weight loss. When total dietary cholesterol is less than 150, progression of plaque development in blood vessels appears to cease even in the presence of other risk factors like smoking, hypertension, obesity, and diabetes.

21. **Answer D.** The DASH Diet has been proven to reduce hypertension.

22. **Answer D.** The Esselstyn diet has been proven to regress CAD and atherosclerosis and coronary event rate was 100 times higher over four years in those who did not adhere versus those who did.

23. **Answer B.** The Ornish Diet and lifestyle intervention has been proven to regress coronary artery disease and atherosclerosis, increase telomere length, and inhibit prostate cancer cells.

24. **Answer A.** The portfolio diet has been proven to be as effective in lowering LDL cholesterol as statins.

25. **Answer: C.** The World Health Organization has not declared red meat a Group 1 carcinogen, but it was labeled as Group 2A. This means it's probably carcinogenic to humans, but insufficient evidence exists to rule out chance or bias as the cause. Processed meats have been labeled Group 1, meaning they are carcinogenic to humans. Coconut oil has not been shown to reduce Alzheimer's disease. Ground flax seed is an excellent source of omega-3 fatty acid. A more optimal fiber recommendation for health benefits would be 40–45 grams per day.

SECTION 5 REFERENCES

1. US Department of Agriculture and US Department of Health and Human Services. *Dietary Guidelines for Americans, 2020-2025*. 9th ed. Washington, DC: US Department of Agriculture; 2020.
2. US Department of Agriculture. Dietary Guidelines Advisory Committee. *Scientific Report of the 2020 Dietary Guidelines Advisory Committee: Advisory Report to the Secretary of Agriculture and the Secretary of Health and Human Services*. Washington, DC: U.S. Department of Agriculture; 2020.
3. US Department of Agriculture and US Department of Health and Human Services. Dietary Guidelines for Americans, 2015-2020. 8th Ed. Washington, DC: US Department of Agriculture; 2015. https://health.gov/our-work/food-and-nutrition/2015-2020-dietary-guidelines/.
4. Iacobucci G. Food and soft drink industry has too much influence over US dietary guidelines, report says. *BMJ*. 2020;369:m1666.
5. National Academies of Sciences Engineering, Medicine. *Redesigning the Process for Establishing the Dietary Guidelines for Americans*. Washington, DC: The National Academies Press; 2017.
6. US Department of Agriculture. Choose my plate. https://www.choosemyplate.gov/. Accessed September 2020.
7. Yu E., Hu F. B. Dairy products, pairy fatty acids, and the prevention of cardiometabolic disease: a review of recent evidence. *Curr Atheroscler Rep*. 2018;20(5):24.
8. US Department of Agriculture. Food availability (per capita) data system. 2016. https://www.ers.usda.gov/data-products/food-availability-per-capita-data-system/ . Accessed September 25, 2020.
9. US Department of Agriculture, Agricultural Research Service. *What We Eat in America*. NHANES 2007-2010 for average intakes by age-sex group. https://data.nal.usda.gov/dataset/what-we-eat-america-wweia-database. Accessed September, 2020.
10. Lee M., Lee H., Kim J. Dairy food consumption is associated with a lower risk of the metabolic syndrome and its components: a systematic review and meta-analysis. *Br J Nutr*. 2018;120(4):373-384.
11. Sochol K. M., Johns T. S., Buttar R. S., et al. The effects of dairy intake on insulin resistance: a systematic review and meta-analysis of randomized clinical trials. *Nutrients*. 2019;11(9).
12. Chen M., Li Y., Sun Q., et al. Dairy fat and risk of cardiovascular disease in 3 cohorts of US adults. *Am J Clin Nutr*. 2016;104(5):1209-1217.
13. de Lamas C., de Castro M. J., Gil-Campos M., Gil Á, Couce M. L., Leis R. Effects of dairy product consumption on height and bone mineral content in children: a systematic review of controlled trials. *Adv Nutr*. 2019;10(suppl_2):S88-s96.
14. van den Heuvel Ellen G. H. M., Steijns Jan M. J. M. Dairy products and bone health: how strong is the scientific evidence? Nutrition research reviews. 2018;31(2):164-178.
15. Tai V., Leung W., Grey A., Reid I. R., Bolland M. J. Calcium intake and bone mineral density: systematic review and meta-analysis. *BMJ*. 2015;351:h4183.
16. Gadotti T. N., Norde M. M., Rogero M. M, et al. Dairy consumption and inflammatory profile: a cross-sectional population-based study, São Paulo, Brazil. *Nutrition*. 2018;48:1-5.
17. Cavero-Redondo I., Alvarez-Bueno C., Sotos-Prieto M., Gil A., Martinez-Vizcaino V., Ruiz J. R. Milk and dairy product consumption and risk of mortality: an overview of systematic reviews and meta-analyses. *Adv Nutr*. 2019;10(suppl_2):S97-s104.
18. Malmir H., Larijani B., Esmaillzadeh A. Consumption of milk and dairy products and risk of osteoporosis and hip fracture: a systematic review and meta-analysis. *Crit Rev Food Sci Nutr*. 2020;60(10):1722-1737.
19. Schlesinger S., Neuenschwander M., Schwedhelm C., et al. Food groups and risk of overweight, obesity, and weight gain: a systematic review and dose-response meta-analysis of prospective studies. *Adv Nutr*. 2019;10(2):205-218. https://www.ncbi.nlm.nih.gov/pubmed/30801613.
20. Hu F. B., Stampfer M. J., Manson J. E., et al. Dietary fat intake and the risk of coronary heart disease in women. *N Engl J Med*. 1997;337(21):1491-1499. http://www.ncbi.nlm.nih.gov/pubmed/9366580.
21. Kratz M. Dietary cholesterol, atherosclerosis and coronary heart disease. *Atherosclerosis: Diet and Drugs*. Springer; 2005:195-213.
22. Hu F. B., Stampfer M. J., Rimm E. B., et al. A prospective study of egg consumption and risk of cardiovascular disease in men and women. *JAMA*. 1999;281(15):1387-1394.
23. Díez-Espino J., Basterra-Gortari F. J., Salas-Salvadó J., et al. Egg consumption and cardiovascular disease according to diabetic status: The PREDIMED study. *Clin Nutr*. 2017;36(4):1015-1021.
24. Zhong V. W., Van Horn L., Cornelis M. C. Associations of dietary cholesterol or egg consumption with incident cardiovascular disease and mortality. *JAMA*. 2019 Mar 19;321(11):1081-1095.
25. Shin J. Y., Xun P., Nakamura Y., He K. Egg consumption in relation to risk of cardiovascular disease and diabetes: a systematic review and meta-analysis. *Am J Clin Nutr*. 2013;98(1):146-159.
26. Djoussé L., Khawaja O. A., Gaziano J. M. Egg consumption and risk of type 2 diabetes: a meta-analysis of prospective studies. *Am J Clin Nutr*. 2016;103(2):474-480.
27. Sabaté J., Burkholder-Cooley N. M., Segovia-Siapco G., et al. Unscrambling the relations of egg and meat consumption with type 2 diabetes risk. *Am J Clin Nutr*. 2018;108(5):1121-1128. https://doi.org/10.1093/ajcn/nqy213.
28. US Department of Agriculture Agricultural Research Service. FoodData Central; 2019. fdc.nal.usda.gov.
29. Rouhani M. H., Rashidi-Pourfard N., Salehi-Abargouei A., Karimi M., Haghighatdoost F. Effects of egg consumption on blood lipids: a systematic review and meta-analysis of randomized clinical trials. *J Am Coll Nutr*. 2018;37(2):99-110.

30. Khalighi S. M., Soltani S., Kolahdouz-Mohammadi R., et al. The responses of different dosages of egg consumption on blood lipid profile: An updated systematic review and meta-analysis of randomized clinical trials. *J Food Biochem.* 2020;44(8):e13263.
31. US Department of Agriculture and US Department of Health and Human Services. *Dietary Guidelines for Americans, 2010-2015.* 7th ed. Washington, DC: US Department of Agriculture; 2010.
32. World Health Organization. *Guideline: Sugars Intake for Adults and Children.* Geneva, Switzerland: World Health Organization; 2015. https://www.who.int/publications/i/item/9789241549028.
33. Drewnowski A., Rehm C. D. Consumption of added sugars among US children and adults by food purchase location and food source. *Am J Clin Nutr.* 2014;100(3):901-907. https://www.ncbi.nlm.nih.gov/pubmed/25030785.
34. Johnson R. K., Appel L. J., Brands M., et al. Dietary sugars intake and cardiovascular health: a scientific statement from the American Heart Association. *Circulation.* 2009;120(11):1011-1020. https://www.ncbi.nlm.nih.gov/pubmed/19704096.
35. Bailey R. L., Fulgoni V. L., Cowan A. E., Gaine P. C. Sources of added sugars in young children, adolescents, and adults with low and high intakes of added sugars. *Nutrients.* 2018;10(1):102.
36. US Department of Agriculture. Nutrient lists from standard reference legacy (2018). 2018. https://www.nal.usda.gov/fnic/nutrient-lists-standard-reference-legacy-2018
37. Xu Z., McClure S. T., Appel L. J. Dietary cholesterol intake and sources among US adults: results from National Health and Nutrition Examination Surveys (NHANES), 2001–2014. *Nutrients.* 2018;10(6):771.
38. Carson J. A. S., Lichtenstein A. H., Anderson C. A. M., et al. Dietary cholesterol and cardiovascular risk: a science advisory from the American Heart Association. *Circulation.* 2020;141(3):e39-e53.
39. Sacks F. M., Lichtenstein A. H., Wu J. H. Y, et al. Dietary fats and cardiovascular disease: a presidential advisory from the American Heart Association. *Circulation.* 2017;136(3):e1-e23.
40. O'Neil C. E., Keast D. R., Fulgoni V. L., Nicklas T. A. Food sources of energy and nutrients among adults in the US: NHANES 2003-2006. *Nutrients.* 2012;4(12):2097-2120. http://www.ncbi.nlm.nih.gov/pubmed/23363999.
41. Harnack L. J., Cogswell M. E., Shikany J. M., et al. Sources of sodium in US adults from 3 geographic regions. *Circulation.* 2017;135(19):1775-1783.
42. US Food and Drug Administration. Final determination regarding partially hydrogenated oils (removing trans fat). May 18, 2018. https://www.fda.gov/food/food-additives-petitions/final-determination-regarding-partially-hydrogenated-oils-removing-trans-fat.
43. Mozaffarian D., Aro A., Willett W. C. Health effects of trans-fatty acids: experimental and observational evidence. *Eur J Clin Nutr.* 2009;63 Suppl 2:S5-21.
44. Arnett D. K., Blumenthal R. S., Albert M. A., et al. 2019 ACC/AHA guideline on the primary prevention of cardiovascular disease: executive summary: a report of the American College of Cardiology/American Heart Association Task Force on Clinical Practice Guidelines. *J Am Coll Cardiol.* 2019;74(10):1376-1414.
45. US Food and Drug Administration, Center for Food Safety and Applied Nutrition. *A Food Labeling Guide: Guidance for Industry.* Washington, DC: US Department of Health and Human Services; 2013.
46. US Food and Drug Administration. 21CFR101.54: Nutrient content claims for "good source," "high," "more," and "high potency." Updated April 1, 2020. www.accessdata.fda.gov.
47. Heaney R. P., Weaver C. M. Calcium absorption from kale. *Am J Clin Nutr.* 1990;51(4):656-657.
48. Oliveira R. Getting clarity about calcium. May 21, 2015. https://www.forksoverknives.com/wellness/milk-myth-why-you-dont-need-dairy-for-calcium/.
49. Melse-Boonstra A. Bioavailability of micronutrients from nutrient-dense whole foods: zooming in on dairy, vegetables, and fruits. *Front Nutr.* 2020;7:101-101. https://pubmed.ncbi.nlm.nih.gov/32793622
50. Melina V., Craig W., Levin S. Position of the Academy of Nutrition and Dietetics: vegetarian diets. *J Acad Nutr Diet.* 2016;116(12):1970-1980.
51. Anderson J. W., Baird P., Davis R. H. Jr., et al. Health benefits of dietary fiber. *Nutr Rev.* 2009;67(4):188-205.
52. Abdelhamid A. S., Brown T. J., Brainard J. S., et al. Omega-3 fatty acids for the primary and secondary prevention of cardiovascular disease. *Cochrane Database Syst Rev.* 2020;3(2):Cd003177.
53. National Institutes of Health, Office of Dietary Supplements. *Vitamin D: Fact Sheet for Professionals.* Bethesda, MD: National Institutes of Health; 2014.
54. Nair R., Maseeh A. Vitamin D: The "sunshine" vitamin. *J Pharmacol Pharmacother.* 2012;3(2):118-126. https://pubmed.ncbi.nlm.nih.gov/22629085.
55. Afshin A., Sur P. J., Fay K. A., et al. Health effects of dietary risks in 195 countries, 1990–2017: a systematic analysis for the Global Burden of Disease Study 2017. *Lancet.* 2019;393(10184):1958-1972.
56. Chung R. T. M. Detoxification effects of phytonutrients against environmental toxicants and sharing of clinical experience on practical applications. *Environ Sci Pollut Res.* 2017;24:8946–8956. https://doi.org/10.1007/s11356-015-5263-3
57. Pollan M. *In Defense of Food: An Eater's Manifesto.* New York, NY: Penguin Publishing Group; 2008.
58. Middleton E. Jr., Kandaswami C., Theoharides T. C. The effects of plant flavonoids on mammalian cells: implications for inflammation, heart disease, and cancer. *Pharmacol Rev.* 2000;52(4):673-751.
59. Ali B., Khandaker L., Oba S. Comparative study on functional components, antioxidant activity and color parameters of selected colored leafy vegetables as affected by photoperiods. *J Food Agric Environ.* 2009;7(3-4):392-398.
60. Karlsen M. C., Rogers G., Miki A., et al. Theoretical food and nutrient composition of whole-food plant-based and vegan diets compared to current dietary recommendations. *Nutrients.* 2019;11(3):625. https://www.ncbi.nlm.nih.gov/pubmed/30875784.
61. Tuso P. J., Ismail M. H., Ha B. P., Bartolotto C. Nutritional update for physicians: plant-based diets. *Perm J.* 2013;17(2):61-66. http://www.ncbi.nlm.nih.gov/pubmed/23704846.

62. Jenkins D. J., Kendall C. W., Marchie A., et al. Effects of a dietary portfolio of cholesterol-lowering foods vs lovastatin on serum lipids and C-reactive protein. *JAMA.* 2003;290(4):502-510.
63. Jenkins D. J., Kendall C. W., Faulkner D. A., et al. Assessment of the longer-term effects of a dietary portfolio of cholesterol-lowering foods in hypercholesterolemia. *Am J Clin Nutr.* 2006;83(3):582-591.
64. Appel L. J., Moore T. J., Obarzanek E., et al. A clinical trial of the effects of dietary patterns on blood pressure. DASH Collaborative Research Group. *N Engl J Med.* 1997;336(16):1117-1124.
65. Sacks F. M., Svetkey L. P., Vollmer W. M., et al. Effects on blood pressure of reduced dietary sodium and the Dietary Approaches to Stop Hypertension (DASH) diet. DASH-Sodium Collaborative Research Group. *N Engl J Med.* 2001;344(1):3-10.
66. Ornish D., Scherwitz L. W., Billings J. H., et al. Intensive lifestyle changes for reversal of coronary heart disease. *JAMA.* 1998;280(23):2001-2007. http://www.ncbi.nlm.nih.gov/pubmed/9863851.
67. Ornish D., Brown S. E., Scherwitz L. W., et al. Can lifestyle changes reverse coronary heart disease? The Lifestyle Heart Trial. *Lancet.* 1990;336(8708):129-133.
68. Ornish D., Magbanua M. J., Weidner G., et al. Changes in prostate gene expression in men undergoing an intensive nutrition and lifestyle intervention. *Proc Natl Acad Sci USA.* 2008;105(24):8369-8374.
69. de Lorgeril M., Salen P., Martin J. L., Monjaud I., Delaye J., Mamelle N. Mediterranean diet, traditional risk factors, and the rate of cardiovascular complications after myocardial infarction: final report of the Lyon Diet Heart Study. *Circulation.* 1999;99(6):779-785.
70. de Lorgeril M., Renaud S., Mamelle N., et al. Mediterranean alpha-linolenic acid-rich diet in secondary prevention of coronary heart disease. *Lancet.* 1994;343(8911):1454-1459.
71. Esselstyn C. B. A plant-based diet and coronary artery disease: a mandate for effective therapy. *J Geriatr Cardiol.* 2017;14(5):317-320.
72. Esselstyn C. B., Jr., Gendy G., Doyle J., Golubic M., Roizen M. F. A way to reverse CAD? *J Fam Pract.* 2014;63(7):356-364b. http://www.ncbi.nlm.nih.gov/pubmed/25198208.
73. Shurney D., Hyde S., Hulsey K., Elam R., Cooper A., Groves J. CHIP lifestyle program at Vanderbilt University demonstrates an early ROI for a diabetic cohort in a workplace setting: a case study. *J Man Care Med.* 2012;15(4):5-15.
74. Barnard N. D., Cohen J., Jenkins D. J., et al. A low-fat vegan diet improves glycemic control and cardiovascular risk factors in a randomized clinical trial in individuals with type 2 diabetes. *Diabetes Care.* 2006;29(8):1777-1783. http://www.ncbi.nlm.nih.gov/pubmed/16873779.
75. Lianov L., Johnson M. Physician competencies for prescribing lifestyle medicine. *JAMA.* 2010;304(2):202-203.
76. US Preventive Services Task Force. Grade definitions. 2018; https://www.uspreventiveservicestaskforce.org/Page/Name/grade-definitions. Accessed August 25, 2017.
77. US Preventive Services Task Force. Healthy diet and physical activity for cardiovascular disease prevention in adults with cardiovascular risk factors: behavioral counseling interventions. November 24, 2020; https://www.uspreventiveservicestaskforce.org/uspstf/recommendation/healthy-diet-and-physical-activity-counseling-adults-with-high-risk-of-cvd. Accessed 2021 .
78. US Preventive Services Task Force. Healthful diet and physical activity for cardiovascular disease prevention in adults without known risk factors: behavioral counseling. July 11, 2017; https://www.uspreventiveservicestaskforce.org/uspstf/recommendation/healthful-diet-and-physical-activity-for-cardiovascular-disease-prevention-in-adults-without-known-risk-factors-behavioral-counseling. Accessed 2021.
79. Heber D, Li Z. *Primary Care Nutrition: Writing the Nutrition Prescription.* Boca Raton, FL: CRC Press, Taylor & Francis Group; 2017.
80. Grandes G., Sanchez A., Sanchez-Pinilla R. O., et al. Effectiveness of physical activity advice and prescription by physicians in routine primary care: a cluster randomized trial. *Arch Intern Med.* 2009;169(7):694-701.
81. Ash S., Campbell K. L., Bogard J., Millichamp A. Nutrition prescription to achieve positive outcomes in chronic kidney disease: a systematic review. *Nutrients.* 2014;6(1):416-451.
82. Norgan N. G. Laboratory and field measurements of body composition. Public Health *Nutrition.* 2005;8(7a):1108-1122. https://pubmed.ncbi.nlm.nih.gov/16277823/.
83. Duren D. L., Sherwood R. J., Czerwinski S. A., et al. Body composition methods: comparisons and interpretation. *J Diabetes Sci Technol.* 2008;2(6):1139-1146. https://pubmed.ncbi.nlm.nih.gov/19885303.
84. National Institutes of Health, National Cancer Institute. Automated Self-Administered 24-Hour (ASA24®) dietary assessment tool. Updated October 5, 2020; https://epi.grants.cancer.gov/asa24/. Accessed 2021.
85. Johnson R. K., Driscoll P., Goran M. I. Comparison of multiple-pass 24-hour recall estimates of energy intake with total energy expenditure determined by the doubly labeled water method in young children. *J Am Diet Assoc.* 1996;96(11):1140-1144.
86. Nestlé Nutrition Institute. *MNA Mini Nutritional Assessment*. Nestlé Nutrition Institute; 2009: http://www.mna-elderly.com/.
87. US Department of Agriculture, Food and Nutrition Information Center. Individual dietary assessment. https://www.nal.usda.gov/fnic/individual-dietary-assessment. Accessed 2018.
88. NutritionQuest. Web-based wellness solutions: fat intake screener. 2019; https://nutritionquest.com/wellness/free-assessment-tools-for-individuals/fat-intake-screener/. Accessed 2021.
89. NutritionQuest. Web-based wellness solutions: fruit/vegetable/fiber screener. 2019; https://nutritionquest.com/wellness/free-assessment-tools-for-individuals/fruit-vegetable-fiber-screener/. Accessed 2021.
90. Ask the Dietitian. Healthy body calculator. https://www.dietitian.com/healthy-body-calculator/. Accessed 2021.
91. US Department of Agriculture, Food and Nutrition Information Center. Calculators and counters. https://www.nal.usda.gov/fnic/calculators-and-counters. Accessed 2018.
92. Institute of Medicine. *Dietary Reference Intakes for Energy, Carbohydrate, Fiber, Fat, Fatty Acids, Cholesterol, Protein, and Amino Acids*. Washington, DC: The National Academies Press; 2015. https://doi.org/10.17226/10490.

93. Kumar V., Sharma A., Kohli S. K., et al. Amino acids distribution in economical important plants: a review. *Biotechnol Res Innovation.* 2019;3(2):197-207. http://www.sciencedirect.com/science/article/pii/S2452072119300449.

94. Gropper S. A. S., Smith J. L., Groff J. L. *Advanced Nutrition and Human Metabolism.* Australia; United States: Wadsworth/Cengage Learning; 2009.

95. Brosnan J. T., Brosnan M. E. The sulfur-containing amino acids: an overview. *J Nutr.* 2006;136(6 Suppl):1636s-1640s.

96. Millward D. J. Optimal intakes of protein in the human diet. *Proc Nutr Soc.* 1999;58(2):403-413.

97. Darling A. L., Millward D. J., Lanham-New S. A. Dietary protein and bone health: towards a synthesised view. *Proc Nutr Soc.* 2020:1-8.

98. Shams-White M. M., Chung M., Fu Z., et al. Animal versus plant protein and adult bone health: a systematic review and meta-analysis from the National Osteoporosis Foundation. *PloS one.* 2018;13(2):e0192459.

99. Young V. R., Pellett P. L. Plant proteins in relation to human protein and amino acid *nutrition. Am J Clin Nutr.* 1994;59(5 Suppl):1203S-1212S. https://www.ncbi.nlm.nih.gov/pubmed/8172124.

100. Gardner C. D., Hartle J. C., Garrett R. D., Offringa L. C., Wasserman A. S. Maximizing the intersection of human health and the health of the environment with regard to the amount and type of protein produced and consumed in the United States. *Nutr Rev.* 2019;77(4):197-215.

101. Liu A. G., Ford N. A., Hu F. B., Zelman K. M., Mozaffarian D., Kris-Etherton P. M. A healthy approach to dietary fats: understanding the science and taking action to reduce consumer confusion. *Nutr J.* 2017;16(1):53-53.

102. Astrup A., Bertram H. C. S., Bonjour J., et al. WHO draft guidelines on dietary saturated and trans fatty acids: time for a new approach? *BMJ.* 2019;366:l4137.

103. Virtanen J. K., Mursu J., Voutilainen S., Tuomainen T. The associations of serum n-6 polyunsaturated fatty acids with serum C-reactive protein in men: the Kuopio Ischaemic Heart Disease Risk Factor Study. *Eur J Clin Nutr.* 2018;72(3):342-348.

104. Wang X., Lin H., Gu Y. Multiple roles of dihomo-γ-linolenic acid against proliferation diseases. *Lipids Health Dis.* 2012;11(1):25-25.

105. Innes J. K., Calder P. C. Omega-6 fatty acids and inflammation. *Prostaglandins Leukot Essent Fatty Acids.* 2018;132:41-48.

106. Bersch-Ferreira Â. C., Sampaio G. R., Gehringer M. O., et al. Association between polyunsaturated fatty acids and inflammatory markers in patients in secondary prevention of cardiovascular disease. *Nutrition.* 2016;37:30-36.

107. Johnson G. H., Fritsche K. Effect of dietary linoleic acid on markers of inflammation in healthy persons: a systematic review of randomized controlled trials. *J Acad Nutri Diet.* 2012;112(7):1029-1041.e1015.

108. O'Sullivan T. A., Hafekost K., Mitrou F., Lawrence D. Food sources of saturated fat and the association with mortality: a meta-analysis. *Am J Pub Health.* 2013;103(9):e31-e42. https://pubmed.ncbi.nlm.nih.gov/23865702.

109. Denke M. A., Grundy S. M. Comparison of effects of lauric acid and palmitic acid on plasma lipids and lipoproteins. *Am J of Clin Nutr.* 1992;56(5):895-898. https://doi.org/10.1093/ajcn/56.5.895.

110. Hima Bindu G., Veena S. R., Vijay V. K. Friend turns foe: transformation of anti-inflammatory HDL to proinflammatory HDL during acute-phase response. *Cholesterol.* 2010;2011:274629-274627.

111. Kontush A. HDL particle number and size as predictors of cardiovascular disease. *Front Pharmacol.* 2015;6:218-218.

112. Krauss R. M. Lipoprotein subfractions and cardiovascular disease risk. *Curr Opin Lipidol.* 2010;21(4):305-311.

113. Zong G., Li Y., Wanders A. J, et al. Intake of individual saturated fatty acids and risk of coronary heart disease in US men and women: two prospective longitudinal cohort studies. *BMJ.* 2016;355:i5796. https://www.bmj.com/content/bmj/355/bmj.i5796.full.pdf.

114. Wang D. D., Li Y., Chiuve S. E., et al. Association of specific dietary fats with total and cause-specific mortality. *JAMA Internal Medicine.* 2016;176(8):1134-1145. https://doi.org/10.1001/jamainternmed.2016.2417.

115. Harvey K. A., Walker C. L., Pavlina T. M., Xu Z., Zaloga G. P., Siddiqui R. A. Long-chain saturated fatty acids induce pro-inflammatory responses and impact endothelial cell growth. *Clin Nutr.* 2010;29(4):492-500.

116. Zampetaki A., Kirton J. P., Xu Q. Vascular repair by endothelial progenitor cells. *Cardiovasc Res.* 2008;78(3):413-421. https://doi.org/10.1093/cvr/cvn081.

117. May-Wilson S., Sud A., Law P. J., et al. Pro-inflammatory fatty acid profile and colorectal cancer risk: a Mendelian randomisation analysis. *Euro J Cancer.* 2017;84:228-238. http://www.sciencedirect.com/science/article/pii/S0959804917311541.

118. Mu Y. M., Yanase T., Nishi Y., et al. Saturated FFAs, palmitic acid and stearic acid, induce apoptosis in human granulosa cells. *Endocrinology.* 2001;142(8):3590-3597. https://doi.org/10.1210/endo.142.8.8293.

119. Olivieri O., Speziali G., Castagna A., et al. The positive association between plasma myristic acid and ApoCIII concentrations in cardiovascular disease patients is supported by the effects of myristic acid in HepG2 cells. *J Nutr.* 2020;150(10):2707-2715. https://doi.org/10.1093/jn/nxaa202.

120. Temme E. H., Mensink R. P., Hornstra G. Effects of medium chain fatty acids (MCFA), myristic acid, and oleic acid on serum lipoproteins in healthy subjects. *J Lipid Res.* 1997;38(9):1746-1754.

121. de Souza R. J., Mente A., Maroleanu A., et al. Intake of saturated and trans unsaturated fatty acids and risk of all cause mortality, cardiovascular disease, and type 2 diabetes: systematic review and meta-analysis of observational studies. *BMJ.* 2015;351:h3978.

122. Hermann J. FDA cuts trans fat in processed foods. 2015. https://education.okstate.edu/outreach/fcs/site-files/research/FDA-Cuts-Trans-Fat-in-Processed-Food.pdf.

123. Reynolds A., Mann J., Cummings J., Winter N., Mete E., Te Morenga L. Carbohydrate quality and human health: a series of systematic reviews and meta-analyses. *Lancet.* 2019;393(10170):434-445. https://www.thelancet.com/pdfs/journals/lancet/PIIS0140-6736(18)31809-9.pdf.

124. Liu S. Intake of refined carbohydrates and whole-grain foods in relation to risk of type 2 diabetes mellitus and coronary heart disease. *J Am Coll Nutr.* 2002;21(4):298-306.

125. Kahleova H., Dort S., Holubkov R., Barnard N. D. A plant-based high-carbohydrate, low-fat diet in overweight individuals in a 16-week randomized clinical trial: the role of carbohydrates. *Nutrients.* 2018;10(9). https://res.mdpi.com/d_attachment/nutrients/nutrients-10-01302/article_deploy/nutrients-10-01302.pdf.

126. Bradley P. Refined carbohydrates, phenotypic plasticity and the obesity epidemic. *Med Hypotheses.* 2019;131:109317-109317.

127. Yu D., Shu X. O., Li H., et al. Dietary carbohydrates, refined grains, glycemic load, and risk of coronary heart disease in Chinese adults. *Am J Epidemiol.* 2013;178(10):1542-1549.

128. Sun Q., Spiegelman D., van Dam R. M., et al. White rice, brown rice, and risk of type 2 diabetes in US men and women. *Arch Intern Med.* 2010;170(11):961-969. https://doi.org/10.1001/archinternmed.2010.109.

129. Anderson J. W., Chen W. J. L. Plant fiber, carbohydrate and lipid metabolism. *Am J Clin Nutr.* 1979;32(2):346-363. https://doi.org/10.1093/ajcn/32.2.346.

130. Weickert M. O., Pfeiffer A. F. H. Impact of dietary fiber consumption on insulin resistance and the prevention of type 2 diabetes. *J Nutr.* 2018;148(1):7-12.

131. Veronese N., Solmi M., Caruso M. G., et al. Dietary fiber and health outcomes: an umbrella review of systematic reviews and meta-analyses. *Am J Clin Nutr.* 2018;107(3):436-444.

132. Jenkins D. J., Kendall C. W., Popovich D. G., et al. Effect of a very-high-fiber vegetable, fruit, and nut diet on serum lipids and colonic function. *Metabolism.* 2001;50(4):494-503.

133. Hervik A. K., Svihus B. The role of fiber in energy balance. *J Nutr Metab.* 2019;2019:4983657-4983657. https://pubmed.ncbi.nlm.nih.gov/30805214.

134. Parada V. D., De la Fuente M. K., Landskron G., et al. Short chain fatty acids (SCFAs)-mediated gut epithelial and immune regulation and its relevance for inflammatory bowel diseases. *Front Immunol.* 2019;10(277). https://www.frontiersin.org/article/10.3389/fimmu.2019.00277.

135. Camilleri M. Leaky gut: mechanisms, measurement and clinical implications in humans. *Gut.* 2019;68(8):1516-1526.

136. Haber G. B., Heaton K. W., Murphy D., Burroughs L. F. Depletion and disruption of dietary fibre. Effects on satiety, plasma-glucose, and serum-insulin. *Lancet.* 1977;2(8040):679-682.

137. Brown L., Rosner B., Willett W. W, Sacks F. M. Cholesterol-lowering effects of dietary fiber: a meta-analysis. *Am J Clin Nutr.* 1999;69(1):30-42. https://doi.org/10.1093/ajcn/69.1.30.

138. Riccardi G., Rivellese A. A. Effects of dietary fiber and carbohydrate on glucose and lipoprotein metabolism in diabetic patients. *Diabetes Care.* 1991;14(12):1115-1125.

139. Ohlsson B., Darwiche G., Roth B., Bengtsson M., Höglund P. High fiber fat and protein contents lead to increased satiety reduced sweet cravings and decreased gastrointestinal symptoms independently of anthropometric hormonal and metabolic factors. *J Diabetes Metab.* 2017;8:3.

140. Ocvirk S., Wilson A. S., Appolonia C. N., Thomas T. K., O'Keefe S. J. D. Fiber, fat, and colorectal cancer: new insight into modifiable dietary risk factors. *Curr Gastroenterol Rep.* 2019;21(11):62.

141. Institute of Medicine. *Dietary Reference Intakes: The Essential Guide to Nutrient Requirements.* Washington, DC: The National Academies Press; 2006.

142. Carlsen M. H., Halvorsen B. L., Holte K., et al. The total antioxidant content of more than 3100 foods, beverages, spices, herbs and supplements used worldwide. *Nutr J.* 2010;9:3.

143. Burton-Freeman B., Sesso H. D. Whole food versus supplement: comparing the clinical evidence of tomato intake and lycopene supplementation on cardiovascular risk factors. *Adv Nutr.* 2014;5(5):457-485.

144. Riso P., Soldati L. Food ingredients and supplements: is this the future? *J Transl Med.* 2012;10:227.

145. Ford E. S., Bergmann M. M., Kröger J., Schienkiewitz A., Weikert C., Boeing H. Healthy living is the best revenge: findings from the European Prospective Investigation Into Cancer and Nutrition-Potsdam study. *Arch Intern Med.* 2009;169(15):1355-1362.

146. Littleton R. M., Miller M., Hove J. R. Whole plant based treatment of hypercholesterolemia with Crataegus laevigata in a zebrafish model. *BMC Complement Altern Med.* 2012;12:105.

147. Hlebowicz J., Persson M., Gullberg B., et al. Food patterns, inflammation markers and incidence of cardiovascular disease: the Malmö Diet and Cancer study. *J Intern Med.* 2011;270(4):365-376.

148. Bouvard V., Loomis D., Guyton K. Z., et al. Carcinogenicity of consumption of red and processed meat. *Lancet Oncol.* 2015;16(16):1599-1600.

149. López-Moreno J., García-Carpintero S., Jimenez-Lucena R., et al. Effect of dietary lipids on endotoxemia influences postprandial inflammatory response. *J Agric Food Chem.* 2017;65(35):7756-7763.

150. Morrison M. C., Mulder P., Stavro P. M., et al. Replacement of dietary saturated fat by PUFA-rich pumpkin seed oil attenuates non-alcoholic fatty liver disease and atherosclerosis development, with additional health effects of virgin over refined oil. *PLoS One.* 2015;10(9):e0139196.

151. Peña-Orihuela P., Camargo A., Rangel-Zuñiga O. A., et al. Antioxidant system response is modified by dietary fat in adipose tissue of metabolic syndrome patients. *J Nutr Biochem.* 2013;24(10):1717-1723.

152. American Cancer Society. Known and probable human carcinogens. Updated August 14, 2019. https://www.cancer.org/cancer/cancer-causes/general-info/known-and-probable-human-carcinogens.html.

153. Uribarri J., Woodruff S., Goodman S., et al. Advanced glycation end products in foods and a practical guide to their reduction in the diet. *J Am Diet Assoc.* 2010;110(6):911-916.e912.

154. Dyer D. G., Blackledge J. A., Katz B. M., et al. The maillard reaction in vivo. *Zeitschrift fur Ernahrungswissenschaft.* 1991;30(1):29-45.

155. Uribarri J., del Castillo M. D., de la Maza M. P., et al. Dietary advanced glycation end products and their role in health and disease. *Adv Nutr.* 2015;6(4):461-473.

156. Hashemzadeh M., Rahimi A., Zare-Farashbandi F., Alavi-Naeini A. M., Daei A. Transtheoretical model of health behavioral change: A systematic review. *Iran J Nurs Midwifery Res.* 2019;24(2):83.

157. Lacagnina S., Tips J., Pauly K., Cara K., Karlsen M. Lifestyle medicine shared medical appointments. *Am J Lifestyle Med.* 2020:1559827620943819.

158. Kelly J., Karlsen M., Steinke G. Type 2 diabetes remission and lifestyle medicine: a position statement from the American College of Lifestyle Medicine. *Am J Lifestyle Med.* 2020:1559827620930962.

159. Orlich M. J., Singh P. N., Sabate J., et al. Vegetarian dietary patterns and mortality in Adventist Health Study 2. *JAMA Intern Med.* 2013;173(13):1230-1238. http://www.ncbi.nlm.nih.gov/pubmed/23836264 http://archinte.jamanetwork.com/data/Journals/INTEMED/927256/ioi130047.pdf.

160. Orlich M. J., Fraser G. E. Vegetarian diets in the Adventist Health Study 2: a review of initial published findings. *Am J Clin Nutr.* 2014;100 Suppl 1:353s-358s.

161. Li Y., Hruby A., Bernstein A. M., et al. Saturated fats compared with unsaturated fats and sources of carbohydrates in relation to risk of coronary heart disease: a prospective cohort study. *J Am Coll Cardiol.* 2015;66(14):1538-1548.

162. Campbell T. C., Parpia B., Chen J. Diet, lifestyle, and the etiology of coronary artery disease: the Cornell China study. *Am J Cardiol.* 1998;82(10):18t-21t.

163. Appel L. J., Espeland M. A., Easter L., Wilson A. C., Folmar S., Lacy C. R. Effects of reduced sodium intake on hypertension control in older individuals: results from the Trial of Nonpharmacologic Interventions in the Elderly (TONE). *Arch Intern Med.* 2001;161(5):685-693. https://doi.org/10.1001/archinte.161.5.685.

164. US Department of Agriculture and US Department of Health and Human Services. Appendix 7 nutritional goals for age-sex groups based on dietary reference intakes and dietary guidelines recommendations. In: *Dietary Guidelines for Americans 2015-2020.* Washington, DC: US Department of Health and Human Services; 2015. https://health.gov/our-work/food-nutrition/2015-2020-dietary-guidelines/guidelines/appendix-7/,.

165. US Food and Drug Administration. Sodium in your diet. Updated April 2, 2020. https://www.fda.gov/food/nutrition-education-resources-materials/sodium-your-diet.

166. Santana N. M. T., Mill J. G., Velasquez-Melendez G., et al. Consumption of alcohol and blood pressure: results of the ELSA-Brasil study. *PloS one.* 2018;13(1):e0190239-e0190239. https://pubmed.ncbi.nlm.nih.gov/29309408.

167. Whelton P. K., Carey R. M., Aronow W. S., et al. 2017 ACC/AHA/AAPA/ABC/ACPM/AGS/APhA/ASH/ASPC/NMA/PCNA guideline for the prevention, detection, evaluation, and management of high blood pressure in adults: a report of the American College of Cardiology/American Heart Association Task Force on Clinical Practice Guidelines. *Hypertension.* 2018;71(6):e13-e115.

168. Moore T. J., Conlin P. R., Ard J., Svetkey L. P. DASH (Dietary Approaches to Stop Hypertension) diet is effective treatment for stage 1 isolated systolic hypertension. *Hypertension.* 2001;38(2):155-158.

169. Ried K. Garlic lowers blood pressure in hypertensive individuals, regulates serum cholesterol, and stimulates immunity: an updated meta-analysis and review. *J Nutr.* 2016;146(2):389S-396S. https://doi.org/10.3945/jn.114.202192.

170. Goldhamer A., Lisle D., Parpia B., Anderson S. V., Campbell T. C. Medically supervised water-only fasting in the treatment of hypertension. *J Manipulative Physiol Ther.* 2001;24(5):335-339.

171. McCarty M. F. A preliminary fast may potentiate response to a subsequent low-salt, low-fat vegan diet in the management of hypertension - fasting as a strategy for breaking metabolic vicious cycles. *Med Hypotheses.* 2003;60(5):624-633.

172. Landau R. L., Rochman H., Blix-Gruber P., Rubenstein A. H. The protein-sparing action of protein feeding: absence of relationship to insulin secretion. *Am J Clin Nutr.* 1981;34(7):1300-1304. https://doi.org/10.1093/ajcn/34.7.1300.

173. Tonstad S., Butler T., Yan R., Fraser G. E. Type of vegetarian diet, body weight, and prevalence of type 2 diabetes. *Diabetes Care.* 2009;32(5):791-796.

174. Lee Y., Park K. Adherence to a vegetarian diet and diabetes risk: a systematic review and meta-analysis of observational studies. *Nutrients.* 2017;9(6).

175. Gross L. S., Li L., Ford E. S., Liu S. Increased consumption of refined carbohydrates and the epidemic of type 2 diabetes in the United States: an ecologic assessment. *Am J Clin Nutr.* 2004;79(5):774-779.

176. Payne A. N., Chassard C., Lacroix C. Gut microbial adaptation to dietary consumption of fructose, artificial sweeteners and sugar alcohols: implications for host-microbe interactions contributing to obesity. *Obes Rev.* 2012;13(9):799-809.

177. Ojo O., Feng Q., Ojo Osarhumwese O., Wang X.. The role of dietary fibre in modulating gut microbiota dysbiosis in patients with type 2 diabetes: a systematic review and meta-analysis of randomised controlled trials. *Nutrients.* 2020;12(11):3239.

178. Greenwald P. Lifestyle and medical approaches to cancer prevention. In: Senn H. J., Morant R., eds., T*umor Prevention and Genetics III. Recent Results in Cancer Research.* Berlin, Heidelberg: Springer; 2005:1-15.

179. Saha S. K., Lee S. B., Won J., et al. Correlation between oxidative stress, nutrition, and cancer initiation. *Int J Mol Sci.* 2017;18(7):1544.

180. Ornish D., Weidner G., Fair W. R., et al. Intensive lifestyle changes may affect the progression of prostate cancer. *J Urol.* 2005;174(3):1065-1070. http://www.sciencedirect.com/science/article/pii/S0022534701685185.

181. Peisch S. F., Van Blarigan E. L., Chan J. M., Stampfer M. J., Kenfield S. A. Prostate cancer progression and mortality: a review of diet and lifestyle factors. *World J Urol.* 2017;35(6):867-874. https://doi.org/10.1007/s00345-016-1914-3.

182. Levine M. E., Suarez J. A., Brandhorst S., et al. Low protein intake is associated with a major reduction in IGF-1, cancer, and overall mortality in the 65 and younger but not older population. *Cell Metabol.* 2014;19(3):407-417. http://www.ncbi.nlm.nih.gov/pubmed/24606898.

183. Campbell T. C., Junshi C. Diet and chronic degenerative diseases: perspectives from China. *Am J Clin Nutr.* 1994;59(5 Suppl):1153S-1161S. http://www.ncbi.nlm.nih.gov/pubmed/8172116.

184. Halliwell B. The antioxidant paradox. *Lancet.* 2000;355(9210):1179-1180. http://www.sciencedirect.com/science/article/pii/S0140673600020754.

185. Aune D, Chan D. S. M., Lau R., et al. Dietary fibre, whole-grains, and risk of colorectal cancer: systematic review and dose-response meta-analysis of prospective studies. *BMJ*. 2011;343:d6617. https://www.bmj.com/content/bmj/343/bmj.d6617.full.pdf.
186. American Gastroenterological Association. American Gastroenterological Association medical position statement: impact of dietary fiber on colon cancer occurrence. *Gastroenterology*. 2000;118(6):1233-1234. http://www.sciencedirect.com/science/article/pii/S0016508500703763.
187. Sales C. H., Fontanelli M. M, Vieira D. A. S, Marchioni D. M., Fisberg R. M. Inadequate dietary intake of minerals: prevalence and association with socio-demographic and lifestyle factors. *Br J Nutr*. 2017;117(2):267-277.
188. Burkitt D. P. The etiological significance of related diseases. *Can Fam Physician*. 1976;22:63-71.
189. Burkitt D. P. Western diseases and their emergence related to diet. *South African Med J*. 1982;61(26):1013-1015.
190. Trowell H. C., Burkitt D. P. The development of the concept of dietary fibre. *Mol Aspects Med*. 1987;9(1):7-15.
191. Frattaroli J., Weidner G., Dnistrian A. M., et al. Clinical events in prostate cancer lifestyle trial: results from two years of follow-up. *Urology*. 2008;72(6):1319-1323. http://www.ncbi.nlm.nih.gov/pubmed/18602144.
192. Barnard R. J., Gonzalez J. H., Liva M. E., Ngo T. H. Effects of a low-fat, high-fiber diet and exercise program on breast cancer risk factors in vivo and tumor cell growth and apoptosis in vitro. *Nutr Cancer*. 2006;55(1):28-34. https://www.tandfonline.com/doi/abs/10.1207/s15327914nc5501_4.
193. Pierce J. P., Stefanick M. L., Flatt S. W., et al. Greater survival after breast cancer in physically active women with high vegetable-fruit intake regardless of obesity. *J Clin Oncol*. 2007;25(17):2345-2351. http://jco.ascopubs.org/content/25/17/2345.full.pdf.
194. Katan M. B., Boekschoten M. V., Connor W. E., et al. Which are the greatest recent discoveries and the greatest future challenges in nutrition? *Eur J Clin Nutr*. 2009;63(1):2-10.
195. Tonstad S., Stewart K., Oda K., Batech M., Herring R. P., Fraser G. E. Vegetarian diets and incidence of diabetes in the Adventist Health Study-2. *Nutr Metab Cardiovasc Dis*. 2013;23(4):292-299.
196. Anderson J. W., Ward K. High-carbohydrate, high-fiber diets for insulin-treated men with diabetes mellitus. *Am J Clin Nutr*. 1979;32(11):2312-2321.
197. Trapp C. B., Barnard N. D. Usefulness of vegetarian and vegan diets for treating type 2 diabetes. *Curr Diab Rep*. 2010;10(2):152-158.
198. Dunaief D. M., Fuhrman J., Dunaief J., Ying G. Glycemic and cardiovascular parameters improved in type 2 diabetes with the high nutrient density (HND) diet. *Open J Prev Med*. 2012;2:364-371.
199. Barnard N. D., Cohen J., Jenkins D. J., et al. A low-fat vegan diet and a conventional diabetes diet in the treatment of type 2 diabetes: a randomized, controlled, 74-wk clinical trial. *Am J Clin Nutr*. 2009;89(5):1588S-1596S. http://www.ncbi.nlm.nih.gov/pubmed/19339401.
200. Pettersen B. J., Anousheh R., Fan J., Jaceldo-Siegl K., Fraser G. E. Vegetarian diets and blood pressure among white subjects: results from the Adventist Health Study-2 (AHS-2). *Public Health Nutr*. 2012;15(10):1909-1916. http://www.ncbi.nlm.nih.gov/pubmed/22230619.
201. McDougall J., Litzau K., Haver E., Saunders V., Spiller G. A. Rapid reduction of serum cholesterol and blood pressure by a twelve-day, very low fat, strictly vegetarian diet. *J Am Coll Nutr*. 1995;14(5):491-496.
202. Appleby P. N., Allen N. E., Key T. J. Diet, vegetarianism, and cataract risk. *Am J Clin Nutr*. 2011;93(5):1128-1135.
203. Walda I. C., Tabak C., Smit H. A., et al. Diet and 20-year chronic obstructive pulmonary disease mortality in middle-aged men from three European countries. *Eur J Clin Nutr*. 2002;56(7):638-643.
204. Keranis E., Makris D., Rodopoulou P., et al. Impact of dietary shift to higher-antioxidant foods in COPD: a randomised trial. *Eur Respir J*. 2010;36(4):774-780.
205. Lin J., Hu F. B., Curhan G. C. Associations of diet with albuminuria and kidney function decline. *Clin J Am Soc Nephrol*. 2010;5(5):836-843.
206. Gibson A., Edgar J. D., Neville C. E., et al. Effect of fruit and vegetable consumption on immune function in older people: a randomized controlled trial. *Am J Clin Nutr*. 2012;96(6):1429-1436. https://watermark.silverchair.com/1429.pdf.
207. Chiba M., Abe T., Tsuda H., et al. Lifestyle-related disease in Crohn's disease: relapse prevention by a semi-vegetarian diet. *World J Gastroenterol*. 2010;16(20):2484-2495.
208. Kadoch M. A. Is the treatment of multiple sclerosis headed in the wrong direction? *Can J Neurol Sci*. 2012;39(3):405.
209. Young D. R., Vollmer W. M., King A. C., et al. Can individuals meet multiple physical activity and dietary behavior goals? *Am J Health Behav*. 2009;33(3):277-286
210. CDC WONDER: Underlying Cause of Death, 1999–2018. Centers for Disease Control and Prevention; 2018. Updated December 3, 2020. https://wonder.cdc.gov/.
211. World Health Organization. Cardiovascular diseases. https://www.who.int/health-topics/cardiovascular-diseases/#tab=tab_1. Accessed 2021.
212. Gaziano T., Reddy K. S., Paccaud F., Horton S., Chaturvedi V. Cardiovascular disease. In: Jamison D. T., Breman J. G., Measham A. R., et al., eds. *Disease Control Priorities in Developing Countries*. Washington, DC, New York, NY: Oxford University Press; 2006.
213. Esselstyn C. B., Jr. Is the present therapy for coronary artery disease the radical mastectomy of the twenty-first century? *Am J Cardiol*. 2010;106(6):902-904.
214. Boudi F. B., Ahsan C. H. Risk factors for coronary artery disease. Medscape emedicine. Updated March 30, 2020. https://emedicine.medscape.com/article/164163-overview.
215. Fryar C. D., Chen T. C., Li X. *Prevalence of uncontrolled risk factors for cardiovascular disease: United States, 1999-2010*. NCHS data brief, 103. Hyattsville, MD: National Center for Health Statistics; 2012.

216. Frattaroli J., Weidner G., Merritt-Worden T. A., Frenda S., Ornish D. Angina pectoris and atherosclerotic risk factors in the multisite cardiac lifestyle intervention program. *Am J Cardiol.* 2008;101(7):911-918.
217. Gould K. L., Ornish D., Kirkeeide R., et al. Improved stenosis geometry by quantitative coronary arteriography after vigorous risk factor modification. *Am J Cardiol.* 1992;69(9):845-853.
218. Koertge J., Weidner G., Elliott-Eller M., et al. Improvement in medical risk factors and quality of life in women and men with coronary artery disease in the Multicenter Lifestyle Demonstration Project. *Am J Cardiol.* 2003;91(11):1316-1322. https://www.ajconline.org/article/S0002-9149(03)00320-5/fulltext.
219. Pischke C. R., Weidner G., Elliott-Eller M., et al. Comparison of coronary risk factors and quality of life in coronary artery disease patients with versus without diabetes mellitus. *Am J Cardiol.* 2006;97(9):1267-1273. https://www.ajconline.org/article/S0002-9149(06)00157-3/pdf.
220. Esselstyn C. B., Jr., Favaloro R. G. More than coronary artery disease. *Am J Cardiol.* 1998;82(10b):5t-9t.
221. Vogel R. A., Corretti M. C., Plotnick G. D. Changes in flow-mediated brachial artery vasoactivity with lowering of desirable cholesterol levels in healthy middle-aged men. *Am J Cardiol.* 1996;77(1):37-40.
222. Pashkow F. J. Oxidative stress and inflammation in heart disease: do antioxidants have a role in treatment and/or prevention? *Int J Inflam.* 2011;2011:514623. https://doi.org/10.4061/2011/514623.
223. Shaper A. G., Jones K. W. Serum-cholesterol, diet, and coronary heart-disease in Africans and Asians in Uganda: 1959. *Int J Epidemiol.* 2012;41(5):1221-1225.
224. De Biase S. G., Fernandes S. F., Gianini R. J., Duarte J. L. Vegetarian diet and cholesterol and triglycerides levels. *Arq Bras Cardiol.* 2007;88(1):35-39.
225. Connor W. E., Cerqueira M. T., Connor R. W., Wallace R. B., Malinow M. R., Casdorph H. R. The plasma lipids, lipoproteins, and diet of the Tarahumara indians of Mexico. *Am J Clin Nutr.* 1978;31(7):1131-1142.
226. Sinnett P. F., Whyte H. M. Epidemiological studies in a total highland population, Tukisenta, New Guinea. Cardiovascular disease and relevant clinical, electrocardiographic, radiological and biochemical findings. *J Chronic Dis.* 1973;26(5):265-290.
227. Higginson J., Pepler W. J. Fat intake, serum cholesterol concentration, and atherosclerosis in the South African Bantu. II. Atherosclerosis and coronary artery disease. *J Clin Invest.* 1954;33(10):1366-1371.
228. Benjamin M. M., Roberts W. C. Facts and principles learned at the 39th Annual Williamsburg Conference on Heart Disease. *Proc (Bayl Univ Med Cent).* 2013;26(2):124-136. https://www.ncbi.nlm.nih.gov/pmc/articles/PMC3603726/pdf/bumc0026-0124.pdf.
229. Javed U., Deedwania P. C., Bhatt D. L., et al. Use of intensive lipid-lowering therapy in patients hospitalized with acute coronary syndrome: An analysis of 65,396 hospitalizations from 344 hospita participating in Get With The Guidelines (GWTG). *Am Heart J.* 2011;161(2):418-424.e411-413.
230. O'Keefe J. H., Jr., Cordain L., Harris W. H., Moe R. M., Vogel R. Optimal low-density lipoprotein is 50 to 70 mg/dl: lower is better and physiologically normal. *J Am Coll Cardiol.* 2004;43(11):2142-2146.
231. Eckel R. H., Jakicic J. M., Ard J. D., et al. 2013 AHA/ACC guideline on lifestyle management to reduce cardiovascular risk: a report of the American College of Cardiology/American Heart Association Task Force on Practice Guidelines. *J Am Coll Cardiol.* 2014;63(25 Pt B):2960-2984. http://www.ncbi.nlm.nih.gov/pubmed/24239922.
232. Trumbo P. R., Shimakawa T. Tolerable upper intake levels for trans fat, saturated fat, and cholesterol. *Nutr Rev.* 2011;69(5):270-278.
233. Roberts W. C. Preventing and arresting coronary atherosclerosis. *Am Heart J.* 1995;130(3 Pt 1):580-600.
234. Ferdowsian H. R., Barnard N. D. Effects of plant-based diets on plasma lipids. *Am J Cardiol.* 2009;104(7):947-956.
235. Castelli W. P. The new pathophysiology of coronary artery disease. *Am J Cardiol.* 1998;82(10b):60t-65t.
236. Ornish D., Scherwitz L. W., Doody R. S., et al. Effects of stress management training and dietary changes in treating ischemic heart disease. *JAMA.* 1983;249(1):54-59.
237. Esselstyn C. B., Jr. Updating a 12-year experience with arrest and reversal therapy for coronary heart disease (an overdue requiem for palliative cardiology). *Am J Cardiol.* 1999;84(3):339-341, A338. http://www.ncbi.nlm.nih.gov/pubmed/10496449.
238. Horrigan B. J. Ornish and Pritikin programs approved by CMS. *Explore (NY).* 2010;6(6):346-348.
239. Bloomfield H. E., Koeller E., Greer N., MacDonald R., Kane R., Wilt T. J. Effects on health outcomes of a Mediterranean diet with no restriction on fat intake. *Ann Intern Med.* 2016;165(7):491-500. https://www.acpjournals.org/doi/abs/10.7326/M16-0361.
240. Liyanage T., Ninomiya T., Wang A., et al. Effects of the Mediterranean diet on cardiovascular outcomes-a systematic review and meta-analysis. *PLoS One.* 2016;11:e0159252. https://link.gale.com/apps/doc/A460426930/AONE?u=mlin_m_tufts&sid=AONE&xid=c1d5a0e0.
241. Palacios O. M., Maki K. C. Vegetarian diet patterns and chronic disease risk: what we know and what we don't. *Nutr Today (Annapolis).* 2019;54(4):132-140.
242. National Heart, Lung, and Blood Institute. DASH eating plan. https://www.nhlbi.nih.gov/health-topics/dash-eating-plan. Accessed 2021.
243. Chiavaroli L., Viguiliouk E., Nishi S. K., et al. DASH dietary pattern and cardiometabolic outcomes: an umbrella review of systematic reviews and meta-analyses. *Nutrients.* 2019;11(2):338.
244. Salehi-Abargouei A. M., Maghsoudi Z. M., Shirani F. M., Azadbakht L. Effects of Dietary Approaches to Stop Hypertension (DASH)-style diet on fatal or nonfatal cardiovascular diseases—incidence: a systematic review and meta-analysis on observational prospective studies. *Nutrition.* 2013;29(4):611-618.
245. Filippou C. D, Tsioufis C. P., Thomopoulos C. G, et al. Dietary Approaches to Stop Hypertension (DASH) diet and blood pressure reduction in adults with and without hypertension: a systematic review and meta-analysis of randomized controlled trials. *Adv Nutr.* 2020;11(5):1150-1160. https://doi.org/10.1093/advances/nmaa041.

246. Soltani S., Shirani F., Chitsazi M. J., Salehi-Abargouei A. The effect of dietary approaches to stop hypertension (DASH) diet on weight and body composition in adults: a systematic review and meta-analysis of randomized controlled clinical trials. *Obes Rev.* 2016;17(5):442-454. https://onlinelibrary.wiley.com/doi/abs/10.1111/obr.12391.
247. Macknin M., Kong T., Weier A., et al. Plant-based, no-added-fat or American Heart Association diets: impact on cardiovascular risk in obese children with hypercholesterolemia and their parents. *J Pediatr.* 2015;166(4):953-959.e951-953.
248. Wright N., Wilson L., Smith M., Duncan B., McHugh P. The BROAD study: A randomised controlled trial using a whole food plant-based diet in the community for obesity, ischaemic heart disease or diabetes. *Nutr Diabetes.* 2017;7(3):e256-e256. https://doi.org/10.1038/nutd.2017.3.
249. Ornish Lifestyle Medicine. Undo it with Ornish. https://www.ornish.com/undo-it/. Accessed 2021.
250. Pritikin Longevity Center. Pritikin health and wellness resort. https://www.pritikin.com/resort-wellness-retreat.Accessed 2021.
251. Esselstyn C. B. *Prevent and Reverse Heart Disease: The Revolutionary, Scientifically Proven, Nutrition-Based Cure.* New York, NY: Avery; 2007.
252. Dr. Esselstyn's prevent & reverse heart disease program. http://www.dresselstyn.com/site/. Accessed 2021.
253. CHIP Lifestyle Medicine Institute. A lifestyle medicine solution. https://chiphealth.com/. Accessed 2021.
254. Feinberg A. P. Epigenetics at the epicenter of modern medicine. *JAMA.* 2008;299(11):1345-1350.
255. Schulz L. C. The Dutch Hunger Winter and the developmental origins of health and disease. *Proc Natl Acad Sci USA.* 2010;107(39):16757-16758.
256. Duhl D. M., Vrieling H., Miller K. A., Wolff G. L., Barsh G. S. Neomorphic agouti mutations in obese yellow mice. *Nat Genet.* 1994;8(1):59-65.
257. Godfrey K. M., Sheppard A., Gluckman P. D., et al. Epigenetic gene promoter methylation at birth is associated with child's later adiposity. *Diabetes.* 2011;60(5):1528-1534.
258. Clausen T. D., Mathiesen E. R., Hansen T., et al. Overweight and the metabolic syndrome in adult offspring of women with diet-treated gestational diabetes mellitus or type 1 diabetes. *J Clin Endocrinol Metab.* 2009;94(7):2464-2470.
259. Villeneuve L. M., Reddy M. A., Natarajan R. Epigenetics: deciphering its role in diabetes and its chronic complications. *Clin Exp Pharmacol Physiol.* 2011;38(7):451-459.
260. Ling C., Groop L. Epigenetics: a molecular link between environmental factors and type 2 diabetes. *Diabetes.* 2009;58(12):2718-2725.
261. Yang Q., Graham T. E., Mody N., et al. Serum retinol binding protein 4 contributes to insulin resistance in obesity and type 2 diabetes. *Nature.* 2005;436(7049):356-362.
262. Möller-Levet C. S., Archer S. N., Bucca G., et al. Effects of insufficient sleep on circadian rhythmicity and expression amplitude of the human blood transcriptome. *Proc Natl Acad Sci USA.* 2013;110(12):E1132-1141.
263. Nilsson E., Jansson P. A., Perfilyev A., et al. Altered DNA methylation and differential expression of genes influencing metabolism and inflammation in adipose tissue from subjects with type 2 diabetes. *Diabetes.* 2014;63(9):2962-2976.
264. Patel A., MacMahon S., Chalmers J., et al. Intensive blood glucose control and vascular outcomes in patients with type 2 diabetes. *N Engl J Med.* 2008;358(24):2560-2572.
265. Indrio F., Martini S., Francavilla R., et al. Epigenetic matters: the link between early nutrition, microbiome, and long-term health development. *Front Pediatr.* 2017;5:178.
266. Panico A., Tumolo M. R., Leo C. G., et al. The influence of lifestyle factors on miRNA expression and signal pathways: a review. *Epigenomics.* 2021;13(2):145-164.
267. Pasman W. J., van Erk M. J., Klöpping W. A., et al. Nutrigenomics approach elucidates health-promoting effects of high vegetable intake in lean and obese men. *Genes Nutr.* 2013;8(5):507-521.
268. Gasser S.M., Li E.. *Epigenetics and Disease: Pharmaceutical Opportunities.* Springer; 2011.
269. Junien C. Impact of diets and nutrients/drugs on early epigenetic programming. *J Inherit Metab Dis.* 2006;29(2-3):359-365.
270. Chang G. Q., Gaysinskaya V., Karatayev O., Leibowitz S. F. Maternal high-fat diet and fetal programming: increased proliferation of hypothalamic peptide-producing neurons that increase risk for overeating and obesity. *J Neurosci.* 2008;28(46):12107-12119.
271. Barrès R., Yan J., Egan B., et al. Acute exercise remodels promoter methylation in human skeletal muscle. *Cell Metabol.* 2012;15(3):405-411. https://www.cell.com/cell-metabolism/pdf/S1550-4131(12)00005-8.pdf.
272. Zhang B., Gao Y., Li Y., Yang J., Zhao H. Sleep deprivation influences circadian gene expression in the lateral habenula. *Behav Neurol.* 2016;2016:7919534. https://doi.org/10.1155/2016/7919534.
273. Cordero P., Li J., Oben J. A. Epigenetics of obesity: beyond the genome sequence. *Curr Opin Clin Nutr Metab Care.* 2015;18(4):361-366.
274. Centers for Disease Control and Prevention. Prevalence of diagnosed diabetes. In: *National Diabetes Statistics Report, 2020.* Atlanta, GA: Centers for Disease Control and Prevention; 2020.
275. Centers for Disease Control and Prevention. *National Diabetes Statistics Report, 2020.* Atlanta, GA: Centers for Disease Control and Prevention; 2020 https://www.cdc.gov/diabetes/pdfs/data/statistics/national-diabetes-statistics-report.pdf.
276. Centers for Disease Control and Prevention. *National Diabetes Statistics Report, 2017.* Atlanta, GA: Centers for Disease Control and Prevention; 2017. cdc.gov/diabetes/pdfs/data/statistics/national-diabetesstatistics-report.pdf.
277. Lin J., Thompson T. J., Cheng Y. J., et al. Projection of the future diabetes burden in the United States through 2060. *Popul Health Metr.* 2018;16(1):9. https://doi.org/10.1186/s12963-018-0166-4.
278. Saeedi P., Petersohn I., Salpea P., et al. Global and regional diabetes prevalence estimates for 2019 and projections for 2030 and 2045: Results from the International Diabetes Federation Diabetes Atlas, 9th edition. *Diabetes Res Clin Pract.* 2019;157:107843. http://www.sciencedirect.com/science/article/pii/S0168822719312306.
279. American Diabetes Association. Economic costs of diabetes in the U.S. in 2017. *Diabetes Care.* 2018;41(5):917-928. https://www.ncbi.nlm.nih.gov/pmc/articles/PMC5911784/pdf/dci180007.pdf.

280. Association American Diabetes. Standards of medical care in diabetes—2018 abridged for primary care providers. *Clin Diabetes.* 2018;36(1):14.

281. Effect of intensive blood-glucose control with metformin on complications in overweight patients with type 2 diabetes (UKPDS 34). UK Prospective Diabetes Study (UKPDS) Group. *Lancet.* 1998;352(9131):854-865.

282. McDuffie R., Summerson J., Reilly P., et al. The Action to Control Cardiovascular Risk in Diabetes (ACCORD) Trial and Hurricane Katrina: lessons for managing clinical trials during and after a natural disaster. *Contemp Clin Trials.* 2008;29(5):756-761. https://pubmed.ncbi.nlm.nih.gov/18577469.

283. Madonna R., Pandolfi A., Massaro M., Consoli A., De Caterina R. Insulin enhances vascular cell adhesion molecule-1 expression in human cultured endothelial cells through a pro-atherogenic pathway mediated by p38 mitogen-activated protein-kinase. *Diabetologia.* 2004;47(3):532-536.

284. Taylor R. Putting insulin resistance into context by dietary reversal of type 2 diabetes. *J R Coll Physicians Edinb.* 2017;47(2):168-171.

285. Taylor R. Pathogenesis of type 2 diabetes: tracing the reverse route from cure to cause. *Diabetologia.* 2008;51(10):1781-1789.

286. Boucher J., Kleinridders A., Kahn C. R. Insulin receptor signaling in normal and insulin-resistant states. *Cold Spring Harb Perspect Biol.* 2014;6(1):a009191. https://pubmed.ncbi.nlm.nih.gov/24384568.

287. Mahadev K., Zilbering A., Zhu L., Goldstein B. J. Insulin-stimulated hydrogen peroxide reversibly inhibits protein-tyrosine phosphatase 1b in vivo and enhances the early insulin action cascade. *J Biol Chem.* 2001;276(24):21938-21942.

288. Pan H., Guo J., Su Z. Advances in understanding the interrelations between leptin resistance and obesity. *Physiol Behav.* 2014;130:157-169.

289. Granic I., Dolga A. M., Nijholt I. M., van Dijk G., Eisel U. L. Inflammation and NF-kappaB in Alzheimer's disease and diabetes. *J Alzheimers Dis.* 2009;16(4):809-821.

290. Eshak E. S., Iso H., Maruyama K., Muraki I., Tamakoshi A. Associations between dietary intakes of iron, copper and zinc with risk of type 2 diabetes mellitus: A large population-based prospective cohort study. *Clin Nutr.* 2018;37(2):667-674.

291. Zelber-Sagi S., Ivancovsky-Wajcman D., Fliss Isakov N., et al. High red and processed meat consumption is associated with non-alcoholic fatty liver disease and insulin resistance. *J Hepatol.* 2018;68(6):1239-1246.

292. Liu Q., Sun L., Tan Y., Wang G., Lin X., Cai L. Role of iron deficiency and overload in the pathogenesis of diabetes and diabetic complications. *Curr Med Chem.* 2009;16(1):113-129.

293. Cnop M., Hannaert J. C., Grupping A. Y., Pipeleers D. G. Low density lipoprotein can cause death of islet beta-cells by its cellular uptake and oxidative modification. *Endocrinology.* 2002;143(9):3449-3453.

294. Roehrich M. E., Mooser V., Lenain V., et al. Insulin-secreting beta-cell dysfunction induced by human lipoproteins. *J Biol Chem.* 2003;278(20):18368-18375.

295. Maedler K., Sergeev P., Ehses J. A., et al. Leptin modulates beta cell expression of IL-1 receptor antagonist and release of IL-1beta in human islets. *Proc Natl Acad Sci USA.* 2004;101(21):8138-8143.

296. Kolb H., Martin S. Environmental/lifestyle factors in the pathogenesis and prevention of type 2 diabetes. *BMC Med.* 2017;15(1):131-131.

297. Tuomilehto J., Lindstrom J., Eriksson J. G., et al. Prevention of type 2 diabetes mellitus by changes in lifestyle among subjects with impaired glucose tolerance. *N Engl J Med.* 2001;344(18):1343-1350. https://www.ncbi.nlm.nih.gov/pubmed/11333990.

298. Booth F. W., Gordon S. E., Carlson C. J., Hamilton M. T. Waging war on modern chronic diseases: primary prevention through exercise biology. *J Appl Physiol (1985).* 2000;88(2):774-787. https://journals.physiology.org/doi/pdf/10.1152/jappl.2000.88.2.774.

299. Pan X. R., Li G. W., Hu Y. H., et al. Effects of diet and exercise in preventing NIDDM in people with impaired glucose tolerance. The Da Qing IGT and Diabetes Study. *Diabetes Care.* 1997;20(4):537-544.

300. Katula J. A., Vitolins M. Z., Morgan T. M., et al. The Healthy Living Partnerships to Prevent Diabetes study: 2-year outcomes of a randomized controlled trial. *Am J Prev Med.* 2013;44(4 Suppl 4):S324-332.

301. Ali M. K., Echouffo-Tcheugui J., Williamson D. F. How effective were lifestyle interventions in real-world settings that were modeled on the Diabetes Prevention Program? *Health Aff (Millwood).* 2012;31(1):67-75.

302. Herman W. H. The cost-effectiveness of diabetes prevention: results from the Diabetes Prevention Program and the Diabetes Prevention Program Outcomes Study. *Clin Diabetes Endocrinol.* 2015;1:9.

303. Poti J. M., Mendez M. A., Ng S. W., Popkin B. M. Is the degree of food processing and convenience linked with the nutritional quality of foods purchased by US households? *Am J Clin Nutr.* 2015;101(6):1251-1262.

304. US Department of Agriculture, Economic Research Service. Average daily intake of food by food source and demographic characteristics 2007-10. Updated June 27 2014. www.ers.usda.gov/data-products/food-consumption-and-nutrient-intakes/.

305. Johnson R. J., Segal M. S., Sautin Y., et al. Potential role of sugar (fructose) in the epidemic of hypertension, obesity and the metabolic syndrome, diabetes, kidney disease, and cardiovascular disease. *Am J Clin Nutr.* 2007;86(4):899-906.

306. Putnam J. Major trends in U.S food supply, 1909-99. *Food Review/National Food Review.* 2000;23(1):8-15. http://ageconsearch.umn.edu/record/205508/files/Food%20Review%20Vol.%2023%20Issue%201-2.pdf.

307. Buse J. B., Caprio S., Cefalu W. T., et al. How do we define cure of diabetes? *Diabetes Care.* 2009;32(11):2133-2135.

308. Lim E. L., Hollingsworth K. G, Aribisala B. S., Chen M. J., Mathers J. C., Taylor R. Reversal of type 2 diabetes: normalisation of beta cell function in association with decreased pancreas and liver triacylglycerol. *Diabetologia.* 2011;54(10):2506-2514. https://www.ncbi.nlm.nih.gov/pmc/articles/PMC3168743/pdf/125_2011_Article_2204.pdf.

309. Steven S., Lim E. L., Taylor R. Population response to information on reversibility of type 2 diabetes. *Diabet Med.* 2013;30(4):e135-138. https://www.ncbi.nlm.nih.gov/pubmed/23320491.

310. Sarathi V., Kolly A., Chaithanya H. B., Dwarakanath C. S. High rates of diabetes reversal in newly diagnosed Asian Indian young adults with type 2 diabetes mellitus with intensive lifestyle therapy. *J Nat Sci Biol Med.* 2017;8(1):60. http://www.jnsbm.org/article.asp?issn=0976-9668;year=2017;volume=8;issue=1;spage=60;epage=63;aulast=Sarathi.
311. Gow M. L., Baur L. A., Johnson N. A., Cowell C. T., Garnett S. P. Reversal of type 2 diabetes in youth who adhere to a very-low-energy diet: a pilot study. *Diabetologia.* 2017;60(3):406-415. https://link.springer.com/content/pdf/10.1007/s00125-016-4163-5.pdf.
312. Cheng C. W., Villani V., Buono R., et al. Fasting-mimicking diet promotes Ngn3-Driven beta-cell regeneration to reverse diabetes. *Cell.* 2017;168(5):775-788 e712. https://www.ncbi.nlm.nih.gov/pubmed/28235195.
313. MacDonald K. G. Jr., Long S. D., Swanson M. S., et al. The gastric bypass operation reduces the progression and mortality of non-insulin-dependent diabetes mellitus. *J Gastrointest Surg.* 1997;1(3):213-220; discussion 220.
314. Singh A. K., Singh R., Kota S. K. Bariatric surgery and diabetes remission: who would have thought it? *Indian J Endocrinol Metab.* 2015;19(5):563-576.
315. Schauer P. R., Bhatt D. L., Kirwan J. P., et al. Bariatric surgery versus intensive medical therapy for diabetes - 5-year outcomes. *N Engl J Med.* 2017;376(7):641-651.
316. Sjöström L. Review of the key results from the Swedish Obese Subjects (SOS) trial - a prospective controlled intervention study of bariatric surgery. *J Intern Med.* 2013;273(3):219-234.
317. Parker B., Noakes M., Luscombe N., Clifton P. Effect of a high-protein, high-monounsaturated fat weight loss diet on glycemic control and lipid levels in type 2 diabetes. *Diabetes Care.* 2002;25(3):425-430.
318. Salas-Salvadó J., Bulló M., Babio N., et al. Reduction in the incidence of type 2 diabetes with the Mediterranean diet: results of the PREDIMED-Reus nutrition intervention randomized trial. *Diabetes Care.* 2011;34(1):14-19.
319. Nicholson A. S., Sklar M., Barnard N. D., Gore S., Sullivan R., Browning S. Toward improved management of NIDDM: a randomized, controlled, pilot intervention using a lowfat, vegetarian diet. *Prev Med.* 1999;29(2):87-91.
320. Schulze M. B., Manson J. E., Willett W. C., Hu F. B. Processed meat intake and incidence of type 2 diabetes in younger and middle-aged women. *Diabetologia.* 2003;46(11):1465-1473.
321. Hu F. B., Manson J. E., Stampfer M. J., et al. Diet, lifestyle, and the risk of type 2 diabetes mellitus in women. *N Engl J Med.* 2001;345(11):790-797.
322. Snowdon D. A., Phillips R. L. Does a vegetarian diet reduce the occurrence of diabetes? *Am J Public Health.* 1985;75(5):507-512.
323. Sluijs I., Beulens J. W., van der A. DI, Spijkerman A. M., Grobbee D. E., van der Schouw Y. T. Dietary intake of total, animal, and vegetable protein and risk of type 2 diabetes in the European Prospective Investigation into Cancer and Nutrition (EPIC)-NL study. *Diabetes Care.* 2010;33(1):43-48.
324. Kahleova H., Matoulek M., Malinska H., et al. Vegetarian diet improves insulin resistance and oxidative stress markers more than conventional diet in subjects with Type 2 diabetes. *Diabet Med.* 2011;28(5):549-559.
325. Pan A., Sun Q., Bernstein A. M., et al. Red meat consumption and risk of type 2 diabetes: 3 cohorts of US adults and an updated meta-analysis. *Am J Clin Nutr.* 2011;94(4):1088-1096.
326. Satija A., Bhupathiraju S. N., Rimm E. B., et al. Plant-based dietary patterns and incidence of type 2 diabetes in US men and women: results from three prospective cohort studies. *PLoS Med.* 2016;13(6):e1002039.
327. Knowler W. C., Barrett-Connor E., Fowler S. E., et al. Reduction in the incidence of type 2 diabetes with lifestyle intervention or metformin. *N Engl J Med.* 2002;346(6):393-403. https://www.ncbi.nlm.nih.gov/pubmed/11832527.
328. Robertson M. D., Currie J. M., Morgan L. M., Jewell D. P., Frayn K. N. Prior short-term consumption of resistant starch enhances postprandial insulin sensitivity in healthy subjects. *Diabetologia.* 2003;46(5):659-665.
329. Crane M. G., Sample C. Regression of diabetic neuropathy with total vegetarian (vegan) diet. *J Nutr Med.* 1994;4(4):431-439. https://doi.org/10.3109/13590849409003592.
330. Kempner W., Peschel R. L., Schlayer C. Effect of rice diet on diabetes mellitus associated with vascular disease. *Postgrad Med.* 1958;24(4):359-371. https://www.tandfonline.com/doi/abs/10.1080/00325481.1958.11692236.
331. Fuhrman J., Sarter B., Glaser D., Acocella S. Changing perceptions of hunger on a high nutrient density diet. *Nutr J.* 2010;9:51.
332. US Department of Health and Human Services and US Department of Agriculture. Chapter 1: a-closer-look-inside-healthy-eating-patterns. In: *Dietary Guidelines for Americans 2015-2020,* 8th ed. Washington, DC; 2015. https://health.gov/dietaryguidelines/2015/guidelines/chapter-1/a-closer-look-inside-healthy-eating-patterns/

SECTION 6
Physical Activity Science and Prescription

Objective 1 Describe the relationship between physical activity and health **185**

Objective 2 Define physical activity and exercise........................... **186**

Objective 3 List the components of exercise **187**

Objective 4 Describe the major evidence for the physical activity components (aerobic, strength, flexibility, and balance) **188**

Objective 5 List the components of writing an exercise prescription........... **190**

Objective 6 Describe the US Physical Activity Guidelines for Americans **191**

Objective 7 Describe the role of personal behavior and role modeling **196**

Objective 8 Explain the use of metabolic equivalents of tasks in assessing fitness **196**

Objective 9 Describe the impact of exercise on weight....................... **197**

Objective 10 Identify the minimum and maximum levels of exercise........... **198**

Objective 11 List key physical activity assessment tools **201**

Objective 12 Medical screening before exercise and recommended progression of physical activity **206**

Objective 13 Describe how to collaborate with your patients to promote physical activity change **210**

Objective 14 Identify resources for sustainable behavior change **214**

Objective 15 Describe the treatment of disease with exercise as compared with medication **217**

Objective 16 List evidence-based physical activity recommendations for healthy older adults, pregnancy, obesity, heart disease, diabetes, cancer, disability, and stroke **218**

Section 6 Glossary **223**
Section 6 Review Questions **224**
Section 6 Review Question Answers and Summaries **227**
Section 6 References **229**

OBJECTIVE 1

Describe the relationship between physical activity and health

1) **Physical inactivity is the fourth leading risk factor for global mortality.[1,2]**

   a) Low cardiorespiratory fitness (CRF) was the number one cause of preventable deaths from all-cause mortality among 40,842 men and women enrolled in the Aerobics Center Longitudinal Study (see Table 6.1).[3]

Table 6.1 Attributable Fraction (%) of All-Cause Mortality

	Men	Women
Poor cardiorespiratory fitness as measured by maximum on treadmill test	16%	17%
Smoking	8%	9%
Hypertension	15%	7%
High cholesterol	4%	1%
Diabetes	4%	1%
Obesity	2%	3%

Note: the attributable fraction is the estimated number of deaths in the study population that could have been avoided if the health behavior had not been present.

2) **Physical activity and all-cause mortality[4]**

   a) Physical inactivity is the cause of approximately 1 in 10 premature deaths.
      1. In the US, it is estimated that 8.3% of deaths are attributed to physical inactivity.[5]

   b) If worldwide physical inactivity decreased by 25%, then over 1.3 million deaths could be averted every year.

   c) The percent of burden of disease attributed to physical inactivity in a worldwide population:[4]
      1. 6% of coronary heart diseases
      2. 7% of type 2 diabetes
      3. 10% of breast cancers
      4. 10% of colon cancers

3) **Years of life lost in inactive individuals who were normal weight to overweight[6]**

   a) People who get the most exercise have the least number of years of life lost, whether they are normal weight, overweight, or obesity class 1 or 2.

   b) Physically active individuals in obesity class 2 have slightly fewer years of life lost (4.5 vs 4.7) than inactive normal weight subjects.

4) **Sitting and sedentary behavior**

   a) Sedentary behavior is a distinct class of behavior.[7,8]
      1. Has specific determinants and effects on disease risk
      2. Independently increases disease risk despite leisure time exercise
      3. Increases mortality and disease risk further in individuals with insufficient physical activity

   b) Only one in three adults achieve the recommended amount of physical activity each week. This means nearly 66% of Americans are physically inactive, whereas only 13.7% of the population smokes cigarettes.[9,10] Sedentary behavior is associated with increased mortality and morbidity.

1. A study evaluating sitting time and all-cause mortality evaluated 222,497 people, age 45 or older, and followed them for an average of 2.8 years. The results showed that 6.9% of all-cause mortality was attributable to sitting.[11]
    a. The results were consistent across gender, age groups, body mass index (BMI), physical activity level and healthy participants compared with those who had preexisting cardiovascular disease or diabetes mellitus.
    b. Portions of the population were meeting physical activity guidelines but sitting was still an independent risk factor.
2. Another study assessed the risk of prolonged sitting when it is broken up by activity. The study included 19 overweight or obese adults who were 45–65 years old. The participants were divided into three groups:[12]
    a. Group 1: uninterrupted sitting as controls
    b. Group 2: seated with 2-minute bouts of light-intensity walking every 20 minutes
    c. Group 3: seated with 2-minute bouts of moderate-intensity walking every 20 minutes
    d. Results on blood glucose and insulin levels:
        (1) Blood glucose and insulin levels were reduced with both light and moderate activity breaks compared to uninterrupted sitting.
        (2) Benefits were gained with the walking break, regardless of intensity of walking. Neither intensity showed more benefits than the other.
3. Sedentary behavior during television watching[13]
    a. Television viewing increased (hazard ratio [HR] ~1.5) of all-cause mortality even in those getting 7 hours of exercise per week. This increased risk of all-cause mortality was equivalent to those who never exercised but never watched television.
    b. Television has also been associated with eating unhealthy foods and prolonged sitting.

OBJECTIVE 2

Define physical activity and exercise

1) Definitions

- **a)** Physical activity: any movement of the body done through skeletal muscle contraction that causes the energy expenditure to be beyond its baseline.[14]
- **b)** Physical inactivity: the absence of physical activity; usually reflected as the amount or proportion of time not engaged in physical activity of some predetermined intensity.[8]
- **c)** Exercise: purposeful physical activity that is organized, planned, and reoccurring and that is done with the intent of improving or maintaining one or more components of one's health.[14]
- **d)** Non-Exercise Activity Thermogenesis (NEAT): the energy expended for everything we do that is not sleeping, eating, or exercise.[15]
- **e)** Sedentary Behavior: a distinct class of behaviors (e.g., sitting, watching TV, and driving) characterized by little physical movement and low energy expenditure (≤1.5 METs) in a sitting or reclining posture requiring low levels of energy expenditure for a prolonged period of time.[8]

f) Fitness: the ability to perform one's activities of daily life, respond to emergencies, and enjoy leisure time activities with sufficient energy and vitality and without excess fatigue. It is the outcome of exercise.[14]

g) Physical fitness includes fitness in the following categories:[14]
   1. Cardiorespiratory endurance
   2. Muscle strength
   3. Muscle endurance
   4. Body composition
   5. Flexibility

h) Deconditioning[16]
   1. A state of health that occurs from being consistently physically inactive and lacking exercise in one's daily life, all of which results in functional loss.
   2. Deconditioning is a common preventable cause of morbidity and mortality.
   3. If deconditioning were recognized as a disease, it would be more common than hypertension or diabetes.

2) Overall benefits of physical activity on health include:[1]

a) Increased muscular and cardiovascular fitness

b) Improved bone health and less risk of falls and vertebral fractures

c) Reduced risk of chronic diseases such as hypertension, cardiovascular disease, diabetes, some cancers like breast and colon, and depression

d) Higher control and maintenance of a healthy weight

3) Health care savings from physical activity

a) Activity level and health claims[17]
   1. Health care spending increases as activity levels decrease and vice-versa. Each additional day of physical activity decreased median health care costs by 4.7%.
   2. An inactive person costs $1,543 more per year than an active person.

b) The cost effectiveness of physical activity interventions in primary care and the community were assessed in a systematic review of 12 studies, which found that:[18]
   1. The cost to change one person from the physically "inactive" to physically "active" category was between $500 and $5,000.
   2. Most interventions to increase physical activity were cost-effective.
      a. Brief advice given in person, by phone, or by mail were more cost-effective than supervised activities, such as gym classes or exercise.

OBJECTIVE 3

List the components of exercise

1) Types of exercise[19]

a) Aerobic/endurance exercise (cardiovascular): the body's large muscles move in a rhythmic manner for a sustained period of time.

b) Strength or resistance exercise: any exercise that causes muscles to contract against an external resistance with the goal of increasing lean body mass and improving muscular strength and endurance.

c) Flexibility: the range of motion that is possible at a joint.
   1. Specific to each joint
   2. Dependent on ligament, tendon, and muscle tightness

d) Balance:
   1. Static and dynamic exercises
   2. Improves one's ability to withstand destabilizing stimuli or postural sway due to self-motion, environment, or objects

e) Other types of exercise exist but are not included here.

OBJECTIVE 4

Describe the major evidence for the physical activity components (aerobic, strength, flexibility, and balance)

1) **Aerobic exercise**

   a) Complete list of benefits is listed in physical activity and health section (see Table 6.4 in Objective 6)

2) **Resistance exercise and strength training benefits**[20]

   a) Reduced injury

   b) Increased basal metabolic rate

   c) Reduced fatigue

   d) Improved sleep

   e) Improved performance and muscle strength

   f) Improved quality of life, strength, endurance, and bone mineral density in early post-menopausal years

   g) Reduced body fat, improved weight maintenance, and improved body aesthetics

   h) Improved cholesterol levels, glucose tolerance, glucose control, and heart muscle function

   i) Decreased pain and disability associated with arthritis

   j) Strength training and non-alcoholic fatty liver disease (NAFLD)[21]
      1. Sedentary adults with clinically defined non-alcoholic fatty liver disease may experience a reduction in hepatic steatosis, despite not having any change in visceral adipose tissue volume or whole-body fat mass.

3) **Table 6.2 compares the benefits from aerobic and resistance training.**

Table 6.2 Comparison of Effects of Aerobic Endurance Training with Strength Training on Health and Fitness Variables[20]

Variable	Aerobic Exercise	Resistance Exercise
Body composition		
Bone mineral density	↑↑	↑↑
Percent body fat	↓↓	↓
Lean body mass	0	↑↑
Muscle strength	↑0	↑↑↑
Glucose metabolism		
Insulin response to glucose challenge	↓↓	↓↓
Basal insulin levels	↓	↓
Insulin sensitivity	↑↑	↑↑
Plasma lipids and lipoproteins		
HDL cholesterol	↑0	↑0
LDL cholesterol	↓0	↓0
Triglycerides	↓↓	↓0

↑ Indicates values increase; ↓ values decrease; 0 values remain unchanged; 1 arrow, small effect; 2 arrows, moderate effect; 3 arrows, large effect; HDL is high-density lipoprotein cholesterol; and LDL is low-density lipoprotein cholesterol[20]

4) **Introducing strength training or resistance exercises to an exercise prescription**
   - **a)** It is common, even for active patients, to not engage in resistance training.
   - **b)** Muscle-strengthening activity components
     1. Frequency: how often
     2. Intensity: the weight or force used relative to a person's ability to lift
        a. For example, 70% of a patient's one repetition maximum is roughly a weight that can be lifted 12 times before muscle failure and inability to do another repetition while maintaining good form.
     3. Repetitions: number of times a weight is lifted
     4. Sets: the number of cycles of repetitions
        a. For example, two sets of 15 repetitions means to perform 15 repetitions, rest, and then perform another 15 repetitions.
   - **c)** Initiating resistance exercises
     1. Work with an intensity of 5 or 6 on a 10-point scale, and complete 8–12 repetitions before fatiguing, which may mean to add weight to reach difficulty level.
     2. Avoid working the same muscle group 2 days in a row to prevent muscle fatigue and allow for growth and recovery. Often workouts are done every 48 hours.
        a. However, those desiring to workout more frequently can train different muscle groups on consecutive days (e.g., upper body one day then lower body the next day).
   - **d)** Patients may benefit more from professional advice (fitness trainers) for resistance exercises than aerobic/cardiovascular exercise.

5) **Flexibility exercises**

a) Enhance the ability of a joint to move through its full range of motion

b) Flexibility exercise benefits

1. There are few studies on the benefits.
   a. Flexibility exercises help increase muscle length and range of motion or align collagen fibers in healing muscles.[22,23] The rat-tail tendon studies first presented the idea that warmer temperatures allow for better stretching.[24]
   b. In elderly adults, daily hip flexor stretching increased gait by increasing stride length and peak hip extension during walking.[25]
   c. When patients with type 2 diabetes engaged in flexibility exercise, there were small but significant improvements in fasting blood glucose, postprandial glucose, hemoglobin A1c (HbA1c), and BMI.[25]

c) Introducing flexibility training

1. Warm up (before flexibility/stretching activities).
2. Hold each stretch for 10–30 seconds.
3. Do two to four repetitions for each muscle group, accumulating 60 seconds total for each stretch.
4. Remember, the goal is to feel some tension but not pain during a stretch.

6) **Balance exercises**

a) Improves ability to withstand postural sway or destabilizing stimuli

b) Balance exercise benefits

1. A systematic review of balance exercises on fall prevention in older patients in an outpatient setting showed:[26]
   a. 37% decrease in injuries from falls
   b. 30% decrease in injuries resulting in medical care
   c. 43% decrease in severe injury falls
   d. 61% decrease in falls resulting in fractures

c) Introducing balance training

1. Start with hand-hold support.
2. Increase exercise difficulty by removing support.
3. For further challenge, stand on an unstable surface, such as a foam board.
4. For a quick balance assessment, assess patient's ability to stand on one foot.

OBJECTIVE 5

List the components of writing an exercise prescription

7) **Exercise prescription**

a) Providers can communicate to patients their expectations for physical activity in a specific and meaningful way by using the following exercise prescription format (see Table 6.3). Work with patients to agree on the exercise prescription.

Table 6.3 F.I.T.T.

F	Frequency	# days/week (i.e., 3 days per week)
I	Intensity	Talk Test, rating of percieved exertion (RPE) (i.e., 7–8 out of 10)
T	Time	# of minutes/session (i.e., 30 minutes)
T	Type	Mode of physical activity (i.e., swimming, walking, biking)

American College of Sports Medicine 2018[27]

b) FITT-VP[28]

1. Frequency: number of days
2. Intensity: light, moderate, or vigorous
3. Type (of exercise): aerobic, strength, balance, and flexibility
4. Time (duration): how long? Hours and minutes?
5. Volume (amount): how much total exercise per week or per month?
6. Progression (start slow and build incrementally): when to adjust/increase exercise will be based on an individual's tolerance and preference.

c) Exercise prescription example: Begin walking (type) at 60 steps per minute or a pace where you feel like you are breathing faster than normal (intensity) for 30 minutes (time) 5 days per week (frequency).

d) New exercise prescriptions should continue to meet the physical activity guidelines and reduce sedentary behavior (e.g., limit sitting and TV watching). The guidelines suggest:[29]

1. 150 minutes per week of exercise
2. Resistance training two times per week
3. Avoid prolonged sitting throughout the day, and include 5 minutes of movement once an hour.

OBJECTIVE 6

Describe the US Physical Activity Guidelines for Americans

1) 2018 Physical Activity Guidelines for Americans (PAGA)[2,30]

a) The inaugural guidelines for physical activity were published in 2008.[2,30]

b) These provide evidence-based recommendations on physical activity levels for health promotion and disease prevention.

c) The guidelines are used by policy makers, health care providers, and the general public.

2) Key points to know from the original 2008 PAGA[2,30]

a) Regular physical activity reduces the risk of many adverse health outcomes.

b) Most health benefits are achieved at 150 minutes per week of moderate-intensity physical activity or 75 minutes of vigorous-intensity physical activity or an equivalent combination.

c) Dose response: The more physical activity, the more benefits, and any amount of exercise is better than none. There is no threshold level of physical activity that must be achieved before benefits are seen.

d) Vigorous-intensity physical activity may have modest additional benefits (lower mortality rates and cardiovascular disease risk factors) than moderate-intensity (see Table 6.4)[31]

Table 6.4 Physical Activity-Related Health Benefits for the General Population and Selected Populations Documented by the 2018 Physical Activity Guidelines Advisory Committee

Children	
3 to <6 years of age	**Improved bone health and weight status**
6 to 17 years of age	**Improved cognitive function (ages 6 to 13 years)**
	Improved cardiorespiratory and muscular fitness
	Improved bone health
	Improved cardiovascular risk factor status
	Improved weight status or adiposity
	Fewer symptoms of depression
Adults, All Ages	
All-cause mortality	Lower risk
Cardiometabolic conditions	Lower cardiovascular incidence and mortality (including heart disease and stroke)
	Lower incidence of hypertension
	Lower incidence of type 2 diabetes
Cancer	Lower incidence of **bladder**, breast, colon, **endometrium, esophagus, kidney, stomach, and lung cancers**
Brain health	**Reduced risk of dementia**
	Improved cognitive function
	Improved cognitive function following bouts of aerobic activity
	Improved quality of life
	Improved sleep
	Reduced feelings of anxiety and depression in healthy people and in people with existing clinical syndromes
	Reduced incidence of depression
Weight status	**Reduced risk of excessive weight gain**
	Weight loss and the prevention of weight regain following initial weight loss when a sufficient dose of moderate-to-vigorous physical activity is attained
	An additive effect on weight loss when combined with moderate dietary restriction
Older Adults	
Falls	Reduced incidence of falls
	Reduced incidence of fall-related injuries
Physical function	**Improved physical function in older adults with and without frailty**
Women Who Are Pregnant or Postpartum	
During pregnancy	**Reduced risk of excessive weight gain**
	Reduced risk of gestational diabetes
	No risk to fetus from moderate-intensity physical activity
During postpartum	**Reduced risk of postpartum depression**

Individuals with Preexisting Medical Conditions	
Breast cancer	**Reduced risk of all-cause and breast cancer mortality**
Colorectal cancer	**Reduced risk of all-cause and colorectal cancer mortality**
Prostate cancer	**Reduced risk of prostate cancer mortality**
Osteoarthritis	**Decreased pain**
	Improved function and quality of life
Hypertension	**Reduced risk of progression of cardiovascular disease**
	Reduced risk of increased blood pressure over time
Type 2 diabetes	**Reduced risk of cardiovascular mortality**
	Reduced progression of disease indicators: hemoglobin A1c, blood pressure, blood lipids, and body mass index
Multiple sclerosis	**Improved walking**
	Improved physical fitness
Dementia	**Improved cognition**
Some conditions with impaired executive function (attention deficit hyperactivity disorder, schizophrenia, multiple sclerosis, Parkinson's disease, and stroke)	**Improved cognition**

Note: Benefits in bold font are those added in 2018; benefits in normal font are those noted in the 2008 Scientific Report. Only outcomes with strong or moderate evidence of effect are included in the table.

3) **Updates from the 2018 Guidelines**[2]

   a) Physical activity improves sleep onset, duration, and quality (including a longer amount of deep sleep).
   b) Single episodes of physical activity improve brain executive function, including concentration, attention, emotional regulation, memory, ability to plan and organize, and speed of processing. Single episodes of physical activity also lower blood pressure, improve sleep, lower anxiety, and improve insulin sensitivity.
   c) Within days to weeks of initiating regular exercise, the risk of disease starts decreasing, and physical function scores improve.
   d) Physical activity reduces depressive symptoms in those with and without clinical depression, and it helps lower the risk of ever acquiring clinical depression.
   e) Feelings of anxiety, whether chronically present or momentarily, are reduced with physical activity.
   f) Perceived quality of life is improved with physical activity.
   g) Physical function is improved for both young (as young as 3–5 years of age) and old, allowing for greater physical independence, improved bone health, reduced risk of falls or injuries from falls in elderly, and the ability to more easily complete tasks of daily living.
   h) Physical activity reduces the risk of several diseases and improves health.
   i) Physical activity should be safe for participants. Therefore, these are the recommendations:
      1. Risks or symptoms of uncontrolled or undiagnosed disease should not be ignored. Types of physical activity should be chosen based on the individual. Also, before initiating an exercise program, cardiovascular screening may be required for specific individuals.

2. Activity should be increased slowly and steadily over time. Inactive individuals should begin with low-intensity exercise and increase the intensity and volume slowly.
3. Appropriate protective gear and equipment should be used. Physical activity should be completed in a safe environment.

4) Aerobic exercise activity guidelines[2]

a) Children 3–5 years of age:

1. Should be physically active throughout day to promote growth and development
2. Adults should assist children in physical activity by encouraging a variety of "active play" activities.

b) Children 6–17 years of age:

1. 60 minutes or more per day of physical activity of moderate-to-vigorous intensity
2. Vigorous-intensity physical activity on at least 3 days per week

c) Adults 18–64 years of age:

1. 2.5 hours (150 minutes) of moderate-intensity exercise per week or 1 hour and 15 minutes (75 minutes) of vigorous intensity exercise per week, or a combination of both.
   a. For additional health benefits: 5 hours (300 minutes) of moderate-intensity aerobic activity or 2 hours and 30 minutes (150 minutes) of vigorous activity, or equivalent amounts of both. Additional benefits are gained beyond this amount.
2. One continuous session or multiple smaller sessions are acceptable. Note: the minimum duration of 10 minutes per session in order to "count" was removed in the 2018 guidelines, as evidence shows that even shorter periods have beneficial health effects.

d) Adults age 65 and older:

1. Should follow adult guidelines or, if they are unable, they should be as physically active as possible

e) Women during pregnancy or postpartum without exercise contraindications:

1. 150 minutes of moderate-intensity exercise per week
2. Vigorous activity is okay to continue if it was done regularly before pregnancy occurred. But avoid contact sports and sports or activities that may cause loss of balance or trauma to the mother or fetus.

f) Adults with chronic conditions or diseases:

1. 150–300 minutes per week of moderate physical activity or 75–150 minutes per week of vigorous physical activity, or a combination of both
2. When unable to meet the above guidelines, one should do as much as possible according to their ability and avoid being sedentary.

5) Strength training and resistance exercise guidelines[2,30]

a) Children 6–17 years of age:

1. Children should participate in muscle-strengthening and bone-strengthening activities that place force or impact on bones for at least 1 hour at least 3 days per week.
2. Examples include activities such as tug of war, squat jumps, and climbing.
3. Resistance exercises involving weights or heavy loads should be done under supervision to assure appropriate form and prevent injury.

b) Adults 18–64 years of age:

1. Perform strength training activities two to three times per week on nonconsecutive days (48 hours apart). Some individuals who chose to do resistance exercises daily can do so but should not work the same major muscle groups 2 days in a row. The major muscle groups are muscles of the chest, back, shoulders, biceps, triceps, abdomen, quadriceps, and hamstrings.
2. Healthy adults: one set of 8–2 repetitions for each major muscle group
3. Older or frail individuals: one set of 10–15 repetitions
4. Sets can be completed with free-weights, machines, or one's own body weight.
5. Resistance training exercises should focus on:
    a. Multi-joint or compound exercises that involve more than one muscle group (e.g., push-ups and squats)
    b. Single-joint exercises that target major muscle groups (e.g., biceps curls and calf raises)
    c. Exercises that affect core muscles (e.g., planks and bridges).[32]
    d. Exercises that promote resistance through agonist and antagonist muscle groups to prevent muscle imbalance, such as the chest and upper back

c) Adults age 65 and older:

1. Healthy older adults should do strength training two times per week or can follow the guidelines as much as possible. They should start at very light or light intensity. Weights used for strength training should be light enough to complete a set of 10–15 repetitions.

d) Adults with chronic conditions or disabilities:

1. Strength training should be done two to three times per week on nonconsecutive days or as much as possible if unable to meet recommended amount.

6) Flexibility exercise guidelines[2,33]

a) Stretching can allow people to more easily do activities that require greater flexibility, however, the health benefits and ability to reduce the risk of injury are unproven.

b) Healthy adults stretching exercise program

1. 10 minutes, two to three days per week. The greatest benefits are seen if performed daily.
2. Include all the major muscle-tendon units and stretch for 10–30 seconds each.
3. Complete two to four repetitions for each muscle group, accumulating 60 seconds for each stretch. Older adults may benefit by holding a stretch 30–60 seconds at a time until accumulating 60 seconds per stretch.

c) Stretching exercises can be:

1. Dynamic—gradual transition from one body position to another with a progressive increase in reach and range of motion as a movement is repeated
2. Static—slowly stretching a muscle-tendon unit and holding it
3. Ballistic—repeated bouncing movements to stretch a targeted muscle group

d) There may be discomfort with range of motion, but it should not be painful.

e) Flexibility exercises are most effective when muscles are warm.

f) There is no strong evidence that ballistic stretching is beneficial or harmful, but due to the nature of rapid, high-tension movements it is not generally recommended.

g) Properly performed ballistic stretching is equally as effective as static stretching at increased joint range of motion—particularly in activities that require ballistic movement such as basketball.[34,35]

7) Balance or neuromotor exercise guidelines[2,36]

- **a)** Healthy adults should perform motor skill and proprioceptive skill training to improve their ability to resist internal or external forces that may lead to falls.
    1. The PAGA do not prescribe a specific amount; however, performing these three times per week may prevent or reduce risk of falls.
- **b)** Adults age 65 and older should do balance training three or more days per week.[17]

OBJECTIVE 7

Describe the role of personal behavior and role modeling

1) Physician health behaviors predict physician counseling and patient behaviors (see Section 4)

- **a)** A positive correlation exists between:[37]
    1. Physicians performing aerobic exercise and counseling on it
    2. Physicians performing strength training exercise and counseling on it
- **b)** Israeli Health Study[38]
    1. The Israeli Health Study evaluated if physicians' personal health practices impacted their patients' health practices. Researchers analyzed electronic medical records of 429 physicians and 1,621 of their patients (matched for demographics) for eight screening and vaccination practices.
    2. If physicians were compliant with screening recommendations, their patients' chance of following those recommendations increased at a maximum of 13.7% relative difference. From this study, it appears that physicians' personal health screening and vaccination practices influence the practices of their patients.

OBJECTIVE 8

Explain the use of metabolic equivalents of tasks in assessing fitness

1) Defining metabolic equivalent of a task

- **a)** MET = Metabolic Equivalent of a Task[39]
    1. METs are a ratio of the metabolic rate during a task compared to a standard resting metabolic rate.
        a. The standard resting metabolic rate is the metabolic rate (amount of oxygen consumed) during quiet rest or sitting and is approximately 3.5 ml O_2/kg body weight per minute. This is the value of 1.0 MET.
    2. The ratios of the energy cost of different tasks is the metabolic rate during a task divided by the standard resting metabolic rate of 1.0 MET.
        a. Sleeping = 0.9 METs
        b. 3 mph walking = 3 METs
        c. Climbing two flights of stairs = 5 METs
        d. Running at 10.9 mph (17.5 kmph) = 18 METs

3. Classifying physical activity intensity using METs
    a. Moderate intensity = 3–5.9 METs
    b. Vigorous intensity = ≥6 METs
    c. It is important to note that METs are absolute, meaning they may not be appropriate ways to classify intensity levels as one becomes more fit. As a person adapts to training, they will be able to accomplish more work at a lower heart rate. This means that physical activity that may have been considered vigorous intensity previously, could become moderate intensity based on the individual's heart rate. However, METs would continue to erroneously classify the activity as moderate or vigorous intensity activity, irrespective of fitness levels.
4. MET hour = metabolic equivalents of activity for 1 hour
5. MET hours per week equation
    a. Calculate activity in METs per 1 hour (e.g., brisk walking = 3.3 METs per hour).
    b. Multiply by the number of hours per week the activity is completed (e.g., brisk walking for 4 hours per week).
    c. The equation would be: (3.3 METs per hour) × (4 hours per week) = 13.2 METs in one week, which is described as 13.2 MET hours per week.

OBJECTIVE 9

Describe the impact of exercise on weight

1) Obesity: key guidelines[2]

a) Recommendations from the American College of Sports Medicine[28]

1. Physical activity for weight maintenance
    a. >250 minutes per week of moderate-intensity physical activity (there's some evidence this may prevent weight re-gain)
    b. 60–90 minutes per day of moderate-intensity daily exercise
    c. Include strength or resistance activities twice per week
        (1) Strength training and resistance exercises are not as helpful as aerobic activity for weight maintenance.
        (2) Resistance exercise may enhance muscular strength and physical function in those who are obese or overweight. Additional benefits include improvements in cardiovascular disease and type 2 diabetes risk factors, as well as other chronic disease risk factors.[2]
2. Physical activity and weight loss[36,40, 41, 42]
    a. If physical activity is used alone as a weight loss intervention, the following results can be expected: improved diastolic pressure, triglycerides and fasting glucose, and lowered risk of cardiovascular disease, but often little to no reduction in weight.[43]
    b. The dose prescribed of exercise for weight loss changes the effectiveness of the intervention.

(1) In a study evaluating energy compensation of 36 overweight/obese adults, they found that subjects compensated ~1000 calories, whether they burned 1,500 calories per week (five sessions of 300 calories) or 3,000 calories per week (five sessions of 600 calories). Note: every 1 mile walked or run burns approximately 100 calories.[44]

(a) Participants in the high energy expenditure group lost 2.6 kg over 12 weeks, whereas the lower expenditure group only lost 0.8 kg. Weight loss is possible with physical activity, but requires a much higher dose than is typically prescribed or generally performed by individuals.

c. Dose response relationship between physical activity levels and magnitude of weight loss[45]

(1) <150 min/week promotes minimal weight loss

(2) >150 min/week of physical activity results in modest weight loss of 2–3 kg

(3) >225–420 min/week of physical activity results in a 5–7.5 kg weight loss

d. Physical activity and reduced caloric intake are both needed to control body weight. Diet is typically necessary to lose weight, but physical activity is essential to maintain weight loss.

e. Physical activity levels are a strong predictor of long-term weight maintenance and lead to better weight stabilization than diet alone.

f. Adding in Non-Exercise Activity Thermogenesis (NEAT) can expend an additional 350 calories per day.[15]

g. Regardless of weight loss outcomes:

(1) Obese individuals who exercise regularly have improved cardiovascular function, lower cardiovascular risk, and less loss of muscle mass.[46]

(2) Moderate to high levels of physical activity reduce mortality risk.[47]

3. There is an inverse relationship between physical activity and all-cause mortality.[3]

a. People who are fit experience a protective effect, independent of adiposity.

b. A 2012 large cohort study looking at years of life lost among people who were inactive and overweight found that physical activity increased life expectancy at any activity level and across all BMI ranges.[6]

c. People who were overweight but achieved physical activity guidelines had no years of life lost compared to their normal weight, physically active controls.

d. People who were obese but met the recommended guidelines had the same years of life lost as those who were normal weight but didn't exercise.

4. Physical activity is critical for maintaining a healthy body weight, losing excess body weight, or maintaining weight loss.

5. The amount of physical activity needed to maintain a healthy weight varies person to person.

6. The National Weight Control Registry (NWCR) is an online registry with open enrollment. The NWCR is the largest prospective study of individuals who have been successful at weight loss maintenance, tracking data on over 10,000 individuals who have been able to lose weight (an average of 66 pounds) and maintain that loss (over an average of 5.5 years).[48]

a. Findings from NWCR support that many people need more than 150 minutes of moderate-intensity activity each week to maintain weight loss. On average, members of the NWCR exercise at least 1 hour per day (420 minutes per week).[48]

OBJECTIVE 10

Identify the minimum and maximum levels of exercise

1) The minimum level of exercise

a) Current physical activity guidelines are based on the amount of exercise needed for optimal health. However, doses of exercise much smaller still provide health benefits.[49]

1. The most benefit is gained within 10–20 MET hours per week of physical activity. However, mortality decreases with any increase in MET hours per week. But may plateau around 80 MET hours per week.[50]

b) The minimum amount of exercise for healthy adults to reduce mortality[6]

1. Effort as little as merely standing more shows health benefits
   a. Standing for 2 hours per day is associated with a 10% reduction in mortality of all causes.[51]
2. Benefits with non-exercise activity like standing instead of sitting, taking the stairs, and fidgeting
   a. Shanghai Women's Health Study[52]
      (1) This study examined the benefits of exercise versus non-exercise physical activity in 67,143 women. The group was 40–70 years old, initially without heart disease, history of stroke, or cancer. The women were sedentary at the baseline and were followed for an average of 5.7 years.
      (2) Women were divided into two groups based on whether they engaged in regular exercise versus non-exercise physical activity.
      (3) The hazard ratio improved for both groups, showing decreased all-cause mortality rates with increasing physical activity. There was a 20–40% risk reduction among the most active individuals in both groups.
         (a) Women who walked more than 1 hour per day had a hazard ratio of 0.65 (95% CI 0.45, 0.92).
         (b) Women who had 4 or more non-exercise physical activity hours per day had a hazard ratio of 0.60 (95% CI 0.50-0.71).
      (4) This study concluded that health benefits can be obtained through purposeful exercise, non-exercise physical activity, or a combination of both.
3. Nurses' Health Study[53]
   a. This study showed a significant reduction in all-cause mortality (rest reduction [RR] 0.82) with as little as 1–1.9 hours of moderate to vigorous physical activity per week. At 7 or more hours per week, only slight, non-statistically significant benefits were seen beyond the above RR of 0.82.
4. Cardiovascular disease risk was assessed in 416,175 individuals who were divided into low-active versus inactive groups.
   a. Benefits in cardiovascular disease reduction occurred with 15 minutes per day or 90 minutes per week of moderate-intensity exercise.

> **Non-exercise activity thermogenesis (NEAT)** is the energy expended by all daily activities excluding purposeful exercise, sleeping, or eating. It includes all other activities like sitting, fidgeting, yard work, housework, and typing.[14]

(1) RR 0.86 for all-cause mortality in the low-active versus the inactive group

(2) The low active group had 3 years longer life expectancy than the inactive group.

5. "Weekend warrior" benefits[54]

a. There is decreased all-cause mortality among men performing physical activity 1–2 days per week (RR 0.85) versus sedentary men.

b. However, completing all 150 minutes of physical activity in 1 day may increase the risk of injury.

2) Maximum amount of exercise

a) Additional physical activity has further and more extensive health benefits.[2]

1. All-cause mortality is further reduced beyond what is expected with 150 minutes of moderate-intensity or 75 minutes of vigorous activity at 300 minutes (5 hours) per week of moderate-intensity, or 150 minutes per week of vigorous-intensity aerobic physical activity, or an equivalent combination of both.

2. However, the magnitude of the risk reduction is lower. See Table 6.5 and Figure 6.1 below.[38,50]

Table 6.5 Risk of Dying Prematurely Declines as People Become More Physically Active[38]

Minutes per Week of Moderate- or Vigorous-Intensity Physical Activity	Relative Risk
30	1.0
90 (3x)	0.80
180 (6x)	0.73
330 (10x)	0.64
420 (14x)	0.615

Figure 6.1 Risk of Dying Prematurely Declines with More Moderate- or Vigorous-Intensity Physical Activity

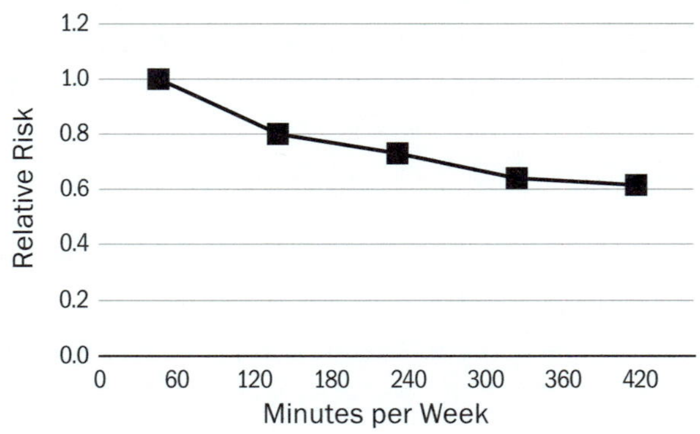

b) Years of life gained by meeting physical activity guidelines compared to sedentary (0 MET hours per week) in individuals age 40 or older[55]

1. 75 minutes of brisk walking per week (0.1–3.74 MET hours per week): ~1.8 years of life gained
2. 90–150 minutes of brisk walking per week (3.75–7.4 MET hours per week): ~2.5 years of life gained
3. 200 minutes per week of brisk walking (7.5–14.9 MET hours per week): ~3 years of life gained
4. 400 minutes per week of brisk walking (15–22.4 MET hours per week): ~4 years of life gained
5. 500 minutes per week of brisk walking (22.5+ MET hours per week): ~4.5 years of life gained

c) Vigorous-intensity physical activity may provide further benefits[31,56]

1. A study evaluating life expectancy, physical activity, race, and gender found 20-year-old Hispanic males had a greater life expectancy if they participated in vigorous- versus moderate-intensity exercise. These men gained 2.6 hours of life per 1 hour of moderate-intensity exercise and earned 5.2 hours of life per 1 hour of vigorous-intensity exercise.[56]

BONUS: High Intensity Interval Training (HIIT)[57]

- HIIT is characterized by brief, intermittent bursts of vigorous activity that are interspersed with periods of rest or low-intensity exercise.
- Example: swimming as fast as you can for 20 seconds, and then swimming slowly for 10 seconds.
- Low-volume HIIT is a potent and time-efficient training for the:
  - Cardiovascular system
  - Skeletal muscle
- Current research
  - Improvement in VO_2 max, endothelial function, hydrogen ion buffering, resting muscle glycogen concentration, time to exhaustion, and a greater loss of abdominal and total fat[58]
  - Studies are currently from short intervention periods (weeks).
  - There is a need for longer-term studies (months to years) and a variety of clinical cohorts (such as people with diabetes or coronary artery disease) to evaluate long-term effects of HIIT exercise.
- Not recommended as a starting point for sedentary individuals
- Best for already fit individuals who are looking to decrease how much time they spend training or to improve cardiovascular conditioning

OBJECTIVE 11

List key physical activity assessment tools

1) Physical activity as a vital sign

a) Health and weight are both directly related to physical activity.[3]

1. Obesity and physical inactivity are linked to increased risk of cardiovascular disease, type 2 diabetes, some cancers, and all-cause mortality in a dose response fashion. The more obese or physically inactive a person is, the higher the risk.
2. Physical activity reduces the risk of all-cause mortality and years of life lost in all individuals regardless of weight.[6]

b) To accurately address someone's future health risks, weight and physical activity should be measured and addressed at each visit.
   1. Recommendations should be made to patients based upon findings (active, sedentary, sit time, etc.)

c) Exercise is Medicine (exerciseismedicine.org) is a health campaign with a vision to make physical activity and exercise a standard part of disease prevention and medical treatment worldwide.
   1. Physical activity vital sign (PAVS) is a tool created to quickly measure one's physical activity level.
      a. PAVS equation: (days per week with physical activity) × (minutes of physical activity per day) = minutes of physical activity per week
         (1) Days per week: On average, how many days do you perform physical activity where your heart is beating faster and your breathing is harder than usual?
         (2) Total minutes: On average, how many total minutes of physical activity or exercise do you perform on those days?'
         (3) Also, it may be helpful to clarify cardiovascular from strength training activities. How many days per week do you perform muscle strengthening exercises, such as body weight exercises or resistance training?

d) The Kaiser Permanente healthcare system in Southern California began tracking physical activity as a vital sign.[59]
   1. 1,793,385 adult patients were seen, and physical activity was documented as a vital sign at 86% of the visits, proving PAVS can be consistently documented in health care.

e) Interpreting PAVs
   1. If the patient is meeting the standard for aerobic and resistance exercises:
      a. Congratulate the patient.
      b. Consider adjusting intensity or incorporating balance or flexibility exercises into their routine.
   2. If the patient is insufficiently active:
      a. Guide them to acknowledge the insufficiency
      b. Assess the physical activity level. What kind of activities does the patient currently engage in? What do they enjoy?
      c. Determine readiness to change. Ask them what it would take to get to the standard (e.g., "Would you be interested in being more active?" "How can we get you more active?").
      d. Establish close and frequent follow-up.
   3. If the patient is sedentary:
      a. Lead the patient to acknowledge his sedentary behavior and have a brief discussion regarding barriers to physical activity.
      b. Relate health problems to physical inactivity, if appropriate.
      c. Offer support (e.g., "What would it take for you to be more active?"). Determine readiness to change.
      d. Assess and follow up at future visits.

2) Exercise intensity assessment tools

a) Talk test
   1. This is the least objective test, but it is also the easiest for measuring intensity. It is completed while an individual is performing physical activity.
      a. Very-light to light-intensity exercise means: heart rate 63% or less of maximum, able to talk and sing

b. Moderate-intensity exercise means: heart rate 64–76% of maximum, able to talk but not sing

c. Vigorous to maximal-intensity exercise means: heart rate is 77–100% of maximum, unable to talk

b) Respiratory rate[60]

1. Overlaps with the talk test
2. Breaths per minute (likely best indicator of perceived exertion)

c) Rating of perceived exertion (RPE)

1. Borg scale of perceived exertion
   a. Used to monitor the intensity of exercise and rates of exercise intensity from 6–20 and is based on a rough calculation of estimated maximum HR/10
   b. A shortened version, the Borg category-ratio scale, uses a scale of 0–10

d) Heart rate reserve (HRR)

1. The difference between maximal heart rate and the resting heart rate (or heart rate upon awakening)
2. HRR = maximal heart rate – resting heart rate
3. Recommended exercise intensity is 40–85% of HRR

e) Maximal heart rate percentage (% max HR)

1. Light intensity: ≤63% of maximal heart rate
2. Moderate: 64–76% of maximal heart rate
3. Vigorous: ≥77% of maximal heart rate

f) Metabolic Equivalents of a Task (METs)[28]

1. <3 METs = light intensity
2. 3–5.9 METs = moderate intensity
3. ≥6 METs = vigorous intensity

3) **Exercise Intensity (see Table 6.6)[61]**

Table 6.6 Exercise Intensity

Method	Range	Moderate Intensity	Vigorous Intensity
Rating of Perceived Exertion (RPE)[2]	0–10	5–6	≥7
Borg Scale of Perceived Exertion[62]	6–20	12–13	≥14
% Max HR (Max HR crude calculation = 220 – age in years)[63]	0–100%	64–76%	≥77%
% Heart Rate Reserve (HRR) (HRR = 220 – resting heart rate)[64]	0–100%	40–59%	≥60%
Metabolic Equivalents (METs)[65]	-	3.0–5.9	≥6
Resistance Training[66]	0–100%	50–74%	≥75%
Talk Test[66]		One can talk, but not sing	Unable to say more than a few words without pausing for a breath

4) **Assessing functional capacity**

a) 6-minute walk test[67]

1. Measures functional capacity
    a. The goal is to walk as far as possible within 6 minutes at the submaximal level.
    b. It's reflective of activities of daily life (may stop, rest ,and resume at any point).
2. It is easily administered. All that is needed is:
    a. A long hallway (30 meters, or 100 feet)
    b. A stopwatch, pulse oximeter, and a measuring device to monitor the patient as they walk as far as possible in 6 minutes.
3. The 6-minute walk test is useful when compared to the patient's own results from the 6-minute walk test before and after an intervention (such as before and after starting an exercise program).
    a. Test results from a single 6-minute walk test are less helpful because there are no standard reference populations for a patient's results to be compared against.

5) Assessing the components of fitness

a) Cardiorespiratory fitness tests

1. Cardiorespiratory fitness can be estimated through indirect testing of the maximum volume of oxygen (VO_2 max) consumed during exercise. VO_2 max is also known as aerobic power.
2. Step testing[68,69]
    a. This test includes a 12-inch step, metronome, and stopwatch. The test subject steps for 3 minutes to the timing of the metronome and then rests for 1 minute. At that time, heart rate is auscultated and palpated. The heart rate can then be compared to calculated norms for age and gender.
    b. Step testing is an effective, validated method that can be completed in a clinic with little equipment. It is more accurate for individuals who are not already fit.
3. Submaximal talk test for ventilatory threshold (VT1)[56]
    a. Testing is complex and requires heart rate telemetry for continuous monitoring.
4. Rockport fitness walking test (1 mile, or 1.6 km)[70]
    a. Testing does not require a heart monitor or equipment. Test subjects complete a one-mile walking course as fast as possible, then pulse is recorded. The VO_2 max is estimated with an equation based on gender, age, body weight, time of course completion, and peak heart rate.
    b. For most individuals, the actual VO_2 max is within 0.33 L/min (±4.4 mL × kg × in) of the Rockport fitness test's predicted VO_2 max.
5. Fitness registry and the importance of exercise national database (FRIEND)
    a. This registry is a national database of reference ranges for maximal oxygen consumption per decade for men and women (20–79 years old) during treadmill testing. Having these references on hand can be helpful in counseling patients about their fitness level.[71]

b) Muscular fitness (muscular strength and endurance)

1. Muscular strength
    a. Muscular strength is difficult to test in a clinic unless the clinic has weights or a way to apply a load to certain movements (e.g., a bench press or leg press). It may be best to refer patients to a medical fitness professional for muscular strength testing.
    b. Typically correlates to few (≤3) repetitions of a task prior to reaching muscular fatigue
    c. The one rep max is a reliable indicator of muscle strength as well.

   d. Grip strength is a simple measurement that can be predictive of mortality and functional status in older individuals.[72]

c) Muscular endurance[28]

1. Helps assess one's ability to perform activities of daily living by testing the ability of muscles to perform repeated or sustained contractions until muscle fatigue occurs.
2. Measured as the maximum number of correctly performed repetitions of squats, push-ups or sit-ups without rest. This number can be compared to established norms based on age and sex.

d) Flexibility[73]

1. The sit and reach test measures flexibility in the hamstrings and low back. The standard sit and reach test is highly consistent (reliability estimates 0.96–0.99), but it is moderately accurate for hamstring flexibility (reliability coefficient, r = 0.64) and has poor accuracy for low back flexibility (r = 0.28). The test is not accurate for those with low back pain. The test assumes that those with higher scores have better hamstring and back flexibility. This type of flexibility is believed to protect against acute and chronic musculoskeletal injuries, risk of falls, postural issues, and low back problems. However, this belief is not well documented in the literature.
2. The standard sit and reach test is performed using a standard sit and reach box and marking the right angle with tape at 38 cm (15 in). The participant extends their legs so that their heels are against the box, with palms down and arms extended the participant reaches as far as possible without bending the knees. Three trials are performed, and the average distance is used.

e) Body composition[28]

1. Skin-fold thickness testing with calipers
   a. Evaluation of body composition can be done through skin-fold thickness measurement with calipers because subcutaneous fat is proportional to the total amount of body fat. Approximately one-third of body fat is subcutaneous fat, but this varies based on sex, age, and gender. With proper technique, the accuracy of skin-fold testing for percent total body fat percentage is within ± 3.5%.
   b. Testing is completed with calipers that measure standard skin-fold sites while the patient stands at typically three to seven sites. Measurements are taken on the right side of body at the abdomen, tricep, bicep, chest/pectoral muscle, medial calf, midaxillary, subscapular, suprailiac, and thigh. Note: men and women have different sites.
2. A consensus on exact body composition has not been established, but the American College of Sports Medicine has created accepted normal ranges using skin fold testing. Norms for body fat percentage associated with optimal health include 10–22% for men and 20–32% for women.
3. Densitometry
   a. Body fat percentage is estimated using the ratio of body mass to body volume and is used as the standard for assessing body composition. Current methods for measuring densitometry are hydrodensitometry (underwater weighing) and dual-energy X-ray absorptiometry (DEXA) scans and multicompartment measuring.
   b. These are considered the most accurate body composition measures and are the "gold standard" body composition tests.

OBJECTIVE 12

Medical screening before exercise and recommended progression of physical activity

1) Medical screening for exercise by a health care provider

- **a)** General screening considerations
  1. Screening should not present a barrier for low-level physical activity.
     - a. Risk of death during physical activity is very rare. Estimated occurrence is 1 in every 1.5 million episodes of vigorous exercise for men and 1 in 36.5 million hours of moderate- to vigorous-intensity exercise in (women) and is usually restricted to:
       - (1) Individuals with known disease signs or symptoms, such as cardiac disease (CAD, CHF, valvular disease, HTN), peripheral vascular disease, and cerebrovascular disease
       - (2) Sudden intense activities
     - b. Risk of acute myocardial infarction during or immediately following vigorous intensity exercise was 50 times higher for the habitually sedentary compared to those who exercise regularly.[74]
     - c. Instead of focusing on if exercise is safe for a patient, consider: "Are my patients safe to remain sedentary?"
     - d. The risks of sedentary behavior are universal and far greater than exercising.
     - e. However, it is important to continue to take caution when prescribing exercise to a high-risk individual in order to prevent sudden complications.
  2. 2015 Exercise Screening Guidelines from the American College of Sports Medicine (ACSM)[75]
     - a. Screening identifies two groups of individuals who should receive medical clearance before initiating exercise or increasing intensity.
       - (1) Group 1: Those with clinically significant disease(s) who would benefit from medically supervised exercise programs.
       - (2) Group 2: Those with uncontrolled medical conditions that require treatment or control before further exercise should be initiated.
     - b. The goal of screening is to reduce exercise-related cardiovascular events.
     - c. Screening is based on three factors known to modulate exercise-related cardiovascular events:
       - (1) Current level of physical activity
       - (2) Presence of signs/symptoms or known cardiovascular, metabolic, or renal disease
       - (3) Desired level of physical activity
     - d. Preparticipation health screening by a self-screening tool should be done for all individuals wanting to initiate an exercise program.

Quick Tip

Low-level physical activity is an intensity level at which when one would be able to sing and talk while exercising.

Real work application: Patients who have walked into the office and are not symptomatic can engage in low-level physical activity.

(1) The ACSM recommends the Physical Activity Readiness Questionnaire for Everyone (PAR-Q+), which provides several follow up questions to guide preparticipation recommendations (see Figure 6.2)

(2) Developed to reduce barriers for exercise and false positive screenings[76,77]

Figure 6.2

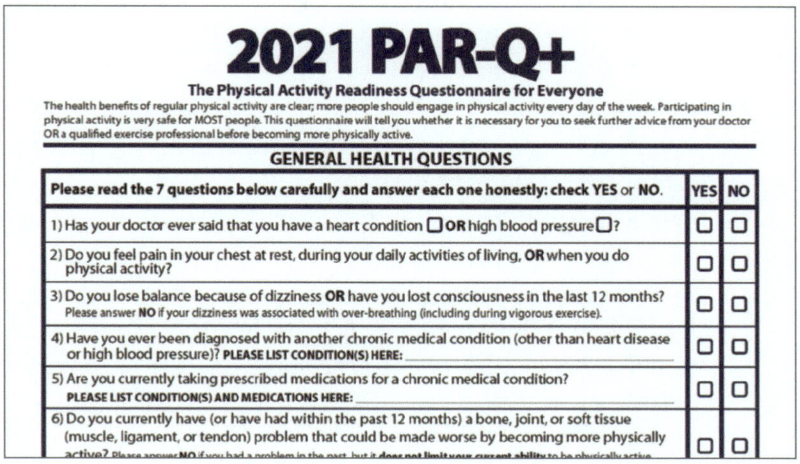

2021 PAR-Q+

The Physical Activity Readiness Questionnaire for Everyone

The health benefits of regular physical activity are clear; more people should engage in physical activity every day of the week. Participating in physical activity is very safe for MOST people. This questionnaire will tell you whether it is necessary for you to seek further advice from your doctor OR a qualified exercise professional before becoming more physically active.

GENERAL HEALTH QUESTIONS

Please read the 7 questions below carefully and answer each one honestly: check YES or NO.	YES	NO
1) Has your doctor ever said that you have a heart condition ☐ **OR** high blood pressure ☐?	☐	☐
2) Do you feel pain in your chest at rest, during your daily activities of living, **OR** when you do physical activity?	☐	☐
3) Do you lose balance because of dizziness **OR** have you lost consciousness in the last 12 months? Please answer **NO** if your dizziness was associated with over-breathing (including during vigorous exercise).	☐	☐
4) Have you ever been diagnosed with another chronic medical condition (other than heart disease or high blood pressure)? **PLEASE LIST CONDITION(S) HERE:** ______	☐	☐
5) Are you currently taking prescribed medications for a chronic medical condition? **PLEASE LIST CONDITION(S) AND MEDICATIONS HERE:** ______	☐	☐
6) Do you currently have (or have had within the past 12 months) a bone, joint, or soft tissue (muscle, ligament, or tendon) problem that could be made worse by becoming more physically active?	☐	☐

3. 2015 ACSM guidelines for risk classification and medical clearance

   a. Referral to a health provider should be made based on current physical activity levels and presence of signs or symptoms and/or known cardiovascular, metabolic, or renal disease.[78]

      (1) If a person is physically inactive and has signs or symptoms of cardiovascular, metabolic, or renal disease, medical clearance is recommended before initiating moderate- to vigorous-intensity physical activity.

         (a) Pulmonary disease does not require medical clearance, however, those with uncontrolled lung disease should be evaluated to determine if accommodations during exercise or changes in medical therapy are needed.

         (b) The medical provider ultimately decides what evaluation is needed for medical clearance before initiation of moderate- to vigorous-intensity exercise. Note: there is a lack of evidence that medical clearance mitigates risk and there are no universal recommendations.[75]

2) Exercise stress testing

a) The American College of Cardiology recommends exercise testing in individuals who are at an increased risk of cardiovascular disease before they engage in moderate to vigorous physical activity. The college acknowledges their recommendations are based on conflicting evidence and expert opinions.

b) The US Preventive Services Task Force (USPSTF) recommends against routine testing or exercise electrocardiography testing in asymptomatic individuals before initiating exercise program due to insufficient evidence that it's helpful in reducing cardiac events.

c) Indications for clinical exercise testing fall into three broad categories: diagnosing disease, determining risk for adverse event, and evaluating the physiologic response to exercise.

1. Exercise stress testing is best used to assess intermediate risk patients. Common indications include:[79]

a. Assessing symptoms suggestive of ischemic heart disease such as chest pain or dyspnea on exertion in intermediate risk patients
b. Evaluating patients who present to the emergency department with chest pain but negative cardiac enzymes
c. It may also be used to evaluate heart function in at-risk patients with syncope, valvular disease, arrhythmias, medical or surgical interventions, or other heart disease.
d. Note: some patients are unable to exercise. In this case, only a nuclear myocardial perfusion test is ordered in place of the exercise stress test.

2. Exercise stress testing is not recommended for patients who are low risk or high risk.[78]
   a. It should not be used for detection of ischemia in asymptomatic patients with no prior history of revascularization.
   b. It is not a benign procedure, as 1 in 10,000 exercise stress tests results in sudden cardiac death or hospitalization.
   c. It is contraindicated in those with a recent myocardial infarction (<2 days), hypertensive emergency, acute infections near or in the heart, decompensated heart failure, unstable angina, severe symptomatic aortic stenosis, uncontrolled arrhythmias, or aortic dissection.

3) Algorithm for pre-participation screening process (see Table 6.7)

Table 6.7 Exercise Preparticipation Health Screening Recommendations[28]

		Participates in Regular Exercise		Does Not Participate in Regular Exercise	
		Medical Clearance	**Recommendations**	**Medical Clearance**	**Recommendations**
Asymptomatic	No known cardiovascular, metabolic, or renal disease	No	May continue or progress to moderate or vigorous activity	No	Light to moderate exercise is recommended, and may progress to higher intensities per ACSM guidelines.
	Known cardiovascular, metabolic, or renal disease	No, moderate intensity Yes, vigorous intensity	Medical clearance (within the last 12 months) necessary before progressing to vigorous intensity exercise	Yes	If cleared, light to moderate exercise is recommended, and may progress to higher intensities per ACSM guidelines.
Symptomatic	Regardless of disease state	Yes	Discontinue exercise, seek medical clearance; if cleared, may return to exercise and progress per ACSM guidelines	Yes	If cleared, light to moderate exercise is recommended, and may progress to higher intensities per ACSM guidelines.

Regular exercise: planned, structured physical activity, ≥30 minutes of moderate intensity, ≥3 days/week for ≥3 months.

Signs and symptoms: occur at rest or during activity, includes discomfort or pain in chest, neck, jaw, arms or other areas that may result from ischemia; dizziness or syncope; orthopnea or paroxysmal nocturnal dyspnea; ankle edema; palpitations or tachycardia; intermittent claudication; heart murmur; unusual fatigue or shortness of breath with usual or mild exertion.

Medical clearance: approval from a health care professional to engage in exercise.

a) The patient currently participates in regular exercise.
   1. Asymptomatic with no known cardiovascular, metabolic, or renal disease:
      a. No medical clearance needed.
      b. May participate in moderate- or vigorous-intensity exercise and progress per ACSM guidelines
   2. Asymptomatic with known cardiovascular, metabolic, or renal disease:
      a. Medical clearance for moderate intensity exercise is not needed.
      b. Medical clearance is not needed with gradual progression to vigorous intensity if one remains asymptomatic and has been medically cleared in the past 12 months.
      c. Medical clearance is required if signs or symptoms occur.
   3. Symptomatic, regardless of known disease status:
      a. Discontinue exercise and seek medical clearance.
      b. If cleared, patient may return to exercise and progress per ACSM guidelines.

b) The patient currently does not participate in regular exercise.
   4. Asymptomatic with no known cardiovascular, metabolic, or renal disease:
      a. No medical clearance is needed.
      b. Light to moderate exercise is recommended, and patient may progress to higher intensities per the ACSM guidelines.
   5. Asymptomatic with known cardiovascular, metabolic, or renal disease:
      a. Medical clearance is required.
      b. If cleared, light to moderate exercise is recommended, and patient may progress to higher intensities per the ACSM guidelines.
   6. Symptomatic, regardless of known disease status.
      a. Medical clearance is required.
      b. If cleared, light to moderate exercise is recommended, and patient may progress per ACSM guidelines.

4) ACSM guidelines recommend progressing from inactivity to physical activity by duration and intensity in the following increments:[28]

a) The ACSM's three stages of exercise progression
   1. Initial stage (1–6 weeks): designed to minimize muscle soreness, discomfort, and injury and to prepare individuals for exercise at the next stage.
      a. Intensity: moderate-intensity (40–60% of heart rate reserve [HRR] aerobic activities in an interval format.)
      b. Duration: start at 15 minutes and progress to 30 minutes
      c. Frequency: three to four times per week
   2. Improvement stage (4 to 8 months):
      a. Intensity: dependent upon the individual and changes with fitness level
         (1) Intensity is usually increased after target duration and frequency have been achieved.
         (2) Can be measured in multiple ways as described in this section. When basing progression of physical intensity from a patient's heart rate, the maximum heart rate during exercise should be increased no more than 5% of one's heart rate reserve every sixth session, providing the prior increase was tolerated.

(a) HRR is equal to maximum heart rate (MHR) minus resting heart rate (RHR): HHR = MHR − RHR

(b) MHR is equal to 220 minus a person's age: MHR = 220 - age.

(c) Example: 40-year-old male MHR should be 180 bpm (MHR = 220 - 40 = 180bpm). His RHR is = 80 bpm (RHR = 80 bpm). The HRR is then equal to 100 bpm, it's his maximum heart rate minus his resting heart rate (HRR = 180 - 80 = 100). 5% of a HRR of 100 = 5 bpm. Therefore, for this patient with an MHR of 180, RHR of 80, and HRR of 100, the highest heart rate during a workout should increase by 5 bpm every sixth exercise session if tolerated well.

b. Duration: steadily increased at no more than 20% more each week until 20–30 minutes of continuous moderate- to vigorous-intensity exercise is achieved.

3. Maintenance stage (indefinitely): this begins once the participant has reached pre-established fitness goals. The patient should be in at least the 50th percentile in all health-related fitness parameters.

Table 6.8 Training Progression for the Sedentary Low-Risk Participants

Program Stage	Week	Exercise Frequency (sessions per week)	Exercise Intensity (%HRR)	Exercise Duration (min)
Initial Stage	1	3	40–50	15–20
	2	3–4	40–50	20–25
	3	3–4	50–60	20–25
	4	3–4	50–60	25–30
Improvement Stage	5-7	3-4	60-70	25-30
	8–10	3–4	60–70	30–35
	11–13	3–4	65–75	30–35
	14–16	3–5	65–75	30–35
	17–20	3–5	70–85	35–40
	21–24	3–5	70–85	35–40
Maintenance Stage	24+	3–5	70–85	20–60

Note: This is for reference and does not need to be memorized.

OBJECTIVE 13

Describe how to collaborate with your patients to promote physical activity change

1) Physical activity counseling

a) The US Preventive Services Task Force encourages health care providers to counsel on lifestyle modification for patients with known risk factors.[81] However, it does not specifically mention physical activity.

b) Activity Counseling Trial (ACT)[82]

1. 54 primary care providers were trained to give 3–4 minutes of physical activity advice to sedentary patients.

2. Results
    a. 99% of patients received initial physician advice
    b. 86% of providers spent less than 5–6 minutes
    c. 46% spent the recommended 3–4 minutes
    d. 63% reported little or no increase in length of patient visit
    e. 83% reported participation was an asset to the clinic

c) Efficacy of physical activity counseling[83]

1. A 2009 cluster randomized trial evaluated the effectiveness of physicians' physical activity advice and physical activity prescriptions for individual patients in routine primary care.
    a. The study, "Effectiveness of Physical Activity Advice and Prescription by Physicians in Routine Primary Care: A Cluster Randomized Trial," included 56 family physicians (29 intervention, 27 control) who treated 4,317 physically inactive patients (2,248 intervention, 2,069 controls).
2. Intervention
    a. Physicians in the intervention group provided physical activity counseling to all patients, and a subgroup (30%) of these patients also received an exercise prescription.
    b. Physical activity was measured with 7-day physical activity recall 6 months from the visit.
3. Results
    a. Physical activity increased by 18 minutes per week in the intervention versus the control group.
    b. The advice-only intervention showed a small effect in older adults and no significant effect in younger adults.
    c. Greater effects were seen in the subgroup with a physical activity prescription.
    d. Older adults, ≥50 years of age
        (1) Increased physical activity by 131 minutes per week compared to controls (95% CI, 105–157)
        (2) Doubled the minutes of moderate to vigorous physical activity compared to controls (difference 67 minutes per week, 95% CI, 47–87)
    e. Younger adults <50 years of age
        (1) Increased physical activity compared to controls by 31.5 minutes per week (95% CI, 11.2–51.8)
        (2) Had a 7% higher probability of meeting physical activity guidelines (95% CI, 2.2–12.8%)
    f. Number needed to treat (NNT) is 26, meaning 26 patients must be given intervention of physical activity counseling to get one sedentary individual to meet the physical activity guidelines
4. Meta-analysis of office-based physical activity counseling[84,85]
    a. The analysis looked at 13 papers on primary care provider counseling with self-reported physical activity by patients.
        (1) Counseling on physical activity by primary care providers significantly increases physical activity at 12 months by self-report (OR 1.42).
        (2) NNT is 12, meaning 12 sedentary adults had to receive counseling to get one to meet the physical activity guidelines at 12 months.

2) **Need and importance for provider counseling for physical activity**

a) Providers giving advice to patients assessed by NHANES-III 1988–1994:[86]

1. Only 33% of hypertensive patients received counseling for physical activity from their physicians. But among that 33%, 71% followed the recommendations, resulting in a decrease of blood pressure by 3–4 mmHg.

b) Prevalence of lifestyle counseling among diabetic patients[87]

1. Nutritional counseling/referral: 36% of visits
2. Exercise counseling: 18% of visits
3. Positive predictors for adherence to nutritional counseling:
    a. Younger patient age
    b. Private insurance
4. Lesson to be learned: very few physicians are counseling on nutrition and exercise

c) Physician barriers to counseling on physical activity[88]

1. Heavy workload and lack of time
2. No reimbursement
3. Lack of consensus about recommendations
4. Doubts about effectiveness
5. Lack of clarity on which professional in primary care is responsible
6. Physician's personal health habits

3) **Practical resources for counseling patients on physical activity**

a) 5A's in practice: assess, advise, agree, assist, arrange.[89,90]

b) Assess: beliefs, behaviors, knowledge

1. Is the patient exercising?
2. How does the patient feel about exercise?

c) Advise: provide specific information about health benefits of change.

1. Match the patient's stage of change (transtheoretical model; see Box).
2. Tailor advice to the patient's specific health problems.
    a. Example: if a patient has obesity, prescribe non-weight bearing activities, such as swimming or biking.
    b. Example: if a patient has arthritis in their knees, prescribe lower body weight resistance training or yoga or tai chi.
    c. Example: if patient has trouble sleeping, prescribe regular cardiovascular exercise.

d) Agree: collaboratively set goals based on the patient's interest and confidence in their ability to change behavior.

Transtheoretical Stages of Change

Translated into five stages of physical exercise:

1. **Precontemplative:** couch potato (no thoughts about becoming active)
2. **Contemplative:** inactive thinker (thinking about becoming active)
3. **Preparation:** planning to start within the next month (joined a gym, purchased shoes)
4. **Action:** activator (beginning to exercise now)
5. **Maintenance:** active exerciser
6. **Relapse:** stopped exercising

1. SMART goal
    a. Another option for goal setting along with or in place of exercise prescription:
        (1) Specific
        (2) Measurable
        (3) Achievable
        (4) Relevant
        (5) Time frame
    b. Example: I will walk 2 miles, twice per week on Tuesdays and Thursdays by the end of the month.

e) Assist: identify personal barriers, strategies, problem-solving techniques and social or environmental support.

1. Assist the patient with realistic goal setting, appropriate accountability, and follow-up.
2. Work with the patient to gain social support and affirmation, begin self-monitoring, problem solve, and find alternatives to past activities.
3. Brainstorm ideas to incorporate physical activity
    a. Instead of using the elevator, take the stairs.
    b. When watching TV, move during commercials (e.g., ride a stationary bike, do squats, or do jumping jacks).
    c. Instead of going out for lunch, take a lunch and use the extra time to go for a short walk.
    d. Purposefully park far away and walk more.
    e. Avoid using the drive-through.
    f. Run errands, if possible.
4. Social support
    a. Help patients engage their family, friends, and neighbors.
    b. Reassure patients that one person cannot provide all the support they will need. Instead, they should focus on building a "team of supporters."
    c. Questions to ask when building a team
        (1) What do I need help with?
        (2) Who could help me?
        (3) How could they help?
        (4) How could I reward them for helping me?
5. Discuss relapse prevention

f) Arrange a follow-up plan.

1. Plan follow-up session.
2. Discuss whether interim support would be helpful (e.g., telephone, email, online group, or newsletter).
3. Refer to support staff (medical fitness professionals and community resources).
    a. The provider's job is to start the process, and the team can assist in regularly connecting with patients.
    b. Follow-up will assist with continued changes.
    c. Having medical fitness professionals involved is beneficial for resistance training program implementation and design.

OBJECTIVE 14

Identify resources for sustainable behavior change

1) **Self-monitoring**

   a) Provides feedback during behavior change, allowing the patient to see whether they are meeting their set goals

   b) Record physical activity goals with objective measures, such as: pedometer, fitness device/ wearables (e.g., Fitbit, Apple Watch, etc.), mobile health applications, GPS, heart rate monitor, or phone

   c) Create physical activity reminders including having an alarm on the pedometer/phone, having an accountability partner, sleeping in workout clothes before a morning workout, placing shoes in a strategic place, using calendar reminders, signing up for a 5K or race and following a training plan, using apps and frequently reviewing the purpose for making health behavior change

2) **Problem-solve**

   a) Identify barriers as to why goals were not met.

      1. What happened?
      2. What did you do?
      3. What did you learn?
      4. It may be helpful to use the antecedent/behavior/consequence (ABC) chart as a tool for observing and identifying problems (see Table 6.9)[91]

         a. Antecedent: events/interactions that occur directly before event
         b. Behavior: observable behavior (not internal states/emotions)
         c. Consequence: what occurs directly after (verbal and physical interactions, promptings, actions).

Table 6.9 Antecedent/Behavior/Consequence (ABC) chart

Component	Description
A - Antecedent	Events/interactions that occur directly before event
B - Behavior	Observable behavior (not internal states/ emotions)
C - Consequence	What occurs directly afterward (verbal and physical interactions, promptings, actions)

   b) Develop potential solutions.

      1. Remaining consistent with the coach approach, help facilitate problem solving but try to avoid giving the solution.
      2. Remember that each person is the expert in their life.
      3. Be willing to help brainstorm with the patient, as they may need assistance with generating ideas and overcoming barriers.

   c) Act and assess.

      1. Practice the potential solution with patient.
      2. Evaluate how the solution worked.

3) **Relapse prevention**

   a) Identify high-risk situations.

1. Travel, holidays, illness, or periods of stress

b) Plan for potential lapses.

1. What skills could be used to get people back to meeting their goal?

c) Cognitive restructuring

1. Encourage patients not to abandon goals when they experience a lapse.
2. Identify unhelpful thought patterns (e.g., all or nothing, avoidance, or shame).

4) Resources for sustainable change in physical activity

a) Health promotion clinics[92]

1. One study looked at 66 primary care providers in 23 practices and compared that group with a control community group.
2. In the study, an intervention of brief physical activity counseling was offered to primary care physicians. Physical activity promotion resources, including print materials and pedometers, were given to the providers to share with patients. Primary care providers were asked to educate patients on physical activity and follow-up with questionnaires.
3. Study results: There was a 31% increase in patient recall of being advised by their primary care provider on physical activity. Compare that to a slight decrease (that was not significant) in patient recall of physical activity advice given by their provider in the control community group.
4. The results showed that physical activity counseling and resources can be administered in a primary care practice.

5) Working as a team

a) Health care providers who can assist with patient care behavioral change include:

1. Physical therapists
    a. They usually work in post-injury, pre- or post-surgery, therapeutic exercise, and training with machinery/modalities.
    b. Pros: Physical therapists are highly trained and have established communication via medical records.
    c. Cons: A limited number of visits are covered by insurance, copays may be high, physical therapy requires a medical diagnosis and is time consuming.
2. Exercise physiologists
    a. They are certified health professionals.
    b. They prescribe and supervise exercises.
    c. Pros: highly trained, experienced, and credentialed
    d. Cons: limited availability, cost, or limited insurance coverage, if at all
3. Coaches[93]
    a. Fitness coaches: credentialed exercise professionals
    b. Wellness coaches: credentialed health, fitness, and mental health professionals
    c. Health coach: credentialed health care professional
    d. Pros: Accessibility is high (these coaches may work by phone or online), and they can target specific behaviors. In 2017, a National Board Certification for Health & Wellness Coaches was created to standardize and uphold the practice, and now over 4,100 coaches have become National Board-Certified Health and Wellness Coaches
    e. Cons: Costly, as coaches are not covered by insurance, and they have variable experience/ knowledge

4. Personal trainers
    a. A total of 18 accrediting bodies for personal trainers exist, but the top four organizations with the most rigorous standards are:
        (1) American Council on Exercise (ACE)
        (2) American College of Sports Medicine (ACSM)
        (3) National Academy of Sports Medicine (NASM)
        (4) National Strength and Conditioning Association (NSCA)
    b. Pros: Accessible, variety of activities
    c. Cons: Private pay, variable knowledge, no established communication

6) External resources

a) Wellness programs

1. Multi-dimensional programs that use in-person meetings together with websites and apps
    a. The National Physical Activity Plan, which is a plan for all Americans to one day be physically active and have an environment that promotes this goal: http://www.physicalactivityplan.org
    b. Walk with a Doc: http://walkwithadoc.org/
    c. Silver Sneakers: https://tools.silversneakers.com
    d. Let's Move: http://www.letsmove.gov
    e. The President's Challenge: https://www.presidentschallenge.org
    f. Exercise Is Medicine: https://www.exerciseismedicine.org
    g. ACE: https://www.acefitness.org/education-and-resources/lifestyle/exercise-library/

b) Worksite wellness

1. Worksite wellness programs have been shown to improve employee health, increase productivity, and yield a return on investment.[94]
    a. Among health promotion and disease management programs, the average return on investment for every $1 spent ranged from $1.49 to $4.91, with the median amount being $3.14.
    b. Disease management programs produced the highest returns on investment.
    c. Educational and disease prevention programs produced the lowest returns.
2. Motorola's wellness program experience, based on a 3-year study of 56,000 employees and their dependents[94,95]
    a. Intervention included health screenings, education, and gym access.
    b. Results:
        (1) In 2000, every $1 invested saved $3.93, leading to a total savings of $6,479,673.
        (2) Although employees who participated in the program had a 2.5% increase in annual health costs, this was compared to an 18% rise for non-participants.
        (3) Participating employees saved $6.5 million annually in medical expenses for lifestyle- related diagnoses versus non-participants.
3. Onsite workplace programs help track health parameters[94]
    a. Tracks parameters: weight, blood pressure, body fat, etc.
    b. Tracks activity: pedometers and questionnaires
    c. Goals: individual/team
    d. Incentives: usually monetary

c) Devices
   1. Strength and flexibility devices: resistance bands, weights, fitness balls, and resistance machines
   2. Aerobic: jump ropes, gliders, rebounders, steps, cardio machines (e.g., treadmill, elliptical, stair climbers, stationary bikes, etc.)
   3. Measurement devices/wearables: pedometers, smart phones, Fitbits, Apple Watches, Garmins, etc. Consumer-based wearable activity trackers may help increase physical activity participation and provide ongoing support to wearers.[96]

d) Gyms or health clubs
   1. Pros: great resource for many patients, especially for resistance training and group activities (yoga, Pilates, spinning, Zumba, etc.)
   2. Cons: cost, hours, locations, childcare

e) Parks (local, state, and national)
   1. Pros: typically free
   2. Sports fields, tennis and basketball courts, open fields, pools
   3. Hiking and walking trails, nature preserves, bike trails
   4. Can improve mood and help people obtain vitamin D from the sun
   5. Cons: location may be less accessible, weather can be a barrier, potential for injury (e.g., cuts, scrapes, allergies, thorns, insect bites, etc.)

OBJECTIVE 15

Describe the treatment of disease with exercise as compared with medication

1) Exercise as a medication

a) A landmark randomized controlled trial by the Diabetes Prevention Program Research Group involving 3,234 patients with prediabetes for more than 2.8 years compared lifestyle-modification program to metformin or placebo (https://www.nejm.org/doi/full/10.1056/NEJMoa012512)
   1. Lifestyle program goal was 7% weight loss and 150 mins of physical activity per week.
   2. When compared to placebo, metformin decreased incidence of diabetes by 31%, whereas lifestyle intervention was significantly more effective and reduced incidence by 58%.
   3. Number needed to treat to prevent one case of diabetes in 3 years for metformin was 13.9 persons but 6.9 persons for lifestyle.

b) A meta-analysis of 305 randomized controlled trials including 339,274 participants, evaluated the effect of exercise on mortality outcomes. Trials compared the effectiveness of exercise and drug interventions with each other or with control (placebo or usual care). Exercise offered similar mortality reduction benefits in the secondary prevention of coronary heart disease, rehabilitation of stroke, and prevention of diabetes but was less effective in treating heart failure. However, further direct comparisons between treatment with exercise to pharmacotherapy is needed.[97]
   1. Results
      a. No statistical difference was evident between physical activity and drug interventions for secondary prevention of coronary heart disease and prediabetes.

b. Physical activity interventions versus anticoagulants and antiplatelet therapy in reducing mortality favored exercise, respectfully OR 0.09, 95% (0.01 to 0.70) and OR 0.10, 95% (0.01 to 0.62).
c. Treatment comparing exercise to pharmacologic interventions, specifically diuretics, was inferior for reducing mortality, OR 4.11 (1.17 to 24.76).

2. Important to note:
a. Adverse events in the exercise trials were not reported consistently, but overall exercise appeared safe.
b. Some of the exercise trials included drug interventions, meaning the observed benefit of exercise may represent the added benefit of exercise to the benefit of pharmacotherapy. Conversely, the benefit of exercise may be under-represented as statins in combination with exercise may cause fatigue, decreased athletic performance, and myalgias.[98]

c) Studying the effects of exercise on blood pressure, a meta-analysis of 391 randomized controlled trials confirmed modest but consistent reductions in systolic blood pressure with exercise compared to placebo, but less than reductions made with anti-hypertensive medications.[99]

OBJECTIVE 16

List evidence-based physical activity recommendations for healthy older adults, pregnancy, obesity, heart disease, diabetes, cancer, disability, and stroke

1) Physical activity guidelines for specific conditions

a) From the 2018 physical activity guidelines[2]

1. There is strong evidence that exercise benefits all the following:
a. All-cause mortality
b. Coronary heart disease
c. Type 2 diabetes
d. Colon cancer
e. Breast cancer

2) Healthy older adults over 65 years old

a) Physical activity guidelines[2]

1. Follow adult guidelines, or as much as possible, for aerobic and resistance exercises. Progression of physical activity should be individualized and tailored to the tolerance and preference of an individual; a conservative approach may be necessary for older adults who are deconditioned or physically limited.
a. 150 minutes of moderate-intensity exercise or 75 minutes of vigorous-intensity exercise, or a combination of both.
b. Resistance exercises at least two times per week
(1) Even 100-year old patients can increase muscle mass.
(2) Benefits from weight resistance exercise in elderly may be greater and more important than in younger adults.

2. Do exercises that maintain and improve balance 3 or more days per week to help prevent falls and injuries.
3. Stretching may also be beneficial to prevent tightness and maintain range of motion. Flexibility exercises should be performed at least 2 days per week.
4. Exercise done in supervised groups, such as tai chi, have been showed to be effective at reducing fall risk[100]

b) Healthy older adults who are obese

1. Weight loss in combination with exercise improves physical function better than either alone.[92]

c) Muscle mass diminution

1. Muscle mass: weight of muscle
2. Muscle quality: Good quality muscle has low amounts of intramuscular fat.
3. Muscles and mortality: Muscle quality is more important than muscle mass in preventing early death.[101]
4. Muscles and mobility limitation: Muscle quality is more important than muscle mass in maintaining mobility.[102]

3) Pregnancy and postpartum key guidelines[2]

a) Healthy women (without contraindications)

1. 150 minutes of moderate intensity aerobic activity per week
2. Preferably spread throughout the week

b) Benefits of exercise during pregnancy[103]

1. Prevention of excessive weight gain
2. Prevention of gestational diabetes
3. Decreased risk of preeclampsia
4. Prevention or improvement of depressive symptoms
5. Decreased risk for surgical delivery
6. Decreased risk for preterm birth and low birth-weight infants

c) Women doing vigorous exercise regularly before pregnancy can continue at this level but should discuss with their health-care provider how and when activity should be adjusted as the pregnancy progresses.

d) Women who are pregnant should avoid exercising in hot, humid environments, be well hydrated, and avoid heat stress.

e) Avoid exercises that require lying on the back after the first trimester of pregnancy, as these exercises can compress the vena cava.

f) Absolute contraindications for exercising during pregnancy

1. Hemodynamically significant heart disease
2. Restrictive lung disease
3. Incompetent cervix or cerclage
4. Multiple gestation at risk for premature labor
5. Persistent second or third trimester bleeding
6. Placenta previa after 26 weeks gestation
7. Premature labor during the current pregnancy

8. Ruptured membranes
9. Preeclampsia or pregnancy induced hypertension

g) Avoid activities that increase the risk of falling or abdominal trauma, including:

1. Contact or collision sports
2. Horseback riding
3. Downhill skiing
4. Soccer
5. Basketball

h) Pregnancy and obesity

1. One-third of women are overweight or obese at the start of pregnancy.
    a. They are twice as likely to gain weight above Institute of Medicine recommendations.
    b. Excess weight is a risk factor for adverse maternal and infant health outcomes.
2. A meta-analysis evaluated physical activity interventions on body weight in overweight or obese women who are pregnant or post-partum.[104]
    a. Pregnant women in the intervention groups gained 2 lbs (0.9 kg) less than controls.
    b. Supervised physical activity and diet interventions were most effective.

4) Physical activity and ischemic heart disease prevention

a) Moderate-intensity physical activity reduces the risk of primary coronary heart disease in active men and women by 20–30% when compared with inactive men and women.[105]

b) A physical activity and coronary heart disease prevention meta-analysis showed that relative risk decreased dramatically as patients moved from sedentary to burning 550 calories per week during leisure time physical activity.[106]

c) The Women's Health Initiative found that the more physically active women are, the less ischemic heart disease they experience.[107]

d) A meta-analysis on physical activity and ischemic heart disease prevention through active commuting (walking/cycling) found:[108]

1. Overall decreased hazard ratio (HR) with active commuting versus inactive, HR = 0.892.
2. The type of activity (walking/cycling) does not seem to be as important as just doing the activity.

e) Patients with coronary heart disease, heart failure, stroke, and peripheral vascular disease who become physically active have fewer complications and lower mortality rates than predicted.[105]

5) Physical activity and type 2 diabetes prevention[2]

a) 150 minutes per week of moderate-intensity physical activity is sufficient to reduce the risk of type 2 diabetes.

b) Cohort studies on physical activity and type 2 diabetes prevention found:[109]

1. 31% decreased risk without accounting for BMI
2. 17% decreased risk accounting for BMI

c) Meta-analysis of structured exercise training regimen[110]

1. Objective: effectiveness of structured exercise (aerobic, resistance, or both) and physical activity advice with or without diet co-intervention
2. Outcome variable: changes in HbA1c levels

3. Results
    a. Physical activity advice is associated with lower HbA1c only when combined with dietary advice.
    b. Structured aerobic exercise, resistance training, and a combination of the two were associated with decreased HbA1c and with greater regression of HbA1c if exercise training exceeded 150 minutes per week.

6) Physical activity and cancer prevention[2,111]

a) Increased physical activity corresponds to a decreased risk in colon and breast cancers.
  1. The amount of physical activity needed to reduce the risk is unclear, but based on the current data, it's likely around 3–4 hours of moderate to vigorous activity each week. There is a clear dose-response relationship between physical activity and reduced cancer risk.

b) Colon cancer has a 17–30% decreased risk with physical activity.[112]

c) Physical activity and breast cancer risk reduction[4]
  1. There is a 25% decreased risk when comparing the most and least active people. This is consistent with other studies showing decreased relative risk of 20–30%.
  2. Physical activity prevents reoccurrence as well as primary onset.
  3. Increasing physical activity decreases the probability of mortality from breast cancer.[113]

d) Associations between physical activity and other cancers is less clear.

7) Physical activity and cancer treatment[2,111]

a) Exercising during and after cancer treatment is important because it:
  1. Improves cardiorespiratory fitness and body composition
  2. Improves symptoms and quality of life during treatment
  3. Improves survival

8) Key guidelines for physical activity and disability

a) Follow adult physical activity guidelines. If one is unable to follow guidelines, be as physically active as possible.

b) Medical mobility impairments include those in balance, strength, power asymmetry, velocity of movement, reaction time, aerobic capacity, range of motion, core muscle integrity, and kyphosis.

c) There's good evidence physical activity is helpful for a diverse group of conditions, including:
  1. Dementia
  2. Intellectual disability
  3. Stroke and spinal cord injury
  4. Multiple sclerosis
  5. Mental illness
  6. Muscular dystrophy
  7. Parkinson's disease
  8. Cerebral palsy and traumatic brain injury
  9. Limb amputations

d) Patients who have physical or mental disabilities would likely benefit from receiving advice from physical activity experts to help the patients with exercise effectiveness and safety.

e) There are strong associations between physical disability and mobility impairments. Medical mobility impairments can increase the risk of mortality.

f) Physical activity and disability: impairments in the short physical performance battery (SPPB) predict mobility.[113]

1. The SPPB includes:
    a. Gait speed test
    b. Balance test
    c. Chair rise test
2. A structured exercise program can improve the SPPB, prevent physical decline, allow people to maintain their independence longer, and lead to an 18% reduction in physical disability.

9) Parkinson's and disability: exercise improves physical function, including walking, balance, muscle strength, and disease-specific motor scores.

a) Parkinson's treatment

1. One study included 195 Parkinson's patients who ranged from stage 1 to stage 4.[114]
2. The intervention divided participants into three groups who were assigned either tai chi, resistance training, or stretching for 60 minutes two times per week for 24 weeks.
3. The results showed that stability improved with tai chi more than with stretching or resistance training.

SECTION 6 GLOSSARY

5A's: a method for counseling patients, including on physical activity. The 5A's include assess, advise, agree, assist, and arrange.

Aerobic/endurance exercise (cardiovascular): the body's large muscles move in rhythmic manner for a sustained period of time.

Balance: the ability to withstand destabilizing stimuli (especially important with age).

Body composition: the percentages of body water, bone, muscle, and fat.

Borg scale: a rating of perceived exertion (RPE) used to monitor intensity of exercise. The short version ranges from 1 to 10.

Cardiorespiratory endurance: the ability to continue aerobic exercise like walking or running.

Exercise Tolerance Test (ETT): an exercise stress test that tests for cardiovascular fitness.

Deconditioning: a state of health that occurs from being consistently physically inactive and lacking exercise in one's daily life, all of which results in functional losses.

Exercise: purposeful physical activity that is organized, planned, reoccurring, and that is done with the intent of improving or maintaining one or more components of one's health.

Fitness: the ability to perform one's activities of daily life, respond to emergencies and enjoy leisure time activities with sufficient energy and vitality, without excess fatigue.

FITT-VP: a type of exercise prescription that includes recommendations on frequency, intensity, type of exercise, time, volume, and progression.

Flexibility: the ability to move a joint closer to its full range of motion.

Heart Rate Reserve (HRR): a number equal to the Maximum Heart Rate (MHR) minus the Resting Heart Rate (RHR).

High Intensity Interval Training (HIIT): HIIT is characterized by brief, intermittent bursts of vigorous activity that are interspersed with periods of rest or low-intensity exercise.

Metabolic Equivalent of a Task (MET): METs are a ratio of the metabolic rate during a task compared to a standard resting metabolic rate.

Physical activity: any movement of the body done through skeletal muscle contraction that causes the energy expenditure to be beyond its baseline.

Physical Activity Vital Sign (PAVS): PAVS is a tool created to quickly measure one's physical activity level. The equation is (days per week) × (minutes per day) = minutes per week.

Physical fitness: includes fitness in the following categories: cardiorespiratory endurance; skeletal muscle endurance, strength, and power; flexibility; balance; speed and agility; and body composition.

Physical inactivity: the absence of physical activity; usually reflected as the amount or proportion of time not engaged in physical activity of some predetermined intensity.

Reaction time: the time it takes one to react to some stimuli.

Skeletal muscle endurance: the ability to continue holding weight or position.

Skeletal muscle power: the amount of work completed by a muscle in a period of time.

Skeletal muscle strength: the maximum force a muscle or muscle group can produce at a specified velocity. This is equal to one repetition maximum.

SMART goal: another option for goal setting along with or in place of exercise prescription. SMART goals are specific, measurable, achievable, relevant, and include a time frame.

Speed of movement: the distance traveled in a period of time.

Talk test: a commonly used measure of exercise intensity, which includes very-light or light-intensity, moderate intensity and vigorous or maximal intensity.

SECTION 6 REVIEW QUESTIONS

1. **Which of the following statements is most accurate about the benefits of physical activity?**
   - **A.** It increases the risk of developing disabling medical conditions.
   - **B.** It leads to significant weight loss.
   - **C.** Increased physical activity is associated with lower health care costs.
   - **D.** It increases the risk of chronic disease development.

2. **Physical fitness includes which of the following?**
   - **A.** Balance with static and dynamic exercises
   - **B.** Body composition
   - **C.** Muscle hypertrophy
   - **D.** Yoga

3. **The US Physical Activity Guidelines for Americans includes the following:**
   - **A.** At least 150 minutes of exercise per week must be achieved to reduce the risk of developing a chronic disease.
   - **B.** Most health benefits are achieved with 300 minutes per week of moderate-intensity physical activity.
   - **C.** For children 6–17 years old, 60 minutes or more of moderate- to vigorous-intensity physical activity is recommended daily.
   - **D.** Strength training for adults 18–64 years old is recommended at least once per week.

4. **"The Aerobics Center Longitudinal Study," from 1987 to 2003, showed that the number one preventable cause of deaths from all-cause mortality in 40,842 men and women was due to:**
   - **A.** Smoking
   - **B.** Diabetes
   - **C.** Obesity
   - **D.** Poor cardiorespiratory fitness

5. **Which of the following statements is true about sitting and sedentary behavior?**
   - **A.** The prevalence of inactivity is equivalent to that of smoking, hypertension, and hyperlipidemia.
   - **B.** Sitting is estimated to contribute to at least 20% of all-cause mortality.
   - **C.** Breaking up sitting with light- and moderate-intensity walking every 20 minutes reduced blood glucose and insulin levels in obese patients.
   - **D.** Sitting causes more deaths than smoking.

6. **Which prescription best describes the FITT-VP cardiovascular exercise prescription?**
   - **A.** Begin walking at a moderate intensity for 45 minutes at 5 days per week.
   - **B.** Begin running at a vigorous intensity for 30 minutes by the end of the month.
   - **C.** Walk around the block twice daily with your significant other and write it down in a log.
   - **D.** Lift heavy weights for 25 minutes at a vigorous intensity.

7. **When considering prescribing the correct level of intensity, the "talk" test is a commonly used intensity measure and includes which of the following factors?**
   - **A.** With very light-intensity exercise one should be able to talk but not sing.
   - **B.** Moderate exercise is 64–76% of maximal heart rate.
   - **C.** With vigorous-intensity exercise, one should have difficulty talking but be able to sing.
   - **D.** With moderate-intensity exercise, one should be able to talk but not sing.

8. **Which statement best describes a prescription for resistance training?**
   - **A.** Do four toe-touches daily for the next 4 weeks.
   - **B.** Use 3-lb weights in each hand and do 15 bicep curls for three repetitions every other day for the next 4 weeks.
   - **C.** Spend 5 minutes warming-up before and after physical exercise.
   - **D.** Stand for 5 minutes on an unstable surface or a foam board.

9. **__________ is defined as "any bodily movement produced by the contraction of skeletal muscle that increases energy expenditure above a basal level."**
   - **A.** Physical activity
   - **B.** Fitness
   - **C.** Exercise
   - **D.** Isokinetic exercise

10. **Which of the following are considered components of physical fitness?**
    - **A.** Respiratory rate
    - **B.** Cardiorespiratory exercise
    - **C.** Warm-up and cool-down
    - **D.** Squats

11. **What are the recommended aerobic activity guidelines for children?**
    - **A.** 30 minutes or more per day of moderate- to vigorous-intensity physical activity.
    - **B.** 60 minutes or more per day of moderate- to vigorous-intensity physical activity.
    - **C.** 150 minutes of moderate-intensity exercise per week, or 75 minutes of vigorous-intensity exercise per week.
    - **D.** 300 minutes of moderate-intensity exercise per week, or 150 minutes of vigorous-intensity exercise per week.

12. **Current aerobic exercise activity guidelines recommend that bouts of physical activity should be at least the following in length at one time for health benefits to be achieved:**
    - **A.** 10 minutes
    - **B.** 30 minutes
    - **C.** 60 minutes
    - **D.** Any amount

13. **Which of the following is considered part of a FITT-VP prescription for cardiovascular exercise?**
    - **A.** Fitness
    - **B.** Type
    - **C.** Interval
    - **D.** Repetitions

14. **When counseling patients on physical activity, one approach is to use the 5A's. What is the correct order that these steps should be delivered in?**

   A. Ask, assess, assist, agree, arrange

   B. Assess, advise, assist, arrange, agree

   C. Assess, advise, agree, assist, arrange

   D. Ask, advise, assist, agree, arrange

15. **With regard to pre-participation exercise screening, what are the major disease entities one needs to consider when deciding whether additional medical clearance is needed?**

   A. Cardiovascular, pulmonary, and renal disease

   B. Cardiovascular, pulmonary, and metabolic disease

   C. Cardiovascular, renal, and metabolic disease

   D. Pulmonary, renal, and metabolic disease

SECTION 6 REVIEW QUESTION ANSWERS AND SUMMARIES

1. **Answer: C.** Overall benefits of physical activity include:
   a. It improves health-related fitness.
   b. Lower risk of disabling medical conditions
   c. Significant amounts of physical activity can result in weight loss, but it is not a general expectation to lose weight with physical activity alone. It plays an important role in weight maintenance.
   d. Most interventions to increase physical activity are cost effective. Health care spending also increases when physical activity levels decrease.
   e. Physical activity decreases the risk of chronic disease.

2. **Answer: B.** Physical fitness is comprised of the following domains: body composition, cardiorespiratory endurance, muscular strength and endurance, and flexibility. Yoga is a type of activity. Balance is not included as a physical fitness domain.

3. **Answer: C.** Children should achieve 60 minutes of moderate- to vigorous-intensity physical activity daily. Any amount of physical activity can improve health. For adults, most health benefits are achieved at 150 minutes per week of moderate-intensity physical activity, or 75 minutes of vigorous physical activity or an equivalent combination. Beyond 150 minutes there are still benefits, but they are much less in amplitude. The guidelines recommend that adults (not children) engage in two resistance training sessions each week and balance exercises.

4. **Answer: D.** Low cardiorespiratory fitness was the number one cause of preventable deaths from all-cause mortality in 40,842 men and women who were enrolled in the Aerobics Center Longitudinal Study. Physical inactivity is the fourth leading risk factor for global mortality.[115]

5. **Answer: C.** The prevalence of inactivity is at least twice that of smoking, hypertension, and hyperlipidemia. 6.9% of all-cause mortality is attributable to sitting. Breaking up sitting with light- and moderate-intensity walking every 20 minutes reduced blood glucose and insulin levels in obese patients. Smoking is the number one preventable cause of death in the United States.

6. **Answer: A.** The FITT-VP exercise prescription for cardiovascular exercise includes frequency, intensity, type of exercise, time (duration), volume, and progression. For example, begin a slow jog/race walk (type) at a moderate intensity (intensity) for 45 minutes (time) for at least 5 days per week (duration).

7. **Answer: D.** The talk test is a common measure of exercise intensity. Very-light to light-intensity exercise (63% or less of MHR) should allow a person to talk and/or sing. Moderate-intensity exercise (64–76% of MHR) should allow a person to talk but not sing. Vigorous-intensity to maximal exercise (77–100% of maximal HR) will make it difficult to speak or sing.[116]

8. **Answer: B.** Introducing strength training to an exercise prescription should include intensity, frequency, repetitions, and duration.

9. **Answer: A.** Fitness is defined as "the ability to carry out daily tasks with vigor and alertness without undue fatigue, with ample energy to enjoy leisure-time pursuits, and the ability to respond to emergencies." Exercise is a subset of physical activity that is formally defined as "physical activity that is planned, structured, repetitive, and purposeful in the sense that the improvement or maintenance of one or more components." Isokinetic exercise is a type of strength training that uses special machines or dynamometers to maintain a constant (iso) speed (kinetic) of movement.[14]

10. **Answer: B.** Cardiorespiratory exercise, muscular strength and endurance, body composition, and flexibility are considered components of health-related physical fitness.[28]

11. **Answer: B.** The current guidelines recommend 60 minutes or more per day of moderate- to vigorous-intensity physical activity for children. Thirty minutes per day is generally a good goal for most adults, but that's not a specifically recommended amount of time by the CDC.[2]

12. **Answer: D.** Any amount of exercise is beneficial to help reduce risk of disease.

13. **Answer: B.** A FITT-VP prescription includes the frequency, intensity, time, type, volume, and progression of activity.[28]

14. **Answer: C.** The correct order is assess, advise, agree, assist, arrange. The 5A's begin with assessing patient beliefs, behaviors, and knowledge, then advising by providing information about the health benefits of change, and then agreeing on a collaborative goal. Next, the provider assists the patient in identifying barriers, strategies, and problem-solving techniques before finally arranging to follow up on plans.

15. **Answer: C.** Referral to a health provider should be made on current physical activity levels and presence of signs or symptoms and/or known cardiovascular, metabolic, or renal disease. While one might modify an exercise prescription for someone with pulmonary disease, pulmonary disease alone does not require medical clearance, as it has not been shown to increase the risk of cardiovascular complications.[80]

SECTION 6 REFERENCES

1. World Health Organization. *Global Health Risks: Mortality and Burden of Disease Attributable to Selected Major Risks*. Geneva, Switzerland: World Health Organization; 2009; http://www.who.int/healthinfo/global_burden_disease/GlobalHealthRisks_report_full.pdf.
2. US Deptartment of Health and Human Services. *Physical Activity Guidelines for Americans*, 2nd edition. Washington, DC: US Department of Health and Human Services;2018.
3. Blair S. N. Physical inactivity: the biggest public health problem of the 21st century. *Br J Sports Med.* 2009;43(1):1-2.
4. Lee I. M., Shiroma E. J., Lobelo F., Puska P., Blair S. N., Katzmarzyk P. T. Effect of physical inactivity on major non-communicable diseases worldwide: an analysis of burden of disease and life expectancy. *Lancet.* 2012;380(9838):219-229.
5. Carlson S. A., Adams E. K., Yang Z., Fulton J. E. Percentage of deaths associated with inadequate physical activity in the United States. *Prev Chronic Dis.* 2018;15:E38.
6. Moore S. C., Patel A. V., Matthews C. E., et al. Leisure time physical activity of moderate to vigorous intensity and mortality: a large pooled cohort analysis. *PLoS Med.* 2012;9(11):e1001335.
7. Ekblom-Bak E., Hellénius M. L., Ekblom B. Are we facing a new paradigm of inactivity physiology? *Br J Sports Med.* 2010;44(12):834-835.
8. Tremblay M. S., Colley R. C., Saunders T. J., Healy G. N., Owen N. Physiological and health implications of a sedentary lifestyle. *Appl Physiol Nutr Metab.* 2010;35(6):725-740. https://www.researchgate.net/publication/49689425_Physiological_and_health_implications_of_a_sedentary_lifestyle.
9. US Department of Health and Human Services, President's Council on Sports, Fitness & Nutrition. Facts and statistics; physical activity. Updated September 16, 2020. https://www.hhs.gov/fitness/resource-center/facts-and-statistics/index.html#footnote-3.
10. Centers for Disease Control and Prevention. Burden of cigarette use in the US: Current cigarette smoking among us adults aged 18 years and older. November 19, 2020; https://www.cdc.gov/tobacco/campaign/tips/resources/data/cigarette-smoking-in-united-states.html#.
11. van der Ploeg H. P., Chey T., Korda R. J., Banks E., Bauman A. Sitting time and all-cause mortality risk in 222 497 Australian adults. *Arch Intern Med.* 2012;172(6):494-500.
12. Dunstan D. W., Kingwell B. A., Larsen R., et al. Breaking up prolonged sitting reduces postprandial glucose and insulin responses. *Diabetes Care.* 2012;35(5):976-983.
13. Matthews C. E., George S. M., Moore S. C., et al. Amount of time spent in sedentary behaviors and cause-specific mortality in US adults. *Am J Clin Nutr.* 2012;95(2):437-445.
14. Centers for Disease Control and Prevention, US Department of Health and Human Services. NHIS - adult physical activity information - glossary. National Center for Health Statistics. February 17, 2017. https://www.cdc.gov/nchs/nhis/physical_activity/pa_glossary.htm.
15. Levine J. A. Non-exercise activity thermogenesis (NEAT). *Best Pract Res Clin Endocrinol Metab.* 2002;16(4):679-702.
16. Joyner M. J. Standing up for exercise: should deconditioning be medicalized? *J Physiol.* 2012;590(15):3413-3414.
17. Anderson L. H., Martinson B. C., Crain A. L., et al. Health care charges associated with physical inactivity, overweight, and obesity. *Prev Chronic Dis.* 2005;2(4):A09.
18. Garrett S., Elley C. R., Rose S. B., O'Dea D., Lawton B. A., Dowell A. C. Are physical activity interventions in primary care and the community cost-effective? A systematic review of the evidence. *Br J Gen Pract.* 2011;61(584):e125-133.
19. Centers for Disease Control and Prevention. *Gynecologic Cancer Incidence, United States—2012–2016, US Cancer Statistics data brief, no 11.* Atlanta, GA: Centers for Disease Control and Prevention; 2019.
20. Williams M. A., Haskell W. L., Ades P. A., et al. Resistance exercise in individuals with and without cardiovascular disease: 2007 update: a scientific statement from the American Heart Association Council on Clinical Cardiology and Council on Nutrition, Physical Activity, and Metabolism. *Circulation.* 2007;116(5):572-584.
21. Hallsworth K., Fattakhova G., Hollingsworth K. G., et al. Resistance exercise reduces liver fat and its mediators in non-alcoholic fatty liver disease independent of weight loss. *Gut.* 2011;60(9):1278-1283.
22. Page P. Current concepts in muscle stretching for exercise and rehabilitation. *Int J Sports Phys Ther.* 2012;7(1):109-119.
23. Watt J. R., Jackson K., Franz J. R., Dicharry J., Evans J., Kerrigan D. C. Effect of a supervised hip flexor stretching program on gait in elderly individuals. *PM R.* 2011;3(4):324-329.
24. Warren C. G., Lehmann J. F., Koblanski J. N. Heat and stretch procedures: an evaluation using rat tail tendon. *Arch Phys Med Rehabil.* 1976;57(3):122-126.
25. Hegde S. V., Adhikari P., Kotian S., Pinto V. J., D'Souza S., D'Souza V. Effect of 3-month yoga on oxidative stress in type 2 diabetes with or without complications: a controlled clinical trial. *Diabetes Care.* 2011;34(10):2208-2210.
26. El-Khoury F., Cassou B., Charles M. A., Dargent-Molina P. The effect of fall prevention exercise programmes on fall induced injuries in community dwelling older adults: systematic review and meta-analysis of randomised controlled trials. *BMJ.* 2013;347:f6234.
27. Albert C. M., Mittleman M. A., Chae C. U., Lee I. M., Hennekens C. H., Manson J. E. Triggering of sudden death from cardiac causes by vigorous exertion. *N Engl J Med.* 2000;343(19):1355-1361.
28. American College of Sports Medicine . *ACSM's Guidelines for Exercise Testing and Prescription,* 10th ed. Philadelphia, PA: Wolters Kluwer Health; 2018.
29. Singh R., Pattisapu A., Emery M. S. US Physical Activity Guidelines: Current state, impact and future directions. *Trends Cardiovasc Med.* 2020;30(7):407-412.

30. US Department of Health and Human Services. *2008 Physical Activity Guidelines for Americans*. Washington, DC: US Department of Health and Human Services; 2008. https://health.gov/sites/default/files/2019-09/paguide.pdf.
31. Kaminsky L. A., Montoye A. H. Physical activity and health: what is the best dose? *J Am Heart Assoc.* 2014;3(5):e001430.
32. Garber C. E., Blissmer B., Deschenes M. R., et al. American College of Sports Medicine position stand. Quantity and quality of exercise for developing and maintaining cardiorespiratory, musculoskeletal, and neuromotor fitness in apparently healthy adults: guidance for prescribing exercise. *Med Sci Sports Exerc.* 2011;43(7):1334-1359.
33. Jonas S. J., Phillips E. M. *ACSM's Exercise is Medicine: A Clinician's Guide to Exercise Prescription*. Philadelphia, PA: Lippincott Williams & Wilkins; 2009.
34. Woolstenhulme M. T., Griffiths C. M., Woolstenhulme E. M., Parcell A. C. Ballistic stretching increases flexibility and acute vertical jump height when combined with basketball activity. *J Strength Cond Res.* 2006;20(4):799-803.
35. Page P. Current concepts in muscle stretching for exercise and rehabilitation. *Int J Sports Phys Ther.* 2012;7(1):109-119. https://pubmed.ncbi.nlm.nih.gov/22319684.
36. Blair S. N. Evidence for success of exercise in weight loss and control. *Ann Intern Med.* 1993;119(7 Pt 2):702-706.
37. Abramson S., Stein J., Schaufele M., Frates E., Rogan S. Personal exercise habits and counseling practices of primary care physicians: a national survey. *Clin J Sport Med.* 2000;10(1):40-48.
38. Frank E., Dresner Y., Shani M., Vinker S. The association between physicians' and patients' preventive health practices. *CMAJ.* 2013;185(8):649-653.
39. Ainsworth B. E., Haskell W. L., Herrmann S. D., et al. 2011 Compendium of physical activities: a second update of codes and MET values. *Med Sci Sports Exerc.* 2011;43(8):1575-1581.
40. Thomas P. R., ed., Committee to Develop Criteria for Evaluating the Outcomes of Approaches to Rrevent and Treat Obesity. *Weighing the Options: Criteria for Evaluating Weight-Management Programs*. Washington DC: National Academies Press; 1995.
41. Shaw K., Gennat H., O'Rourke P., Del Mar C. Exercise for overweight or obesity. *Cochrane Database Syst Rev.* 2006(4):Cd003817.
42. King A. C., Frey-Hewitt B., Dreon D. M., Wood P. D. Diet vs exercise in weight maintenance. The effects of minimal intervention strategies on long-term outcomes in men. *Arch Intern Med.* 1989;149(12):2741-2746.
43. McTigue K. M., Harris R., Hemphill B., et al. Screening and interventions for obesity in adults: summary of the evidence for the US Preventive Services Task Force. *Ann Intern Med.* 2003;139(11):933-949.
44. Flack K. D., Ufholz K., Johnson L., Fitzgerald J. S., Roemmich J. N. Energy compensation in response to aerobic exercise training in overweight adults. *Am J Physiol Regul Integr Comp Physiol.* 2018;315(4):R619-r626.
45. Donnelly J. E., Blair S. N., Jakicic J. M., Manore M. M., Rankin J. W., Smith B. K. American College of Sports Medicine Position Stand. Appropriate physical activity intervention strategies for weight loss and prevention of weight regain for adults. *Med Sci Sports Exerc.* 2009;41(2):459-471.
46. Aronne L. J., Wadden T., Isoldi K. K., Woodworth K. A. When prevention fails: obesity treatment strategies. *Am J Med.* 2009;122(4 Suppl 1):S24-32.
47. Lee C. D., Blair S. N., Jackson A. S. Cardiorespiratory fitness, body composition, and all-cause and cardiovascular disease mortality in men. *Am J Clin Nutr.* 1999;69(3):373-380.
48. National Weight Control Registry. The National Weight Control Registry. http://www.nwcr.ws/default.htm. Accessed 2018.
49. Wasfy M. M., Baggish A. L. Exercise dose in clinical practice. *Circulation.* 2016;133(23):2297-2313.
50. US Department of Health and Human Services. *2018 Physical Activity Guidelines Advisory Committee Scientific Report*. Washington, DC: Office of Disease Prevention and Health Promotion; 2018. https://health.gov/paguidelines/second-edition/report/.
51. Eijsvogels T. M., Molossi S., Lee D. C., Emery M. S., Thompson P. D. Exercise at the extremes: the amount of exercise to reduce cardiovascular events. *J Am Coll Cardiol.* 2016;67(3):316-329.
52. Matthews C. E., Jurj A. L., Shu X. O., et al. Influence of exercise, walking, cycling, and overall nonexercise physical activity on mortality in Chinese women. *Am J Epidemiol.* 2007;165(12):1343-1350.
53. Wen C. P., Wai J. P., Tsai M. K., et al. Minimum amount of physical activity for reduced mortality and extended life expectancy: a prospective cohort study. *Lancet.* 2011;378(9798):1244-1253.
54. Lee I. M., Sesso H. D., Oguma Y., Paffenbarger R. S., Jr. The "weekend warrior" and risk of mortality. *Am J Epidemiol.* 2004;160(7):636-641.
55. Woodcock J., Franco O. H., Orsini N., Roberts I. Non-vigorous physical activity and all-cause mortality: systematic review and meta-analysis of cohort studies. *Int J Epidemiol.* 2011;40(1):121-138.
56. Janssen I., Carson V., Lee I. M., Katzmarzyk P. T., Blair S. N. Years of life gained due to leisure-time physical activity in the US *Am J Prev Med.* 2013;44(1):23-29.
57. Gibala M. J., Little J. P., Macdonald M. J., Hawley J. A. Physiological adaptations to low-volume, high-intensity interval training in health and disease. *J Physiol.* 2012;590(5):1077-1084.
58. Cress M., Porcari J., Foster C. Interval training. *ACSMs Health Fit J.* 2015;19(6). https://journals.lww.com/acsm-healthfitness/Fulltext/2015/11000/INTERVAL_TRAINING.3.aspx.
59. Coleman K. J., Ngor E., Reynolds K., et al. Initial validation of an exercise "vital sign" in electronic medical records. *Med Sci Sports Exerc.* 2012;44(11):2071-2076.
60. Chen M. J., Fan X., Moe S. T. Criterion-related validity of the Borg ratings of perceived exertion scale in healthy individuals: a meta-analysis. *J Sports Sci.* 2002;20(11):873-899.
61. Office of Disease Prevention and Health Promotion. Physical activity. 2018; https://health.gov/guidelines/. Accessed September, 2020.

62. Centers for Disease Control and Prevention. Perceived exertion (Borg Rating of Perceived Exertion Scale). Updated September 17, 2020. https://www.cdc.gov/physicalactivity/basics/measuring/exertion.htm. Accessed December 10, 2020.
63. Centers for Disease Control and Prevention. Target heart rate and estimated maximum heart rate. Updated October 14, 2020. https://www.cdc.gov/physicalactivity/basics/measuring/heartrate.htm. Accessed December 10, 2020.
64. American College of Sports Medicine. *ACSM's Resource Manual for Guidelines for Exercise Testing and Prescription,* 5th ed. Baltimore, MD: Lippincott Williams & Wilkins; 2006.
65. Sigal R. J., Kenny G. P., Wasserman D. H., Castaneda-Sceppa C. Physical activity/exercise and type 2 diabetes. *Diabetes Care.* 2006;29(6):1433-1438.
66. Centers for Disease Control and Prevention. Measuring physical activity intensity. September 17, 2020. https://www.cdc.gov/physicalactivity/basics/measuring/index.html. Accessed December 10, 2020.
67. ATS Committee on Proficiency Standards for Clinical Pulmonary Function Laboratories. ATS statement: guidelines for the six-minute walk test. *Am J Respir Crit Care Med.* 2002;166(1):111-117.
68. Bleich S. N., Bennett W. L., Gudzune K. A., Cooper L. A. Impact of physician BMI on obesity care and beliefs. *Obesity (Silver Spring).* 2012;20(5):999-1005.
69. Cajochen C., Münch M., Kobialka S., et al. High sensitivity of human melatonin, alertness, thermoregulation, and heart rate to short wavelength light. *J Clin Endocrinol Metab.* 2005;90(3):1311-1316.
70. University of Michigan. *Predicting Aerobic Power (VO_2 max) Using the 1-Mile Walk Test.* Ann Arbor, MI: University of Michigan; 2005. http://www.umich.edu/~exphysio/mvs.241/Assig4.Pred.VOmax.pdf
71. Kaminsky L. A., Arena R., Myers J. Reference standards for cardiorespiratory fitness measured with cardiopulmonary exercise testing: data from the Fitness Registry and the Importance of Exercise National Database. *Mayo Clin Proc.* 2015;90(11):1515-1523.
72. Rijk J. M., Roos P. R., Deckx L., van den Akker M., Buntinx F. Prognostic value of handgrip strength in people aged 60 years and older: A systematic review and meta-analysis. *Geriatr Gerontol Int.* 2016;16(1):5-20.
73. Baltaci G., Un N., Tunay V., Besler A., Gerçeker S. Comparison of three different sit and reach tests for measurement of hamstring flexibility in female university students. *Br J Sports Med.* 2003;37(1):59-61.
74. Franklin B. A. Preventing exercise-related cardiovascular events: is a medical examination more urgent for physical activity or inactivity? *Circulation.* 2014;129(10):1081-1084.
75. Riebe D., Franklin B. A., Thompson P. D., et al. Updating ACSM's recommendations for exercise preparticipation health screening. *Med Sci Sports Exerc.* 2015;47(11):2473-2479.
76. Jamnik V. K., Warburton D. E., Makarski J., et al. Enhancing the effectiveness of clearance for physical activity participation: background and overall process. *Appl Physiol Nutr Metab.* 2011;36 Suppl 1:S3-13.
77. Warburton D. E. R., Jamnik V. K., Bredin S. S. D., Gledhill N. The physical activity readiness questionnaire for everyone (PAR-Q+) and electronic physical activity readiness medical examination (ePARmed-X+). *Health Fitness J Can.* 2011;4(2):3-17. https://hfjc.library.ubc.ca/index.php/HFJC/article/view/103.
78. Garner K. K., Pomeroy W., Arnold J. J. Exercise stress testing: indications and common questions. *Am Fam Physician.* 2017;96(5):293-299.
79. Wackers F. J. Customized exercise testing. *J Am Coll Cardiol.* 2009;54(6):546-548.
80. Riebe D., Franklin B. A., Thompson P. D., et al. Updating ACSM's recommendations for exercise preparticipation health screening. *Med Sci Sports Exerc.* 2015;47(11):2473-2479. http://revdesportiva.pt/files/para_publicar/Updating_ACSM_s_Recommendations_for_Exercise.28.pdf.
81. Lin J. S., O'Connor E., Whitlock E. P., Beil T. L. Behavioral counseling to promote physical activity and a healthful diet to prevent cardiovascular disease in adults: a systematic review for the US Preventive Services Task Force. *Ann Intern Med.* 2010;153(11):736-750.
82. Albright C. L., Cohen S., Gibbons L., et al. Incorporating physical activity advice into primary care: physician-delivered advice within the activity counseling trial. *Am J Prev Med.* 2000;18(3):225-234.
83. Grandes G., Sanchez A., Sanchez-Pinilla R. O., et al. Effectiveness of physical activity advice and prescription by physicians in routine primary care: a cluster randomized trial. *Arch Intern Med.* 2009;169(7):694-701.
84. Orrow G., Kinmonth A., Sanderson S., Sutton S. Effectiveness of physical activity promotion based in primary care: systematic review and meta-analysis of randomised controlled trials. *BMJ.* 2012;344:e1389. http://www.bmj.com/content/344/bmj.e1389.abstract.
85. Orrow G., Kinmonth A. L., Sanderson S., Sutton S. Republished research: effectiveness of physical activity promotion based in primary care: systematic review and meta-analysis of randomised controlled trials. *Br J Sports Med.* 2013;47(1):27.
86. Halm J., Amoako E. Physical activity recommendation for hypertension management: does healthcare provider advice make a difference? *Ethn Dis.* 2008;18(3):278-282.
87. Peek M. E., Tang H., Alexander G. C., Chin M. H. National prevalence of lifestyle counseling or referral among African-Americans and whites with diabetes. *J Gen Intern Med.* 2008;23(11):1858-1864.
88. Brotons C., Björkelund C., Bulc M., et al. Prevention and health promotion in clinical practice: the views of general practitioners in Europe. *Prev Med.* 2005;40(5):595-601.
89. Whitlock E. P., Orleans C. T., Pender N., Allan J. Evaluating primary care behavioral counseling interventions: an evidence-based approach. *Am J Prev Med.* 2002;22(4):267-284.
90. Glasgow R. E., Funnell M. M., Bonomi A. E., Davis C., Beckham V., Wagner E. H. Self-management aspects of the improving chronic illness care breakthrough series: implementation with diabetes and heart failure teams. *Ann Behav Med.* 2002;24(2):80-87.

91. PsychCentral. ABC (antecedent, behavior, consequence) chart form. Education and Behavior. https://www.educationandbehavior.com/wp-content/uploads/2017/12/ABC-Chart.pdf. Accessed March, 2021.
92. Eakin E. G., Brown W. J., Marshall A. L., Mummery K., Larsen E. Physical activity promotion in primary care: bridging the gap between research and practice. *Am J Prev Med.* 2004;27(4):297-303.
93. Moore M., Tschannen-Moran B. *Coaching Psychology Manual.* Philadelphia, PA: Wolters Kluwer Health/Lippincott, Williams & Wilkins; 2010.
94. US Department of Health and Human Services. *Prevention Makes Common "Cents".* Washington, DC: US Department of Health and Human Services; 2003. https://aspe.hhs.gov/pdf-report/prevention-makes-common-cents.
95. The Health Project. 2002 winners. 2002. http://thehealthproject.com/year/2002/.
96. Brickwood K., Watson G., O'Brien J., Williams Andrew D. Consumer-based wearable activity trackers increase physical activity participation: systematic review and meta-analysis. *JMIR Mhealth Uhealth.* 2019;7(4):e11819-e11819. https://pubmed.ncbi.nlm.nih.gov/30977740.
97. Naci H., Ioannidis J. P. Comparative effectiveness of exercise and drug interventions on mortality outcomes: metaepidemiological study. *BMJ.* 2013;347:f5577.
98. Deichmann R. E., Lavie C. J., Asher T., et al. The interaction between statins and exercise: mechanisms and strategies to counter the musculoskeletal side effects of this combination therapy. *Ochsner J.* 2015;15(4):429-437. https://pubmed.ncbi.nlm.nih.gov/26730228.
99. Naci H., Salcher-Konrad M., Dias S., et al. How does exercise treatment compare with antihypertensive medications? A network meta-analysis of 391 randomised controlled trials assessing exercise and medication effects on systolic blood pressure. *Br J Sports Med.* 2019;53(14):859-869.
100. Gillespie L. D., Robertson M. C., Gillespie W. J., et al. Interventions for preventing falls in older people living in the community. *Cochrane Database Syst Rev.* 2012(9):Cd007146.
101. Villareal D. T., Chode S., Parimi N., et al. Weight loss, exercise, or both and physical function in obese older adults. *N Engl J Med.* 2011;364(13):1218-1229.
102. Visser M., Goodpaster B. H., Kritchevsky S. B., et al. Muscle mass, muscle strength, and muscle fat infiltration as predictors of incident mobility limitations in well-functioning older persons. *J Gerontol A Biol Sci Med Sci.* 2005;60(3):324-333.
103. Physical activity and exercise during pregnancy and the postpartum period: ACOG committee opinion, number 804. *Obstet Gynecol.* 2020;135(4):e178-e188.
104. Choi J., Fukuoka Y., Lee J. H. The effects of physical activity and physical activity plus diet interventions on body weight in overweight or obese women who are pregnant or in postpartum: a systematic review and meta-analysis of randomized controlled trials. *Prev Med.* 2013;56(6):351-364.
105. Darden D., Richardson C., Jackson E. A. Physical activity and exercise for secondary prevention among patients with cardiovascular disease. *Curr Cardiovasc Risk Rep.* 2013;7(6).
106. Sattelmair J., Pertman J., Ding E. L., Kohl H. W., 3rd, Haskell W., Lee I. M. Dose response between physical activity and risk of coronary heart disease: a meta-analysis. *Circulation.* 2011;124(7):789-795.
107. Manson J. E., Greenland P., LaCroix A. Z., et al. Walking compared with vigorous exercise for the prevention of cardiovascular events in women. *N Engl J Med.* 2002;347(10):716-725.
108. Hamer M., Chida Y. Active commuting and cardiovascular risk: a meta-analytic review. *Prev Med.* 2008;46(1):9-13.
109. Jeon C. Y., Lokken R. P., Hu F. B., van Dam R. M. Physical activity of moderate intensity and risk of type 2 diabetes: a systematic review. *Diabetes Care.* 2007;30(3):744-752.
110. Umpierre D., Ribeiro P. A., Kramer C. K., et al. Physical activity advice only or structured exercise training and association with HbA1c levels in type 2 diabetes: a systematic review and meta-analysis. *JAMA.* 2011;305(17):1790-1799.
111. Kushi L. H., Doyle C., McCullough M., et al. American Cancer Society Guidelines on nutrition and physical activity for cancer prevention: reducing the risk of cancer with healthy food choices and physical activity. *CA Cancer J Clin.* 2012;62(1):30-67.
112. Wolin K. Y., Yan Y., Colditz G. A., Lee I. M. Physical activity and colon cancer prevention: a meta-analysis. *Br J Cancer.* 2009;100(4):611-616.
113. Holmes M. D., Chen W. Y., Feskanich D., Kroenke C. H., Colditz G. A. Physical activity and survival after breast cancer diagnosis. *JAMA.* 2005;293(20):2479-2486.
114. Li F., Harmer P., Fitzgerald K., et al. Tai chi and postural stability in patients with Parkinson's disease. *N Engl J Med.* 2012;366(6):511-519.
115. Sui X., Li H., Zhang J., Chen L., Zhu L., Blair S. N. Percentage of deaths attributable to poor cardiovascular health lifestyle factors: findings from the Aerobics Center Longitudinal Study. *Epidemiol Res Int.* 2013;2013:437465. https://pubmed.ncbi.nlm.nih.gov/24058738.
116. Persinger R., Foster C., Gibson M., Fater D. C., Porcari J. P. Consistency of the talk test for exercise prescription. *Med Sci Sports Exerc.* 2004;36(9):1632-1636.

SECTION 7
Emotional and Mental Well-Being, Assessment, and Interventions

Objective 1 Use screening tools for stress, depression, and anxiety **235**

Objective 2 Describe the relationship between emotional distress and poor health **238**

Objective 3 Describe the provider's role in facilitating patients' emotional wellness........... **241**

Objective 4 Identify indications for referral to a mental health professional **242**

Objective 5 Identify how to manage depression and anxiety in patients with comorbidities **318**

Objective 6 Describe the components of emotional wellness self-management ... **245**

Objective 7 Identify the role of positive psychology and its use in lifestyle medicine........... **246**

Objective 8 Identify the nature of stress as well as manageable elements of pathogenic stress reactions **248**

Objective 9 Describe the integral and essential elements of mindfulness-based stress reduction programs........... **249**

Objective 10 Report how skills of mindfulness-based stress reduction can help patients intervene in stress reactions and better care for themselves **250**

Objective 11 Report how mindfulness-based stress reduction contributes to medicine and health care **251**

Objective 12 Identify the benefits of physician empathy, attunement, and resonance in the clinical encounter **253**

Objective 13 Describe mindfulness skills that enable presence, clarity, and curiosity in the clinical encounter **254**

Section 7 Glossary **257**
Section 7 Review Questions **258**
Section 7 Review Question Answers and Summaries **260**
Section 7 References **261**

OBJECTIVE 1

Use screening tools for stress, depression, and anxiety

1) Emotional wellness

a) Stress and unhealthy lifestyles

1. 70% of primary care provider visits are related to stress and lifestyle.[1]
    a. When people are stressed and overwhelmed, they are less likely to engage in healthy habits, even though healthy habits can improve mood.[2]
2. Stressful stimuli have a physical (objective component) and a psychological (subjective component). Stress activates a complex series of hormones, adrenaline, and neuropeptides that alter the cardiovascular and metabolic functions of the body. If the noxious (stressful) stimuli is overwhelming or unable to be resolved, stress can become chronic and may lead to suppression of the immune system and long-term organ and tissue damage.[3]

b) Screening for significant stress

1. Screening can be done successfully with a brief stress assessment that will help identify which individuals need closer follow up.[4]
2. A brief discussion on stress and its role in a healthy lifestyle is recommended for all patients.[5]
3. Stress can be treated. Stress management plans can help lower the adverse effects of stress and prevent return of stress symptoms.[6,7]
4. Occupational factors that can affect health
    a. Corporate downsizing increases cardiovascular disease death rates.[8]
    b. One study, including 22,430 Finnish municipal workers, age 19–62, looked at the effect of long work hours (3–4 hours of overtime a day). The study found, at the 7.5-year follow up that long hours increased heart disease risk.[9]
    c. Over a 15-year study, work stressors increased the incidence of type 2 diabetes in women by two-fold. Work stressors were an independent risk factor that was only mildly attenuated by 20% when adjusted for obesity and other health behaviors associated with diabetes.[10]
5. Job characteristics and cardiovascular disease: potential pathways[11,12]
    a. Job characteristics can lead to unhealthy responses, including:
        (1) Stress
        (2) Smoking
        (3) Physical inactivity
        (4) Unhealthy diet
        (5) Heavy alcohol use
    b. These unhealthy behaviors increase the risk of:
        (1) Hypertension
        (2) Obesity
    c. Hypertension and obesity may lead to the following risk factors for developing cardiovascular disease:
        (1) Sleep problems
        (2) Decreased heart rate variability
        (3) Inflammation

(4) Hypercoagulability, atherosclerosis

(5) Decreased immune system functioning

(6) Increased cortisol (HPA axis) and catecholamine production

c) Stress assessment

1. Table 7.1 shows the perceived stress scale assessment, which was originally created by psychologist Dr. Sheldon Cohen in 1983.[4,13]

Table 7.1 Perceived Stress Scale Assessment		
The assessment is a 10-item questionnaire that evaluates symptoms of stress on a scale of 1 (never) to 4 (very often) for the negatively phrased questions (items 1, 2, 3, 6, 9, and 10) and for the positively phrased questions (items 4, 5, 7, and 8) the scoring is reversed, never (4) and often (0). The higher the total score, the more perceived stress one is under.		
1. Upset because of something that happened unexpectedly		
2. Unable to control the important things in your life		
3. Felt nervous and stressed		
4. Felt confident about your ability to handle your personal problems		
5. Felt that things were going your way		
6. Could not cope with all the things that you had to do		
7. Able to control irritations in your life		
8. Felt that you were on top of things		
9. Angered because of things that happened that were outside of your control		
10. Felt difficulties were piling up so high that you could not overcome them		
Scoring of Perceived Stress		
0 -13: low stress	14–26: moderate stress	27–40: high stress

d) Screening for depression[14]

1. Mood disorders can present similarly to stress; therefore, it's important to rule out underlying mood disorders.
2. The Grade B US Preventive Services Task Force (USPSTF) 2016 recommendation is to screen the general adult population including pregnant and postpartum women and adolescents (12–18 years of age) for depression in primary care settings that have adequate support systems in place. If support system staff (those who can provide care for mental health, case management, or care coordination) are not available, then screening should not automatically be done. A Grade B recommendation means there is moderate to high certainty that the net benefit is substantial and should be performed.[15]
3. A simple screen for depression can be done with the patient health questionnaire two-question screening tool (PHQ-2). The questions are rated 0 to 3 (0 = not at all, 1 = several days, 2 = more than half the days, 3 = nearly every day).
   a. PHQ-2 screening questions
      (1) Over the past 2 weeks, have you felt down, depressed, or hopeless?
      (2) Over the past 2 weeks, have you felt little interest or pleasure in doing things?
   b. The screen is positive if the score is ≥3.
   c. Sensitivity is 72%, and specificity is 85%.[16]
   d. A positive screen requires further assessment with the nine question PHQ-9, the Hamilton depression scale (HAM-D), or Beck Depression Inventory (BDI-II).[17]

4. Diagnosis of major depressive disorder (MDD) is made based on American Psychiatric Association *Diagnostic and Statistical Manual* (DSM-5) criteria.
   a. Diagnosis is made if a person has five or more symptoms that have persisted nearly every day for the same 2-week period, and if those symptoms are a change from prior levels of functioning.[18]
      (1) At least one of the following must be present:
         (a) Depressed mood most of the day
         (b) Loss of interest or pleasure
      (2) Four or more of the following must be present:
         (a) Significant weight loss or gain (unintentional), or change in appetite
         (b) Insomnia, hypersomnia
         (c) Psychomotor agitation, retardation, or increased irritability
         (d) Fatigue or loss of energy
         (e) Feelings of worthlessness or excessive guilt
         (f) Trouble concentrating or indecisiveness
         (g) Recurrent thoughts of death, recurrent suicidal ideation with or without a specific plan, or suicide attempt
   b. Note that it may be difficult to delineate between depression, chronic illness somatic symptoms, and severe burnout. Insomnia may present itself both as difficulty falling asleep or waking up too early and being unable to fall back to sleep.
   c. Gender and cultural interpretations may make screening for depression more difficult.[19]
      (1) Gender roles for men may not allow them to describe their emotional feelings.
      (2) Spanish-speaking Latinos are more likely to endorse crying versus English-speaking Latinos.

e) Screening for general anxiety disorder, (GAD)
1. Rule out anxiety before concluding symptoms are due to stress.
2. The USPSTF currently has no recommendations on anxiety screening.
3. The following is a suggestion for brief anxiety screening:
   a. The general anxiety disorder 2-question screening tool (GAD-2). The questions are rated 0 to 3 (0 = not at all, 1 = several days, 2 = more than half the days, 3 = nearly every day). A positive screening test is a score of 3 or above.[20]
      (1) In the last 2 weeks, how often have you felt nervous, anxious, or on edge?
      (2) In the last 2 weeks, how often have you not been able to stop or control worrying?
   b. If positive (score ≥3), on the brief screening questions, follow up with HAM-A, GAD-7, DSM-5, or Beck Anxiety Inventory (BAI) diagnostic criteria.[20,21]
4. Diagnostic criteria for anxiety (from the DSM-5)[18]
   a. Diagnosis is made if a person has the following symptoms more than half the days over at least a 6-month period of time:
      (1) Excessive anxiety
      (2) Worry is difficult to control
      (3) At least three other symptoms
         (a) Restlessness
         (b) Easily fatigued
         (c) Difficulty concentrating

(d) Irritability

(e) Muscle tension

(f) Sleep disturbance

(4) Significant impairment has occurred due to anxiety, worry, or physical symptoms

(5) Symptoms above are not due to substance use

(6) Symptoms are not from another disorder (e.g., obsessive compulsive disorder, anorexia, post-traumatic stress disorder, etc.)

f) The PHQ-4[22]

1. This is a brief screening for depression and anxiety.
2. Questions are rated 0 to 3 (0 = not at all, 1 = several days, 2 = more than half the days, 3 = nearly every day). Patients are asked how often they've experienced the following:
    a. Feeling nervous, anxious, or on edge?
    b. Not being able to stop or control worrying?
    c. Over the past 2 weeks, have you felt down, depressed, or hopeless?
    d. Over the past 2 weeks, have you felt little interest or pleasure in doing things?
3. Scoring
    a. The total score is determined by adding all the scores together
        (1) 0 to 2 = normal
        (2) 3 to 5 = mild
        (3) 6 to 8 = moderate
        (4) 9 to 12 = severe
    b. The higher the score, the greater association with impairment, disability days, and health care use.
    c. Any positive score (score ≥3) should lead to further assessment for depression or anxiety.
    d. People with mild to moderate scores can be given education or resources and rescreened at future visits.

OBJECTIVE 2

Describe the relationship between emotional distress and poor health

1) Mental illness has a complex etiology.[23]

a) Non-modifiable factors include genetics; perinatal infections; exposure to environmental hazards; social, cultural, economic, political, and environmental factors; and more.

b) Modifiable factors include stress, nutrition, environment, sedentary lifestyle, lack of light exposure, addictions, and others. Lifestyle medicine aims to address as many of these modifiable factors as possible.

2) Potential causes of clinical depression and/or anxiety disorders

a) There are over 100 potential causes of clinical depression and/or anxiety disorders that can be categorized into ten categories.[24]

1. If four or more of these ten categories are active, depression and/or an anxiety disorder most often results.[25,26] The more categories involved, the more severe the depression/anxiety tends to be.
2. Finding the causes and eliminating the reversible causes can effectively help in treating depression and anxiety.

b) The Depression and Anxiety Assessment Test (DAAT) can assist the provider in identifying which categories are active in an individual patient.[26] The categories of causes are:[27]

1. Inherited genetic mutations
2. Developmental causes
    a. Adverse childhood experiences, such as sexual abuse
3. Lifestyle causes
    a. Not being on a regular physical exercise program
4. Circadian rhythm causes
    a. Not having regular bed and wake-up times, and/or not being exposed to bright enough light upon awakening
5. Addiction causes
    a. Any substance or non-substance that fits the definition of an addiction
6. Nutritional causes
    a. Not enough folate, tryptophan, tyrosine, antioxidants; deficient in omega-3; or too much arachidonic acid
7. Toxic causes
    a. Mercury, lead, or arsenic
8. Social stress causes
    a. Socially traumatic events or emotionally traumatic loss
9. Medical causes
    a. Advanced cancer, autoimmune disease, hypothyroidism, diabetes, previous head concussion, taking medication that can cause depression, stroke, or other known medical causes
10. Frontal lobe causes
    a. Not habitually taking part in activities that enhance frontal lobe function, such as healthy, melodious music, reading and engaging in spiritual material, or the reading of proverbs[24]
    b. Suppressed frontal lobe function occurs with not consistently living according to your value system.
11. Treating the reversible causes can alleviate and possibly eradicate depression and anxiety.[28,29]

3) The relationship between mental illness and chronic disease

a) Depression is a comorbid illness for many chronic diseases.[24]

1. Depression and diabetes have a bidirectional association (a diagnosis of depression predicts a future diabetes diagnosis and vice-versa).
    a. There is an insulin-mediated mechanism for blood levels of both tryptophan and tyrosine that results in brain serotonin, norepinephrine, and dopamine synthesis. Eating carbohydrate-rich meals in insulin-sensitive individuals may help stimulate the formation of the neurotransmitter serotonin.[30,31,32]

b. Depression alters the hypothalamic-pituitary-adrenal cortex axis, the sympathetic nervous system, and subclinical inflammation.
c. Diabetes alters glucose, insulin, insulin sensitivity, and insulin secretion.

2. Depression is also associated with an increased risk in cardiac diseases, stroke, cancer, and diabetes. Depression is as strong of an independent marker for mortality as smoking.[27]

b) Diabetes and emotional health[33]

1. Anxiety and depression are increased in the presence of lower perceived control over diabetes.
2. Poorer emotional health was associated with negative perceptions of diabetes, including perceptions about the seriousness of the illness and the severity of consequences.
3. Risk factors for suicidal ideation in individuals with diabetes[34]
    a. Insulin therapy
    b. Duration of diabetes
    c. Unsatisfactory glycemic control (HbA1c ≥6.5)

c) Coronary artery disease and emotional health

1. Depression
    a. Is an independent risk factor for cardiac events.[35]
    b. Is a primary risk factor for developing ischemic heart disease and a secondary risk factor for worsened prognosis.[36]
    c. Increases cardiac risk by 15–20% in patients with coronary artery disease.[37]
    d. Doubles cardiac events, even when controlling for ejection fraction and number of blocked arteries.[38]
    e. Major depressive disorder (OR 2.55, 95% CI, 1.38–4.73) and generalized anxiety disorder (OR 2.47, 95% CI, 1.23–4.97) predicted increased risk from cardiac death, myocardial infarctions, cardiac arrest, and non-elective revascularization over a 2-year follow up.[39]
    f. Patients with depression suffer from:[35]
        (1) Increased abnormal platelet adherence
        (2) Endothelial dysfunction
        (3) Lowered heart rate variability
        (4) Worse adherence to lifestyle changes
    g. Depression is a modifiable risk factor for coronary artery disease that generally precedes coronary artery disease by several years.[38]
2. Treatment of depression in patients with coronary artery disease
    a. Treatment improves symptoms and quality of life. However, there are no clear findings that treatment of depression improves survival.[40]
    b. Selective seratonin reuptake inhibitors (SSRI) treatment in patients with coronary artery disease is relatively safe, and early treatment with SSRIs may be beneficial in decreasing cardiac events.[36]
    c. Treatment with tricyclic antidepressants (TCAs) is not recommended due to the risk of QT prolongation (the amount of time needed for the ventricles of the heart to depolarize and contract to the time the ventricles repolarize and relax) and orthostatic hypotension (drop in blood pressure with gravity, such as upon sitting or standing).[36]
    d. Optimal treatment includes medication, psychotherapy, cognitive behavioral therapy, and reversal of associated lifestyle risk factors.[37]

OBJECTIVE 3

Describe the provider's role in facilitating patients' emotional wellness

1) **Screen and diagnose significant stress or underlying mood disorders**
   - a) Clinic practice processes that improve outcomes.[41]
     1. Screen every patient for depression (PHQ-2).
     2. Screen for stress and anxiety as warranted.
     3. Develop proactive emotional wellness action plans with patients who are ready.
     4. Train team member(s) to assist patients with adapting self-management techniques and creating relapse prevention plans for stress management, anxiety, and depression.
     5. Ensure emotional wellness is addressed as a component of developing healthy habits.

2) **Develop nonpharmacologic stress management plans.**
   - a) Encourage nonpharmacologic management strategies and interventions, including:
     1. Light therapy, in particular blue light or medical grade light boxes[42,43]
     2. Abdominal breathing
     3. Expressive and creative pursuits, such as movement or dance, playing a musical instrument, singing, or creating art
     4. Massage
     5. Tai chi
     6. Bibliotherapy (the use of books with the intent to bring medical or psychological healing) and self-help websites
     7. Volunteering for meaningful causes
     8. Spiritual and religious activities
     9. Regular time in nature
     10. Mindfulness exercises, meditation, relaxation, and time for contemplation
     11. Physical exercise

3) **Promote self-management techniques for emotional well-being.**
   - a) Encourage healthy coping skills for emotional well-being
     1. Learning cognitive behavioral skills
     2. Developing problem-solving skills
     3. Improving one's sense of humor
     4. Learning time management techniques
     5. Improving frustration tolerance via cognitive behaviorl therapy (CBT) techniques
     6. Improving emotional intelligence

4) **Encourage the patient to use social support.**
   - a) Encourage the patient to use their social support teams for assistance with behavior changes.
     1. It may be beneficial for the patient to write a list of needs for a particular health behavior change and then write the name of a person who may be able to help support or fulfill that need.
   - b) Help the patient identify gaps that are not addressed by their social network.
     1. Work with patient to troubleshoot how to fill those gaps.

5) **Refer the patient to accessible community and online resources.**

6) **Refer the patient to mental health providers if necessary.**

OBJECTIVE 4

Identify indications for referral to a mental health professional

1) **Referral to a mental health provider may be indicated when a patient has one or more of the following:**
   a) High psychiatric screening scores
   b) Meets DSM-5 criteria for depression or anxiety and appropriate care is beyond one's scope of practice
   c) Has active suicidal or homicidal ideation. This is a medical emergency and requires immediate attention.
   d) Has a history of a prior suicide attempt. Further inquiry should be made to assess patient's present safety.
   e) Has comorbid mood disorders (e.g., bipolar, obsessive compulsive disorder, or personality disorder)
   f) Has an unclear diagnosis
   g) Prefers to be seen by a behavioral health provider (cognitive behavioral therapy should be encouraged on its own or in combination with medications)
   h) Shows no improvement despite treatment
   i) Experiences a relapse of symptoms
   j) The patient should also be referred if the physician judges there is a need.

OBJECTIVE 5

Identify how to manage depression and anxiety in patients with comorbidities

1) **Treatment of depression**
   a) Lifestyle modification nonpharmacologic treatments include:
      1. Physical exercise
      2. Mindfulness, intentional distraction, and relaxation therapy
      3. Bibliotherapy
      4. Light therapy
      5. Computerized interventions
      6. Sleep management
      7. Positive relationships and social support
      8. Addressing lifestyle-related precipitants of depression (e.g., lack of sleep, loneliness, and poor diet)

b) Psychological treatment (use especially if the patient is not responding to nonpharmacological treatments)
   1. Cognitive behavioral therapy (CBT)
   2. Behavioral therapy
   3. Interpersonal therapy
   4. Psychotherapy

c) Pharmacotherapy[44,45]
   1. SSRIs/SNRIs are first-line treatment for depression. One in seven to eight patients treated will see a benefit from using the medication versus treatment with a placebo. Two out of three patients who use the medication will have side effects. Treatment will be stopped in 1 out of 20–90 patients due to side effects. The benefit of SSRI treatment is more prominent as disease severity increases from mild-moderate to severe.
   2. TCAs should be used only if SSRI/SNRIs are not tolerated or if a patient has a specific medical history that would make TCAs more favorable. Seven to 16 patients need to be treated in order to see one patient benefit from the medication compared to treatment with a placebo. Treatment will need to be stopped due to side effects in 1 out of 4–30 patients.
   3. Monoamine oxidase inhibitors (MAOs) have increased side effects and more interactions with food and other medications. They are recommended as third-, fourth-, or fifth-line therapy for depression treatment.[46]

d) Combination of two or three categories of treatment, for example:
   1. Physical activity and CBT
   2. SSRIs and CBT

2) Mental health and physical exercise

a) The impact of physical exercise on treating depression is comparable to CBT.[47]

b) Exercise is slightly more effective overall when compared to no treatment or a control group treatment. However, it is not more effective when compared to treatment with psychological or pharmacological therapies.[48]

c) Exercise is a promising treatment intervention for depressed elderly.[49,50]

d) Exercise may prevent depression in young adults if it is regularly practiced starting in childhood.[51]

3) Mental health and nutrition

a) A healthy dietary pattern is significantly associated with reduced odds of depression[52] and suicide.[53] Reduced risk of depression is strongly and positively correlated with intake of whole grains, olive oil, vegetables, and fruit. More refined grains, sugar, and meat are associated with an increased risk of depression.[54]

b) A plant-based diet with no meat, fish, or eggs in a prospective randomized controlled trial showed significant improvement in depression in just 2 weeks.[52,55]

c) Avoiding processed foods, intake of anti-inflammatory diet (no or little arachidonic acid, which is present in meat, fish, and eggs), and increasing magnesium, folate, and long-chain omega-3 fatty acids (EPA, DHA) are associated with less depression.[56]

d) There's good evidence intensive lifestyle intervention treatment is effective for depression and anxiety.[57,58]

1. Beck Depression Index (BDI) scores, social functioning scores, and mental health scores, improved more over a 6-week period when there was a greater decrease in BMI (odds ratio 1.3 to 1.9).[57]

e) Fried foods, refined grains, and sugary products are associated with increased rates of depression and anxiety.[59]

1. Adults who frequently eat fast food are 40% more likely to develop depression than those who avoid fast food.[60]
2. In the United Kingdom, individuals who reported an unhealthy diet also self-reported higher rates of depression.[61]

f) There is a dose-response effect between types of fat intake and depression rates.[62]

1. Diets higher in *trans* fats were associated with an increased risk of depression.
2. Diets higher in mono- and poly-unsaturated fats were weakly associated with lower rates of depression.

4) Association of mood with nutrients

a) *The Lancet Psychiatry Journal* published an article, in 2015, titled "Nutritional medicine as mainstream in psychiatry" in which they stated, "Although the determinants of mental health are complex, the emerging and compelling evidence for nutrition as a crucial factor in the high prevalence and incidence of mental disorders suggests that diet is as important to psychiatry as it is to cardiology, endocrinology, and gastroenterology."[56]

b) A number of select nutrient-based supplements (alone or in combination) may be beneficial in select groups in the management of mental disorders.[63]

1. Omega-3 fatty acids (mercury-poor sources, such as non-fish sources), which may be helpful in bipolar disorder,[64] post-traumatic stress disorder (PTSD), depression and prevention of psychosis. In pregnant women, there is a positive association between low omega-3 levels and higher incidence of maternal depression.[65] Possible mechanisms include modulation of neurotransmitter (serotonin, norepinephrine, or dopamine) re-uptake and synthesis, enhancement of cell membrane fluidity, and neurogenesis via up-regulation of brain-derived neurotrophic factor (BDNF).[66]
2. S-adenosyl methionine (SAMe), which is responsible for adding the final methyl group in the production of serotonin, norepinephrine, and dopamine. A small double-blind, randomized clinical trial (n = 73) did show SAMe to be an effective antidepressant adjunct to a SSRI and clinically augmenting the effects of pharmaceutical antidepressants.[67]
3. N-acetyl cysteine (NAC) needs further studies, but initial literature shows a potential benefit for bipolar depression, schizophrenia, trichotillomania, and other compulsive and addictive behaviors. NAC augments the production of glutathione, a potent antioxidant, and may have an anti-inflammatory effect.[68]
4. Zinc deficiency has been linked to increased depressive symptoms. Zinc augments hippocampal neurogenesis via upregulation of BDNF. Evidence is emerging that zinc may help symptoms of depression, especially as an augmentation to pharmaceutical antidepressants.[69]
5. Folate, or vitamin B9, can help in the production of serotonin and dopamine. When used with antidepressant medication, it has been shown to improve the efficacy or shorten the response time.[70]
6. Vitamin D is a neurosteroid with data showing low maternal levels are implicated in schizophrenia risk and a deficiency is also linked to increased depressive symptoms.[71]

7. Silexan, an active ingredient in lavender oil, in one multi-centered, double-blind, randomized trial showed reduced anxiety equivalent to lorazepam, but with no sedative effects and no potential for drug abuse.[72,73] It can improve test anxiety, while improving test scores[74] (unlike lorazepam, which worsens test scores due to frontal lobe suppression).[75]
8. In small studies, Saffron has shown benefits in reducing depression (N = 40)[76] and premenstrual dysphoria (N = 50).[77]

c) Links between nutrient deficiency and mood

1. Among child-bearing-age women, deficiencies of folate, vitamin B12, calcium, iron, selenium, zinc, and omega-3 fatty acids were more common among depressed versus non-depressed women.[65,78]
2. Supplementation with folic acid helps treat depression.[65,78]

5) Mental health and meditation

a) Meditation

1. Can decrease some of the negative impacts of stress[79]
2. However, more research is needed on meditation to promote happiness.

6) Patient-provider relationship[80]

a) An ongoing patient-provider relationship can be therapeutic for emotional well-being.

b) Tips for a supportive provider-patient relationship:

1. Acknowledge and reflect patients' views of self-care and quality of life.
2. Support patients' autonomy.
3. Promote patients' self-efficacy.

c) Anxiety and depression self-management

1. Action, Beliefs, Consequences (ABC) model of CBT (For more detail, please see Section 2)[81]
   a. Action → Beliefs (that could be distorted) → emotional Consequences[82]

OBJECTIVE 6

Describe the components of emotional wellness self-management

1) Patient responsibilities for emotional wellness

a) Self-management

1. Connect with others; face-to-face interacting encouraged especially for adolescents.[83]
   a. Spending time with and talking with family and friends
   b. Participating in support groups
2. Get involved in real-life, non-screen activities.
3. Try different, healthy ways to relax (e.g., listen to music, exercise, dance, meditate, do yoga, read books, or learn a new skill).
4. Take time for fun activities and hobbies that draw on creativity.
5. Keep a gratitude journal.
6. Take care of spiritual needs.

b) Cognitive restructuring

1. Look at events from a different angle on purpose
    a. Consider, "Is there another way to look at the situation?"
    b. Remember, it's not helpful to focus on events that cannot be changed.
2. Improve mood by looking at what is going well in life
    a. Focus on accomplishments from the past or what challenges have already been overcome.

2) Treatment activities for emotional well-being[41]

a) Create an action plan.

1. The first step is to create a specific plan that addresses which emotional challenge will be focused on; the lifestyle change one is going to make; the commitment to a timeline and follow up; and the support team one will use.
    a. For example, my first activity to cope with [X emotional challenge] and improve my emotions is to begin exercising (lifestyle change) in one week, three times a week for 20 minutes (commitment). My husband will walk with me and keep me accountable (social support). I will follow up in 2 weeks by phone about how this is going.

b) Create a relapse prevention plan.

1. Help the patient plan for challenging times at work or for family emergencies.
2. Help patients decide ahead of time what to say to or do to stay on track.
3. Encourage patients to reach out to family or friends. Encourage them to find at least one trusted individual they can talk with about stressful life events.
4. Encourage patients to share with like-minded people in groups or social networking groups online.

c) The provider's role in promoting activities for emotional well-being

1. Help patients with self-management, cognitive restructuring, treatment plans, and relapse prevention plans.
2. Celebrate success.
3. Note that positive experiences can still be increased, and well-being can still be improved in patients even while they are dealing with a mental illness.

OBJECTIVE 7

Identify the role of positive psychology and its use in lifestyle medicine

1) Positive psychology[84]

a) Definition: The scientific study of strengths and virtues that enable individuals and communities to thrive. The focus is to produce happiness and fulfillment, not to specifically lessen misery.

b) Components

1. Developing positive emotions and affect
2. Experiencing contentment with the past, happiness in the present, and hope for the future
3. Focusing on individual virtues and strengths (courage, compassion, integrity, curiosity, hope, perseverance, gratitude, self-control, etc.)

c) Positive psychology is not a treatment, as of yet, but it can accompany the treatment of mental illness.

d) The practical techniques of positive psychology include:
    1. Finding and improving one's signature strengths
    2. Counting blessings and expressing appreciation
    3. Establishing short- and long-term goals
    4. Savoring the pleasing things in life
    5. Writing down what one wants to be remembered for
    6. Looking for opportunities to extend kindness, then acting
    7. Thinking about the happiest days in one's life frequently

2) Factors that affect well-being either positively or negatively[84]

- **a)** Family relationships
- **b)** How leisure time is spent
- **c)** Finances
- **d)** Physical health
- **e)** Personal freedom (versus governmental control)
- **f)** Social networks
- **g)** Work situations

3) Positive emotions[85]

- **a)** Positive emotions broaden a person's thoughts in the moment and expand one's personal resources socially, physically, intellectually, and artistically. Positive emotions usually occur in non-life-threatening situations, and they are signs a person is flourishing or experiencing optimal well-being.
- **b)** Although more extensive lists exist, positive emotions include joy, interest, contentment, pride, hope, and love.
    1. Joy encourages playfulness, creativity, and pushing limits.
    2. Interest encourages exploration, learning, and broadening oneself.
    3. Contentment encourages relishing the moment and integrating the experience into one's larger self and into the world.
    4. Pride encourages sharing achievements and exploring what other future feats can also be accomplished.
    5. Hope and optimism lead to increased motivation for achieving goals.
    6. Love, when it's experienced in a safe, close relationship, encourages reoccurring cycles of playfulness, relishing the moment, and a desire to explore with loved ones.
- **c)** Positive emotions are protective.[86]
    1. Experiencing more positive emotions lowers the risk of distressing thoughts of suicide in people who have a chronic medical disease.
    2. Positive emotions increase life satisfaction by building resiliency.[87]
        a. The ideal ratio of positive to negative emotions is 3:1, as negative emotions are more potent than positive ones. This ratio is a measure of resiliency. It can be assessed through an online quiz.
            (1) Resilience tipping point (positive to negative): www.positivityratio.com
                (a) Ratio of 3:1 or above: people have the resources to change.

(b) Below 3:1: it's unlikely people will be able to overcome the obstacle at the current time.

3. Encouraging positive emotions in order to influence well-being can be done by:
    a. Promoting activities and perspectives that increase self-efficacy in managing stress or emotional challenges
    b. Viewing stress not necessarily as a bad influence on mental and physical health, but rather as a signal to find more appropriate ways to satisfactorily react to the stressor

d) Healthy time perspectives, viewed through the light of positive emotions

1. Past: forgiveness, gratitude, satisfaction, thinking of what you've achieved
2. Present: savoring the moment, contentment
3. Future: hope, vision, positive anticipation, optimism

e) Increased awareness of one's virtues and strengths can increase positive emotions.[88]

1. Only about one-third of adults know what their strengths are.
2. Character strengths fall into one of six broad categories of core virtues. Individual testing for core virtues and character strengths can be done at the website https://www.viacharacter.org.
    a. Wisdom and knowledge: creativity, curiosity, open-mindedness, love of learning, and perspective
    b. Courage: authenticity, bravery, persistence, and zest
    c. Humanity: kindness, love, and social intelligence
    d. Justice: fairness, leadership, and teamwork
    e. Temperance: forgiveness, modesty, prudence, and self-regulation (self-control)
    f. Transcendence: appreciation of beauty, gratitude, hope, humor, and religiousness
3. American adults are usually lowest in persistence and self-regulation.

OBJECTIVE 8

Identify the nature of stress as well as manageable elements of pathogenic stress reactions

1) Stress reaction versus stress response

a) Stress reaction: An external event causes an internal event by leading to: alarm; activation of the sympathetic nervous system; overstimulation; and internalization of the situation, all of which leads to maladaptive coping and a breakdown of emotions.

b) Stress response: An external event leads to internal conscious processing that allows a person to be mindful of the situation; to recognize influences and chain of event reactions; and to make a deliberate choice. This conscious response allows a person to maintain better control over her emotions; keep a greater sense of calm and balance; recover mentally; and regain equilibrium faster.

2) Definition of suffering: the state of undergoing pain, distress, loss, damage, disability, hardship, or death.[89]

a) There are two kinds of suffering

1. Necessary suffering: experienced by every human being.
    a. Illness
    b. Old age

c. Separation from those we love
d. Death

2. Unnecessary suffering: does not have to be experienced by every human being. Unnecessary suffering stems from egocentricity: our wants, likes, dislikes, attachments, cravings, and aversions.
   a. Wanting a different outcome than the one that has happened
   b. Anticipatory thinking (imagining the worst)
   c. Repeating stories about the past
   d. Trying to resist pain

> *"Pain is inevitable, suffering is optional."*
> –Haruki Murakami

b) Humans can create extra suffering by judging themselves and others without mercy.

c) Our own suffering is one of the greatest points of connection we have with others.

d) Practical techniques to escape suffering include:
1. Be aware of thoughts and thinking patterns that may be harmful.
2. Practice attention instead of inattention.
3. Intentionally connect rather than disconnect.
4. Aim for order and regulation instead of living in disorder and dysregulation.
5. Think and work towards health instead of disease.

OBJECTIVE 9

Describe the integral and essential elements of mindfulness-based stress reduction programs

1) Mindfulness-based stress reduction (MBSR) was designed by Jon Kabat-Zinn.

a) There are more than 800 mindfulness-based stress reduction programs by trained professionals. See:
1. Guided mindfulness meditation practices: https://www.mindfulnesscds.com/
2. Mindfulness Center, University of Virginia School of Medicine: https://med.virginia.edu/mindfulness-center/

2) MBSR programs

a) MBSR usually includes nine classes structured over 8 weeks. In class, participants experience about 45 minutes of mindfulness practices, complete workbook activities, and participate in group activities.

b) Once the program concludes, students are expected to maintain 45 minutes per day of home mindfulness practices, 6 days per week. Resources are available for continued study and practice.

c) The goal is to teach integration and application of mindfulness into daily living and apply a mindful approach to the mental and physical challenges life brings.

d) Formal and informal mindfulness builds upon already present internal resources in order to cultivate health behaviors.
1. Formal: meditation
2. Informal: attentiveness to routine activities (walking, washing hands)

OBJECTIVE 10

Report how skills of mindfulness-based stress reduction can help patients intervene in stress reactions and better care for themselves[90]

1) **A mindfulness practice investigates the relationship between the mind and body and helps create awareness of the space between the stimulus and the response in a situation. This allows for greater freedom and distance from the situation.**
   - **a)** Physical clues like a tight jaw or clenched fists can give help give people greater awareness of stress and prompt questions: "How often do I experience this?" or, "When do I react like this?"
2) **Mindfulness provides a direct path into experiencing a situation in its entirety by being present.**
   - **a)** Being present through mindfulness means not focusing or striving to get or to do something else or to be somewhere else.
3) **Mindfulness creates the potential for each moment to be fully experienced (with calmness and insight) no matter how difficult or intense.**
4) **The attitudes of mindfulness include:**
   - **a)** Non-judging (witnessing)
     1. Being present without judging
        a. Being right here, right now, with things as they are
        b. This is a state of awareness where one can "witness" his or her own body or situation.
   - **b)** Non-striving (relaxing)
     1. Being present without striving
     2. Experiencing a situation directly in its entirety without trying to get, do or be somewhere else
   - **c)** Acknowledging what is happening
     1. Acknowledgement is different than accepting, because many things people experience are not acceptable.
   - **d)** Patience
   - **e)** Keeping an attitude of self-reliance: "I can rely on myself to be with things as they are and work with things as they are to find my way."
   - **f)** Beginner's mind
     1. Fresh, open, wide-aware, and experimental—not afraid of failure
5) **Mindfulness is different than other meditation practices because it is:**
   - **a)** Not a concentrative practice; rather, it's about viewing the broad picture and maintaining an open field of awareness
   - **b)** An awareness that is kind, accepting, self-compassionate and present
   - **c)** Being fully present where you are at (not meditating to be somewhere else)
   - **d)** Done in every moment, in every place
   - **e)** A way of being in the world
   - **f)** A way of life

OBJECTIVE 11

Report how mindfulness-based stress reduction contributes to medicine and health care

1) **Meditation programs for psychological stress and well-being**

   a) In 2014, a systematic review and meta-analysis (47 trials and 3515 participants) was conducted to exam the current research on meditation programs to help clinicians better understand the current evidence associated health benefits.[79]

   b) Study conclusions

      a. Mindfulness meditation programs had moderate evidence of improved anxiety, depression, and pain.

      b. Low evidence of improved stress/distress and mental health–related quality of life

      c. Low evidence or no effect or insufficient evidence of any effect of meditation programs on positive mood, attention, substance use, eating habits, sleep, and weight

      d. No evidence that meditation programs were better than any active treatment (i.e., drugs, exercise, and other behavioral therapies)

      e. No evidence of any harms from meditation programs

2) **Neuroscience and mindfulness-based stress reduction (MBSR)**

   a) Brain neuroplasticity allows people of any age to create new pathways as old thinking patterns are challenged and re-routed.

      1. Adult humans can grow approximately 700 new neurons a day.[91]

      2. The brain learns, adapts and restructures itself based on thought, attitudes, and emotional experience.[92,93,94]

   b) Conscious thought can retrain and shape the brain and emotional traits.

      1. The brain has two distinct forms of self-awareness: extended self-reference and momentary self-reference.[95]

         a. Extended self-reference links one's experiences across time.

         b. Momentary self-reference is awareness of oneself in the present.

         c. With mindfulness training, individuals can distinctly activate these areas, whereas otherwise the two are habitually linked.

      2. 8 weeks of mindfulness training can:[96]

         a. Increase activation of the left prefrontal cortex, which is responsible for planning, personality and happiness

         b. Increase gray matter density in the hippocampus (which is responsible for learning and memory) and increase other brain structures associated with self-awareness, compassion, and introspection

         c. Reduce gray matter density in the amygdala (the emotion area of brain), which correlates with reduced stress

      3. Mindfulness meditation promotes stronger connections between the prefrontal cortex and amygdala areas that are involved in problem-solving skills and modulating emotional responses.[97]

      4. Mindfulness training modifies attention systems, enhances well-being, and may treat a broad spectrum of disorders.[7,98,99,100]

3) **Benefits of mindfulness in medicine and health care**[7,101,102]

a) Enhances psychological hardiness

b) Leads to lasting decreases in physical and psychological symptoms

1. Reduces or can help alleviate inflammation, response to chronic pain, anxiety, depression, and addiction

c) MBSR helps with relationships.[103]

1. Helps develop compassion and empathy for self and others, tolerance, and resilience

a. Reduces loneliness in older adults[104]

4) **Cognitive behavioral therapy (CBT) is an evidence-based structured psychotherapy effective in treating mental health disorders.**

a) CBT is arguably the gold standard psychotherapy with current evidence-based research.[105]

b) CBT follows structured steps to change thoughts.

1. Changing thoughts helps change emotions, potentially leading to changes in behavior.

c) CBT primarily focuses on client's current life, as opposed to their past.

1. Helps develop awareness of triggers, self-talk, or automatic thoughts, emotions, and behaviors, focuses on reframing negative automatic thoughts, and results in healthier ways to cope with life stressors.

d) CBT can reshape the thoughts and enhance brain connectivity and emotional traits.[106]

1. Benefits of CBT compared with other therapies

a. Thoughts are evaluated in the context of being helpful or harmful, positive or negative. Accomplishes this while maintaining a moral context[107]

b. Judgment is maintained while thoughts are evaluated as helpful or harmful. CBT does not attempt to bring up suppressed or damaging memories.[108]

c. Instead of attempting to neutralize all thoughts, rational positive thoughts may be kept and further developed. It does not encourage false-memory formation or loss of positive thoughts.[109]

d. Improves resilience (reduces anxiety and increases self-esteem)[110]

e. Increases ability to cope with stress[111]

2. CBT training can:

a. Establish healthy connectivity of brain regions[112]

b. Build empathy[113]

c. Increase gray matter in the prefrontal cortex[114]

d. Rewire the neural pathways of the brain and normalize neural reactivity, such as among individuals with anxiety disorders[115]

3. CBT has been associated with:

a. Better prefrontal cortex function and planning abilities[116]

b. Healthier neural response to perceived threats[117]

c. Better problem solving[118]

d. Improvement in a broad spectrum of disorders

e. Improvement in well-being[119]

e) Effectively treats disorders, such as:[120,121]

1. Depression

2. Anxiety disorders (including post-traumatic stress disorder, obsessive-compulsive disorder, panic disorder, generalized anxiety disorder, social anxiety disorder, and specific phobia)
3. Personality disorders
4. Marital issues
5. Substance use disorders

f) Compared with antidepressant medication

1. CBT is as efficacious in treating depression as drug medications.[122,123]
2. There is less incidence of depression relapse among patients treated with CBT compared to antidepressant medication.[124]
3. CBT in combined treatment with antidepressant medication appears to be more effective than treatment with only antidepressant medication for major depression, panic disorder, and obsessive-compulsive disorder.[125]

g) See Section 2 for basic CBT practice and techniques.

OBJECTIVE 12

Identify the benefits of physician empathy, attunement, and resonance in the clinical encounter

1) The patient-physician relationship is important in healing.

a) A positive patient-physician relationship leads to better adherence.[126]

b) Physician responsibilities include:

1. Be present, be real, listen, and be aware of perceptions.
2. Maintain interpersonal engagement (pause, relax, stay open, listen, and be truthful).

2) Compassion is maintaining an attitude of kindness, friendliness and gentleness toward yourself and others.

a) Cultivating compassion for yourself and others is important in life and in the clinical encounter.

1. "RAIN" of compassion is a simple pneumonic to help maintain a compassionate attitude.
   a. Recognition: what's happening
   b. Acceptance: make room for the experience
   c. Investigate: be curious
   d. Non-identification: witness the experience and rest in natural awareness

3) Self-care is important for providers.

a) Compassion fatigue and burnout are real.

1. Burnout is a lack of satisfaction with one's job, which may be due to hours, pay, or stress.
2. Compassion fatigue is like post-traumatic stress disorder, but it's an acute distress or tension. With compassion fatigue, the "helper" is traumatized and preoccupied with suffering, which may lead to the "helper" having poor coping, poor self-care or self-sacrificing tendencies.

b) Self-care can help prevent burnout, enhance empathy, and improve attitudes among primary care providers.[127]

c) Self-care is essential.
   1. The American Medical Association Code of Ethics states that physicians are responsible to maintain their own health and wellness. It is unethical for a provider not to attend to her/his self-care.[128]

d) Self-care is exemplified in the body: before the heart sends blood anywhere else, it sends blood to itself.

OBJECTIVE 13

Describe mindfulness skills that enable presence, clarity, and curiosity in the clinical encounter

1) **The current societal environment is difficult for the prefrontal cortex.**
   a) Things that are not helpful for the brain
      1. Multi-tasking
         a. Only 2.5% of people can multi-task in a simulation of driving and completing an auditory test. All other participants had severely impaired performance.[129]
         b. In general, most people do better with sequential tasking.
      2. Addiction to distractions, such as media, phones, watches, etc.
      3. Stress overdose
      4. Sleep deprivation
      5. Low-octane diet
      6. Too little physical exercise (exercise allows the brain to recover)
      7. Too little healthy recreation (hiking in nature, learning a new skill, swimming, bicycling, etc.)
      8. No mental down time
      9. When focusing, too frequent interruptions or disruptions (often by media devices)
   b) Multitasking or having your brain work too hard/long in one area results in shallow and scattered brain states.

2) **The optimal environment for the brain allows for cognitive agility by focusing deeply on one task and then shifting fully to the next task.**

3) **The mindfulness skills that enable presence, clarity, and curiosity in the clinical encounter[130]**
   a) Ten steps to organize your mind and match the correct brain state with the appropriate task for coaching and assisting patients[131]
      1. A provider's mind must be agile, able to go deep, and easily and quickly cross three dimensions: focus, awareness, and content.[132]
         a. Focus ranges from high control to uncontrolled mind wandering states, and both states are necessary for brain health.
         b. Awareness (inside oneself and outside oneself). Awareness ranges from low or narrow (being aware of something very specific such as a musical song) to high or wide (being aware of many sensations at once, like what can occur while watching a brilliant sunrise and noticing the cool air, chirping birds, and dew on the ground).
         c. Content (ranging from detailed to big picture)

2. Agility allows people to transition fully from one brain state to the next.
    a. Various brain states include present awareness, imagining, thinking and evaluating, flow, collaboration, mind wandering, creative thinking, and strategic thinking.
3. How to upgrade your brain energy
    a. Protect your emotional energy.
    b. Improve your physical energy through physical exercise, which helps with focus and creativity, and nutrition that is good for brain health, including omega-3 fatty acids, antioxidants, and water.
4. Tame the sense of frenzy before entering a patient's room or during a patient encounter
    a. Name the frenzy: Gently stopping and naming the negative emotion enables the prefrontal cortex to notice the emotion and let it go or lay it aside.
    b. Acknowledge the frenzy and stop evaluating and judging. Then practice self-compassion and mindfulness, thinking things like, "Every cell is doing the best it can with the resources it has right now."
    c. Elicit positive emotions (creativity, curiosity, open-mindedness, flexibility, etc.) in yourself and others by focusing on what's going well and what's enjoyable. If the situation is dire (such as a cancer diagnosis or death), use compassion.
5. Prepare
    a. Take a moment to clear your mind before entering a patient's room. This gives the mind an opportunity to be ready to think clearly and objectively and to analyze.
6. Connect with those around you (patients during the clinical encounter).[133]
    a. Connecting with others improves brain function and vagal tone (which means the activity of the vagus nerve, which is an important part of the parasympathetic nervous system). Connecting with others allows for sharing of positive and negative emotions and synchrony of thoughts and behaviors.
    b. Humility fosters connection, but attitudes of "I'm stronger, better, and more competent than you" will harm the connection and activate the inner critic in the other person.
7. Focus and sustain your attention. This is the deepest brain state of clinical encounter.
    a. Work collaboratively in a flow with the patient, without distractions, for peak performance.
    b. Use your working memory, imagine possible outcomes, and strategize with the patient about options.[134]
        (1) Note that working memory can be enhanced by simplifying, de-cluttering, associating, and sleeping.
        (2) With visualization and imagination, the brain becomes like a compass and can begin finding ways to achieve a desired outcome.
        (3) Help patients plug into their own motivation.
    c. Providers need to stay curious, compassionate, non-judgmental, and open-minded. Ask: "What's my intention? Why am I here? What do I want to learn?"
8. Put a brake on distractions.
    a. In order to avoid being distracted and preserve executive function, the brain must exhibit effective inhibition. This inhibition is deficient in attention-deficit/hyperactivity disorder.
    b. If you are distracted, go into awareness and then make a conscious choice to go with the distraction or stay present.

9. Take brain breaks.
    a. The mind needs uncontrolled time to wander. Of note, the brain does continue to work on problems even during breaks from intense mental focus.
10. Be creative.
    a. Creativity is non-linear, divergent thinking that creates room for shifts in perspective.
11. Be strategic.
    a. Strategic thinking provides a big-picture view. Ask questions like, "What is important? What's really happening? What's meaningful here? What's a priority? What's the lesson here?"
        (1) Gratitude is not an official brain state, but it is important for strategic perspective, as it allows people to appreciate and enjoy what is good.

SECTION 7 GLOSSARY

Mindfulness: a way of facing a situation in its entirety by being fully present. It creates the potential for each moment to be experienced as it is.

Mindfulness practice: investigates the relationship between the mind and body and helps create awareness of the space between the stimulus and the response in a situation. This allows for more freedom and distance from the situation.

Positive emotions: emotions that broaden a person's thoughts in the moment and expand one's personal resources socially, physically, intellectually, and artistically. Positive emotions are signs of well-being and include joy, interest, contentment, pride, and love.

Positive psychology: the scientific study of strengths and virtues that enable individuals and communities to thrive. Positive psychology involves developing positive emotions and affect; experiencing contentment with the past, happiness in the present, and hope for future; and focusing on individual virtues and strengths.

Stress reaction: an external event causes an internal event by leading to alarm; activation of the sympathetic nervous system; overstimulation; and internalization of the situation, all of which leads to maladaptive coping and a breakdown of emotions.

Stress response: an external event leads to internal conscious processing that allows a person to be mindful of the situation; to recognize influences and chain of event reactions; and to make a deliberate choice. This conscious response allows a person to maintain better control over her emotions; keep a greater sense of calmness and balance; recover mentally; and regain equilibrium faster.

SECTION 7 REVIEW QUESTIONS

1. **Primary care physicians note that lifestyles contribute greatly to an individual's health. Which of the following observations is true?**
   - **A.** Health habits can be engaged equally by a moderately stressed individual as compared to a mildly stressed individual.
   - **B.** The mood of an individual can be altered and equally impacted by healthy behavior change when engaged by a highly stressed individual as compared to an unstressed individual over the long follow-up period.
   - **C.** Roughly 70% of primary care physician visits are related to stress and lifestyle, despite this being a single-factorial relationship.
   - **D.** Multifactorial lifestyle variables contribute to nearly 70% of primary care provider visits and can be successfully diagnosed and treated.

2. **Well-being and absence of disease is correlated to a healthy mental state. Depression can propagate further disease when it is noted in a primary care setting that:**
   - **A.** A low scoring psychiatric assessment has been completed.
   - **B.** DSM-IV criteria have been met.
   - **C.** A diagnosis of depression has been made and is now under initial medication therapy.
   - **D.** A prior self-harm episode via ingestion of only three pills without hospitalization was not documented in the patient's chart.

3. **Fitness and exercise are comparable to which of the following as it pertains to its effects on mental health?**
   - **A.** Cognitive behavioral therapy (CBT)
   - **B.** Monoamine Oxidases (MAOs)
   - **C.** Increasing omega-3 fatty acids when treating bipolar patients with mania
   - **D.** Reducing omega-3 fatty acids when treating bipolar patients with depression

4. **With stress being identifiable and leading to pathological stress reactions, which of the following is a type of "unnecessary suffering" that can lead to a stress reaction?**
   - **A.** Old age
   - **B.** Separation from those we love
   - **C.** Illness
   - **D.** Egocentricity

5. **Mindfulness-based stress reduction (MBSR) has been noted to increase which of the following?**
   - **A.** Emotional reactions
   - **B.** Resilience
   - **C.** Physical and psychological symptoms
   - **D.** Stress

6. A woman presents to you and appears to be crying. She is a home health aide working 36 hours per week. Her husband is nearly bedridden at home and has been needing increased healthcare daily from her for nearly 5 years, as he has a history of cerebral vascular accident (stroke). She says to you that she is now having panic attacks intermittently when she goes to patient homes for work because she can relate so strongly to the suffering of the families. She feels guilty taking time for herself and has even missed her own doctor's appointments. She hasn't exercised for 4 years. She states, "How can I tell my husband I am exercising when he can barely move?" This is an example of which of the following:
   - **A.** Compassion fatigue
   - **B.** Compassion burnout
   - **C.** Normal compassion stress
   - **D.** Failed cognitive agility

7. Which of the following combinations is correct when describing mindfulness-based skills affecting the prefrontal cortex and its respective task function?
   - **A.** The patient-physician relationship and interpersonal mindfulness
   - **B.** Cognitive agility and deep focus
   - **C.** Tight jaw or "TMJ" and increased fitness daily
   - **D.** Positive psychology and maintaining a journal about spiritual needs

8. According to the philosophy that the provider is a coach facilitating health behavior change, which of the following combinations have nearly the same effectiveness?
   - **A.** In-person coaching and phone coaching
   - **B.** Placebo and phone coaching
   - **C.** Self-awareness reflection by a wellness coach and a nutritionist
   - **D.** In-person coaching and use of medication with psychotherapy

9. The PHQ-2 screening questions for depression include questions on?
   - **A.** Apathy
   - **B.** Appetite
   - **C.** Isolation
   - **D.** Mental focus

10. Which of the following accurately describes cognitive behavioral therapy (CBT)?
   - **A.** CBT is inferior to pharmaceutical therapy in treating depression.
   - **B.** CBT is beneficial in treating depression and/or anxiety but no other mental health conditions.
   - **C.** CBT has been shown to increase gray matter in the prefrontal cortex of the brain.
   - **D.** CBT teaches non-judgmentalism towards thoughts (no thoughts are bad, wrong, or irrational).

SECTION 7 REVIEW QUESTION ANSWERS AND SUMMARIES

1. **Answer: D.** Lifestyle contributes to 70% of primary care provider visits; is multifactorial both in disease generation and treatment; is less likely to be engaged by over-stressed and overwhelmed individuals; and is more likely to be impactful when people in need of close follow up are identified.
2. **Answer: D.** Depression causes more harm when it's untreated, unrecognized, or undocumented in a patient's past medical history. It's diagnosed with DSM-Vs and a high psychometric assessment score upon screening. Depression can be treated with lifestyle modifications rather than pharmaceuticals based on certain screening protocols.
3. **Answer: A.** Fitness and exercise is comparable to cognitive behavioral therapy (CBT), but it's not as directly effective as pharmacotherapies. Increasing omega-3 fatty acids demonstrates a good response with bipolar depression and not mania.
4. **Answer: D.** Unnecessary suffering is wanting a different outcome than the one that has happened. It begins with egocentricity (wants, likes, dislikes, attachments, cravings, and aversions), has anticipatory thinking (imagining the worst), can include repeating stories about the past, and trying to resist pain.
5. **Answer: B.** Mindfulness-based stress reduction helps develop compassion and empathy for self and others, tolerance, and resilience.
6. **Answer: A.** Compassion fatigue is distress and tension in which the helper is traumatized and preoccupied with suffering. Compassion fatigue can lead to poor coping, poor self-care, and self-sacrifice, which is similar to PTSD. Compassion burnout is associated with lack of job satisfaction, to many hours, low pay, and stress.
7. **Answer: B.** Mindfulness skills enable presence, clarity, and curiosity in a clinical encounter. These skills directly affect the prefrontal cortex, thereby decreasing scattered brain states and allowing for deep focus inside of sequential tasking. This kind of focus is how roughly 95% of the population processes information and performs tasks, as opposed to the less than 5% of the population who are able to perform multitasking.
8. **Answer: A.** Phone coaching has a 38% effectiveness rate, while in-person coaching has a 41% effectiveness rate. A placebo has a 19% effectiveness rate.
9. **Answer A.** The PHQ-2 asks two questions about how often bothersome symptoms have occurred over the last 2 weeks: 1) little interest or pleasure in doing things 2) feeling down, depressed, or hopeless. Apathy is the lack of interest, enthusiasm, or concern, and is assessed in the first question.
10. **Answer: C.** Cognitive behavioral therapy (CBT) is arguably the gold standard psychotherapy, following structured steps to change thoughts, which can change emotions and potentially change behavior. It increases gray matter in the prefrontal cortex. It is not inferior to pharmaceutical treatment, but rather works synergistically. CBT is effective for treatment of depression, anxiety, personality disorders, substance abuse, or marital disorders.

SECTION 7 REFERENCES

1. Feldman M. D., Christensen, J. F., eds. *Behavioral Medicine in Primary Care: A Practical Guide*. Appleton & Lange; 1997.
2. American Psychological Association. *Stress in America: Key Findings*. Washington, DC: American Psychological Association; 2010. https://www.apa.org/news/press/releases/stress/2010/key-findings#:~:text=Nearly%20one%2Dthird%20said%20they,or%20motivation%20(38%20percent).
3. Mariotti A. The effects of chronic stress on health: new insights into the molecular mechanisms of brain-body communication. *Future Sci OA*. 2015;1(3):FS023-FS023. https://pubmed.ncbi.nlm.nih.gov/28031896.
4. Cohen S., Kamarck T., Mermelstein R. A global measure of perceived stress. *J Health Soc Behav.* 1983;24(4):385-396.
5. Lianov L., Johnson M. Physician competencies for prescribing lifestyle medicine. *JAMA.* 2010;304(2):202-203.
6. van der Klink J. J., Blonk R. W., Schene A. H., van Dijk F. J. The benefits of interventions for work-related stress. *Am J Public Health.* 2001;91(2):270-276.
7. Grossman P., Niemann L., Schmidt S., Walach H. Mindfulness-based stress reduction and health benefits. A meta-analysis. *J Psychosom Res.* 2004;57(1):35-43.
8. Vahtera J., Kivimäki M., Pentti J., et al. Organisational downsizing, sickness absence, and mortality: 10-town prospective cohort study. *BMJ.* 2004;328(7439):555.
9. Virtanen M., Ferrie J. E., Singh-Manoux A., et al. Overtime work and incident coronary heart disease: the Whitehall II prospective cohort study. *Eur Heart J.* 2010;31(14):1737-1744.
10. Heraclides A., Chandola T., Witte D. R., Brunner E. J. Psychosocial stress at work doubles the risk of type 2 diabetes in middle-aged women: evidence from the Whitehall II study. *Diabetes Care.* 2009;32(12):2230-2235.
11. Siegrist J., Rödel A. Work stress and health risk behavior. *Scand J Work Environ Health.* 2006;32(6):473-481.
12. Belkic K. L., Landsbergis P. A., Schnall P. L., Baker D. Is job strain a major source of cardiovascular disease risk? *Scand J Work Environ Health.* 2004;30(2):85-128.
13. Andreou E., Alexopoulos E. C., Lionis C., et al. Perceived Stress Scale: reliability and validity study in Greece. *Int J Environ Res Public Health.* 2011;8(8):3287-3298.
14. US Preventive Services Task Force. Screening for depression in adults: US Preventive Services Task Force recommendation statement. *Ann Intern Med.* 2009;151(11):784-792.
15. US Preventive Services Task Force. Grade definitions. Updated June, 2018. https://uspreventiveservicestaskforce.org/uspstf/about-uspstf/methods-and-processes/grade-definitions#july2012. Accessed 2021.
16. Williams J. W., Jr., Noël P. H., Cordes J. A., Ramirez G., Pignone M. Is this patient clinically depressed? *JAMA.* 2002;287(9):1160-1170.
17. Ebell M. H. Screening instruments for depression. *Am Fam Physician.* 2008;78(2):244-246.
18. American Psychiatric Association. *Diagnostic and Statistical Manual of Mental Disorders (DSM-5)*. 5th ed. Washington, DC: American Psychiatric Association Publishing; 2013.
19. Kerr L. K., Kerr L. D., Jr. Screening tools for depression in primary care: the effects of culture, gender, and somatic symptoms on the detection of depression. *West J Med.* 2001;175(5):349-352.
20. Ebell M. H. Diagnosis of anxiety disorders in primary care. *Am Fam Physician.* 2008;78(4):501-502.
21. Maier W., Buller R., Philipp M., Heuser I. The Hamilton Anxiety Scale: reliability, validity and sensitivity to change in anxiety and depressive disorders. *J Affect Disord.* 1988;14(1):61-68. http://www.sciencedirect.com/science/article/pii/0165032788900729.
22. Kroenke K., Spitzer R. L., Williams J. B., Lowe B. An ultra-brief screening scale for anxiety and depression: the PHQ-4. *Psychosomatics.* 2009;50(6):613-621.
23. World Health Organization. *Mental Disorders Fact Sheet*, vol 2017. Geneva, Switzerland: World Health Organization; 2017.
24. Tabak A. G., Akbaraly T. N., Batty G. D., Kivimaki M. Depression and type 2 diabetes: a causal association? *Lancet Diabetes Endocrinol.* 2014;2(3):236-245.
25. Rippe J. M. *Lifestyle Medicine,* 3rd ed. Boca Raton, FL: CRC Press; 2019.
26. Nedley N., Ramirez F. E. Nedley Depression hit hypothesis: identifying depression and its causes. *Am J Lifestyle Med.* 2016;10(6):422-428.
27. Voinov B., Richie W. D., Bailey R. K. Depression and chronic diseases: it is time for a synergistic mental health and primary care approach. *Prim Care Companion CNS Disord.* 2013;15(2).
28. Nedley N., Francisco R., Jessica C. lifestyle education program improves depression and anxiety in 8 weeks. Presented at American College of Lifestyle Medicine; October, 2019; Orlando, FL.
29. Nedley N., Ramirez F. E., Payton H. Abstract P215: medical lifestyle residential program reduces anxiety in 10 days. *Circulation.* 2020;141:AP215. https://www.ahajournals.org/doi/10.1161/circ.141.suppl_1.P215.
30. Wurtman R. J., Wurtman J. J., Regan M. M., McDermott J. M., Tsay R. H., Breu J. J. Effects of normal meals rich in carbohydrates or proteins on plasma tryptophan and tyrosine ratios. *Am J Clin Nutr.* 2003;77(1):128-132. https://doi.org/10.1093/ajcn/77.1.128.
31. Markus C. R., Panhuysen G., Tuiten A., Koppeschaar H., Fekkes D., Peters M. L. Does carbohydrate-rich, protein-poor food prevent a deterioration of mood and cognitive performance of stress-prone subjects when subjected to a stressful task? *Appetite.* 1998;31(1):49-65.
32. Hidehiko Y., Wurtman R. J. Meal composition and plasma amino acid ratios: effect of various proteins orcarbohydrates, and of various protein concentrations. *Metabolism.* 1986;35(9):837-842. http://wurtmanlab.mit.edu/static/pdf/670.pdf.

33. Hudson J. L., Bundy C., Coventry P. A., Dickens C. Exploring the relationship between cognitive illness representations and poor emotional health and their combined association with diabetes self-care. A systematic review with meta-analysis. *J Psychosom Res.* 2014;76(4):265-274.
34. Lee H. Y., Hahm M. I., Lee S. G. Risk of suicidal ideation in diabetes varies by diabetes regimen, diabetes duration, and HbA1c level. *J Psychosom Res.* 2014;76(4):275-279.
35. Zellweger M. J., Osterwalder R. H., Langewitz W., Pfisterer M. E. Coronary artery disease and depression. *Eur Heart J.* 2004;25(1):3-9. http://dx.doi.org/10.1016/j.ehj.2003.09.009.
36. Jiang W. Impacts of depression and emotional distress on cardiac disease. *Cleve Clin J Med.* 2008;75 Suppl 2:S20-25.
37. Kop W. J., Ader D. N. Assessment and treatment of depression in coronary artery disease patients. *Ital Heart J.* 2001;2(12):890-894.
38. Frasure-Smith N., Lesperance F. Depression and coronary artery disease. *Herz.* 2006;31 Suppl 3:64-68.
39. Frasure-Smith N., Lesperance F. Depression and anxiety as predictors of 2-year cardiac events in patients with stable coronary artery disease. *Arch Gen Psychiatry.* 2008;65(1):62-71.
40. Wang J. T., Hoffman B., Blumenthal J. A. Management of depression in patients with coronary heart disease: association, mechanisms, and treatment implications for depressed cardiac patients. *Expert Opin Pharmacother.* 2011;12(1):85-98.
41. Lianov L. 8B emotional wellness: part 2. In: Lianov L., ed. *Lifestyle Medicine Competencies*. American College of Lifestyle Medicine; 2014.
42. Tsikirai T. M., Ramirez F., Nedley N. SUN-006 light and exercise therapy improves depression in women with premenstrual syndrome. *J Endocr Soc.* 2020;4(Supplement_1). https://doi.org/10.1210/jendso/bvaa046.1929.
43. Lieverse R., Van Someren E. J., Nielen M. M., Uitdehaag B. M., Smit J. H., Hoogendijk W. J. Bright light treatment in elderly patients with nonseasonal major depressive disorder: a randomized placebo-controlled trial. *Arch Gen Psychiatry.* 2011;68(1):61-70.
44. DeJong A., Kovich H. Common questions about the pharmacologic management of depression in adults. *Am Fam Physician.* 2021;92(2):94-100. https://www.aafp.org/afp/2015/0715/p94.pdf.
45. Guirguis-Blake J. Effectiveness of antidepressants compared with placebo for depression in primary care. *Am Fam Physician.* 2010;82(1):42.
46. Thase M. E. The role of monoamine oxidase inhibitors in depression treatment guidelines. *J Clin Psychiatry.* 2012;73 Suppl 1:10-16.
47. Rimer J., Dwan K., Lawlor D. A., et al. Exercise for depression. *Cochrane Database Syst Rev.* 2012(7):Cd004366.
48. Cooney G. M., Dwan K., Greig C. A., et al. Exercise for depression. *Cochrane Database Syst Rev.* 2013(9):Cd004366.
49. Mura G., Carta M. G. Physical activity in depressed elderly. A systematic review. *Clin Pract Epidemiol Ment Health.* 2013;9:125-135.
50. Blake H., Mo P., Malik S., Thomas S. How effective are physical activity interventions for alleviating depressive symptoms in older people? A systematic review. *Clin Rehabil.* 2009;23(10):873-887.
51. McKercher C., Sanderson K., Schmidt M. D., et al. Physical activity patterns and risk of depression in young adulthood: a 20-year cohort study since childhood. *Soc Psychiatry Psychiatr Epidemiol.* 2014;49(11):1823-1834.
52. Lai J. S., Hiles S., Bisquera A., Hure A. J., McEvoy M., Attia J. A systematic review and meta-analysis of dietary patterns and depression in community-dwelling adults. *Am J Clin Nutr.* 2014;99(1):181-197.
53. Nanri A., Mizoue T., Poudel-Tandukar K., et al. Dietary patterns and suicide in Japanese adults: the Japan Public Health Center-based Prospective Study. *Br J Psychiatry.* 2013;203(6):422-427.
54. Adjibade M., Julia C., Allès B., et al. Prospective association between ultra-processed food consumption and incident depressive symptoms in the French NutriNet-Santé cohort. *BMC Med.* 2019;17(1):78.
55. Beezhold B. L., Johnston C. S. Restriction of meat, fish, and poultry in omnivores improves mood: a pilot randomized controlled trial. *Nutr J.* 2012;11:9.
56. Sarris J., Logan A. C., Akbaraly T. N., et al. Nutritional medicine as mainstream in psychiatry. *Lancet Psychiatry.* 2015;2(3):271-274.
57. Thieszen C. L., Merrill R. M., Aldana S. G., et al. The Coronary Health Improvement Project (CHIP) for lowering weight and improving psychosocial health. *Psychol Rep.* 2011;109(1):338-352.
58. Kelly J., Shull J. A comprehensive clinical lifestyle medicine specialty fellowship program: what intensive lifestyle treatment can do. *Am J Lifestyle Med.* 2017;11(5):414-418. https://doi.org/10.1177/1559827617696293.
59. Jacka F. N., Mykletun A., Berk M., Bjelland I., Tell G. S. The association between habitual diet quality and the common mental disorders in community-dwelling adults: the Hordaland Health study. *Psychosom Med.* 2011;73(6):483-490.
60. Sanchez-Villegas A., Toledo E., de Irala J., Ruiz-Canela M., Pla-Vidal J., Martinez-Gonzalez M. A. Fast-food and commercial baked goods consumption and the risk of depression. *Public Health Nutr.* 2012;15(3):424-432.
61. Akbaraly T. N., Brunner E. J., Ferrie J. E., Marmot M. G., Kivimaki M., Singh-Manoux A. Dietary pattern and depressive symptoms in middle age. *Br J Psychiatry.* 2009;195(5):408-413.
62. Sanchez-Villegas A., Verberne L., De Irala J., et al. Dietary fat intake and the risk of depression: the SUN Project. *PLoS One.* 2011;6(1):e16268.
63. Rucklidge J. J., Kaplan B. J. Broad-spectrum micronutrient formulas for the treatment of psychiatric symptoms: a systematic review. *Expert Rev Neurother.* 2013;13(1):49-73. https://doi.org/10.1586/ern.12.143.
64. Stoll A. L., Severus W. E., Freeman M. P., et al. Omega 3 fatty acids in bipolar disorder: a preliminary double-blind, placebo-controlled trial. *Arch Gen Psychiatry.* 1999;56(5):407-412.
65. Leung B. M., Kaplan B. J. Perinatal depression: prevalence, risks, and the nutrition link–a review of the literature. *J Am Diet Assoc.* 2009;109(9):1566-1575.

66. Mischoulon D., Freeman M. P. Omega-3 fatty acids in psychiatry. *Psychiatr Clin North Am.* 2013;36(1):15-23.
67. Papakostas G. I., Mischoulon D., Shyu I., Alpert J. E., Fava M. S-adenosyl methionine (SAMe) augmentation of serotonin reuptake inhibitors for antidepressant nonresponders with major depressive disorder: a double-blind, randomized clinical trial. *TAm J Psychiatry.* 2010;167(8):942-948.
68. Berk M., Malhi G. S., Gray L. J., Dean O. M. The promise of N-acetylcysteine in neuropsychiatry. *Trends Pharmacol Sci.* 2013;34(3):167-177.
69. Lai J., Moxey A., Nowak G., Vashum K., Bailey K., McEvoy M. The efficacy of zinc supplementation in depression: systematic review of randomised controlled trials. *J Affect Disord.* 2012;136(1-2):e31-e39.
70. Fava M., Mischoulon D. Folate in depression: efficacy, safety, differences in formulations, and clinical issues. *J Clin Psychiatry.* 2009;70 Suppl 5:12-17.
71. Eyles D. W., Burne T. H., McGrath J. J. Vitamin D, effects on brain development, adult brain function and the links between low levels of vitamin D and neuropsychiatric disease. *Front Neuroendocrinol.* 2013;34(1):47-64.
72. Ramirez F., Nedley, N. Use of oral lavander oil for anxiety in a depression medical residential program. Presented at: Annual Meeting International Neuropsychological Society; February 3-6, 2016; Boston, MA. https://nedleyhealth.com/media/wysiwyg/infortis/nhs/Lavander_oil_for_anxiety.jpg.
73. Woelk H., Schläfke S. A multi-center, double-blind, randomised study of the Lavender oil preparation Silexan in comparison to Lorazepam for generalized anxiety disorder. *Phytomedicine.* 2010;17(2):94-99.
74. McCaffrey R., Thomas D. J., Kinzelman A. O. The effects of lavender and rosemary essential oils on test-taking anxiety among graduate nursing students. *Holist Nurs Pract.* 2009;23(2):88-93.
75. Kasper S., Gastpar M., Müller W. E., et al. Silexan, an orally administered Lavandula oil preparation, is effective in the treatment of 'subsyndromal' anxiety disorder: a randomized, double-blind, placebo controlled trial. *Int Clin Psychopharmacol.* 2010;25(5):277-287.
76. Noorbala A. A., Akhondzadeh S., Tahmacebi-Pour N., Jamshidi A. H. Hydro-alcoholic extract of Crocus sativus L. versus fluoxetine in the treatment of mild to moderate depression: a double-blind, randomized pilot trial. *J Ethnopharmacol.* 2005;97(2):281-284.
77. Agha-Hosseini M., Kashani L., Aleyaseen A., et al. Crocus sativus L. (saffron) in the treatment of premenstrual syndrome: a double-blind, randomised and placebo-controlled trial. *BJOG.* 2008;115(4):515-519.
78. Bodnar L. M., Wisner K. L. Nutrition and depression: implications for improving mental health among childbearing-aged women. *Biol Psychiatry.* 2005;58(9):679-685.
79. Goyal M., Singh S., Sibinga E. M., et al. Meditation programs for psychological stress and well-being: a systematic review and meta-analysis. *JAMA Intern Med.* 2014;174(3):357-368.
80. Llorca P. M. Severe depression: the doctor/patient relationship. *L'Encephale.* 2009;35 Suppl 7:S310-313.
81. Lam D., Gale J. Cognitive behaviour therapy: teaching a client the ABC model — the first step towards the process of change. *J Adv Nurs.* 2000;31(2):444-451. https://onlinelibrary.wiley.com/doi/abs/10.1046/j.1365-2648.2000.01280.x.
82. Lam D., Cheng L.. Cognitive behaviour therapy approach to assessing dysfunctional thoughts. *Couns Psychol Q.* 2001;14(3):255-265. https://doi.org/10.1080/09515070110092325.
83. Twenge J. M., Spitzberg B. H., Campbell W. K. Less in-person social interaction with peers among US adolescents in the 21st century and links to loneliness. *J Soc Pers Relat.* 2019;36(6):1892-1913. https://doi.org/10.1177/0265407519836170.
84. Egger G., Binns A., Rossner S. *Lifestyle Medicine: Managing Diseases of Lifestyle in the 21st Century.* McGraw-Hill; 2010.
85. Fredrickson B. L. The role of positive emotions in positive psychology. The broaden-and-build theory of positive emotions. *Am Psychol.* 2001;56(3):218-226.
86. Hirsch J. K., Duberstein P. R., Unützer J. Chronic medical problems and distressful thoughts of suicide in primary care patients: mitigating role of happiness. *Int J Geriatr Psychiatry.* 2009;24(7):671-679.
87. Fredrickson B. *Positivity: Groundbreaking Research Reveals How to Embrace the Hidden Strength of Positive Emotions, Overcome Negativity, and Thrive.* New York, NY: Three Rivers Press; 2009.
88. Peterson C., Seligman M. *Character Strengths and Virtues: A Handbook and Classification.* Washington, DC: American Psychological Association Publishing; 2004. https://www.apa.org/pubs/books/4317046.
89. Merriam-Webster. Suffer. September 9, 2017.https://www.merriam-webster.com/dictionary/suffer
90. Flowers S. Mindfulness-based stress reduction. American College of Lifestyle Medicine webinar. August 5, 2014. Accessed March 16, 2021.
91. Spalding K. L., Bergmann O., Alkass K., et al. Dynamics of hippocampal neurogenesis in adult humans. *Cell.* 2013;153(6):1219-1227.
92. Garland E. L., Fredrickson B., Kring A. M., Johnson D. P., Meyer P. S., Penn D. L. Upward spirals of positive emotions counter downward spirals of negativity: insights from the broaden-and-build theory and affective neuroscience on the treatment of emotion dysfunctions and deficits in psychopathology. *Clin Psychol Rev.* 2010;30(7):849-864.
93. Davidson R. J., McEwen B. S. Social influences on neuroplasticity: stress and interventions to promote well-being. *Nat Neurosci.* 2012;15(5):689-695.
94. Chang Y. Reorganization and plastic changes of the human brain associated with skill learning and expertise. *Front Hum Neurosci.* 2014;8:35.
95. Farb N. A., Segal Z. V., Mayberg H., et al. Attending to the present: mindfulness meditation reveals distinct neural modes of self-reference. *Soc Cogn Affect Neurosci.* 2007;2(4):313-322.
96. Hölzel B. K., Carmody J., Vangel M., et al. Mindfulness practice leads to increases in regional brain gray matter density. *Psychiatry Res.* 2011;191(1):36-43.

97. Way B. M., Creswell J. D., Eisenberger N. I., Lieberman M. D. Dispositional mindfulness and depressive symptomatology: correlations with limbic and self-referential neural activity during rest. *Emotion.* 2010;10(1):12-24.
98. Jha A. P., Krompinger J., Baime M. J. Mindfulness training modifies subsystems of attention. *Cogn Affect Behav Neurosci.* 2007;7(2):109-119.
99. Brown K. W., Ryan R. M. The benefits of being present: mindfulness and its role in psychological well-being. *J Pers Soc Psychol.* 2003;84(4):822-848.
100. Baer R. A. Mindfulness training as a clinical intervention: A conceptual and empirical review. *Clin Psychol (New York).* 2003;10(2):125-143.
101. Davis D. M., Hayes J. A. What are the benefits of mindfulness? A practice review of psychotherapy-related research. *Psychotherapy (Chic).* 2011;48(2):198-208.
102. Merkes M. Mindfulness-based stress reduction for people with chronic diseases. *Aust J Prim Health.* 2010;16(3):200-210.
103. Davis D. M, Hayes J. A. What are the benefits of mindfulness? A practice review of psychotherapy-related research. *Psychotherapy.* 2011;48(2):198.
104. Creswell J. D., Irwin M. R., Burklund L. J., et al. Mindfulness-Based Stress Reduction training reduces loneliness and pro-inflammatory gene expression in older adults: a small randomized controlled trial. *Brain Behav Immun.* 2012;26(7):1095-1101.
105. David D., Cristea I., Hofmann S. G. Why cognitive behavioral therapy is the current gold standard of psychotherapy. *Front Psychiatry.* 2018;9:4.
106. Yoshino A., Okamoto Y., Jinnin R., Takagaki K., Mori A., Yamawaki S. Role of coping with negative emotions in cognitive behavioral therapy for persistent somatoform pain disorder: is it more important than pain catastrophizing? *Psychiatry Clin Neurosci.* 2019;73(9):560-565.
107. Clark L. *SOS Help for Emotions: Managing Anxiety, Anger, and Depression*. Bowling Green, KY: SOS Programs & Parents Press; 2001.
108. Nedley N. *The Lost Art of Thinking: How to Improve Emotional Intelligence and Achieve Peak Mental Performance.* Nedley Publishing; 2013.
109. Backus W., Chapian M. *Telling Yourself the Truth: Find Your Way Out of Depression, Anxiety, Fear, Anger, and Other Common Problems By Applying the Principles of Misbelief Therapy.* Bethany House; 2000.
110. Stallard P., Simpson N., Anderson S., Carter T., Osborn C., Bush S.. An evaluation of the FRIENDS programme: a cognitive behaviour therapy intervention to promote emotional resilience. *Arch Dis Child.* 2005;90(10):1016-1019.
111. Hofmann S. G., Asnaani A., Vonk I. J., Sawyer A. T., Fang A. The efficacy of cognitive behavioral therapy: a review of meta-analyses. *Cognit Ther Res.* 2012;36(5):427-440
112. Yoshimura S., Okamoto Y., Matsunaga M., et al. Cognitive behavioral therapy changes functional connectivity between medial prefrontal and anterior cingulate cortices. *J Affect Disord*. 2017;208:610-614.
113. Song M. K., Choi S. H., Lee D. H., Lee K. J., Lee W. J., Kang D. H. Effects of cognitive-behavioral therapy on empathy in patients with chronic pain. *Psychiatry Investig.* 2018;15(3):285-291.
114. Seminowicz D. A., Shpaner M., Keaser M. L., et al. Cognitive-behavioral therapy increases prefrontal cortex gray matter in patients with chronic pain. *J Pain.* 2013;14(12):1573-1584.
115. Månsson K. N., Salami A., Frick A., et al. Neuroplasticity in response to cognitive behavior therapy for social anxiety disorder. *Transl Psychiatry.* 2016;6(2):e727.
116. van der Straten A., Huyser C., Wolters L., Denys D., van Wingen G. Long-term effects of cognitive behavioral therapy on planning and prefrontal cortex function in pediatric obsessive-compulsive disorder. *Biol Psychiatry Cogn Neurosci Neuroimaging.* 2018;3(4):320-328.
117. Lueken U., Straube B., Konrad C., et al. Neural substrates of treatment response to cognitive-behavioral therapy in panic disorder with agoraphobia. *Am J Psychiatry.* 2013;170(11):1345-1355.
118. Warmerdam L., van Straten A., Jongsma J., Twisk J., Cuijpers P. Online cognitive behavioral therapy and problem-solving therapy for depressive symptoms: Exploring mechanisms of change. *J Behav Ther Exp Psychiatry.* 2010;41(1):64-70.
119. Green L. S., Oades L. G., Grant A. M. Cognitive-behavioral, solution-focused life coaching: enhancing goal striving, well-being, and hope. *J Posit Psychol.* 2006;1(3):142-149. https://doi.org/10.1080/17439760600619849.
120. Song M. K., Choi S. H., Lee D. H., Lee K. J., Lee W. J., Kang D. H. Effects of cognitive-behavioral therapy on empathy in patients with chronic pain. *Psychiatry Investig.* 2018;15(3):285-291. https://doi.org/10.30773/pi.2017.07.03. http://www.psychiatryinvestigation.org/journal/view.php?number=851.
121. Kaczkurkin A. N., Foa E. B. Cognitive-behavioral therapy for anxiety disorders: an update on the empirical evidence. *Dialogues Clin Neurosci*. 2015;17(3):337-346. https://pubmed.ncbi.nlm.nih.gov/26487814.
122. DeRubeis R. J., Siegle G. J., Hollon S. D. Cognitive therapy versus medication for depression: treatment outcomes and neural mechanisms. *Nat Rev Neurosci.* 2008;9(10):788-796. https://pubmed.ncbi.nlm.nih.gov/18784657.
123. American Psychological Association. What is cognitive behavioral therapy? July, 2017. https://www.apa.org/ptsd-guideline/patients-and-families/cognitive-behavioral.
124. DeRubeis R. J., Siegle G. J., Hollon S. D. Cognitive therapy versus medication for depression: treatment outcomes and neural mechanisms. *Nat Rev Neurosci.* 2008;9(10):788-796.
125. Cuijpers P., Sijbrandij M., Koole S. L., Andersson G., Beekman A. T., Reynolds C. F., 3rd. Adding psychotherapy to antidepressant medication in depression and anxiety disorders: a meta-analysis. *World Psychiatry.* 2014;13(1):56-67.
126. Han W. T., Collie K., Koopman C., et al. Breast cancer and problems with medical interactions: relationships with traumatic stress, emotional self-efficacy, and social support. *Psycho-oncology.* 2005;14(4):318-330.

127. Krasner M. S., Epstein R. M., Beckman H., et al. Association of an educational program in mindful communication with burnout, empathy, and attitudes among primary care physicians. *JAMA.* 2009;302(12):1284-1293.
128. American Medical Association. Chapter 9: Opinions on professional self-regulation. In: *AMA Principles of Medical Ethics.* Chicago, IL; American Medical Association; 2016. https://www.ama-assn.org/sites/default/files/media-browser/code-of-medical-ethics-chapter-9.pdf.
129. Watson J. M., Strayer D. L. Supertaskers: profiles in extraordinary multitasking ability. *Psychon Bull Rev.* 2010;17(4):479-485.
130. Hammerness P., Moore M. *Organize Your Mind, Organize Your Life.* Ontario, Canada: Harvard Health Books; 2012.
131. Carson S. *Your Creative Brain: Seven Steps to Maximize Imagination, Productivity, and Innovation in Your Life.* San Francisco, CA: Jossey-Bass; 2010.
132. Koutstaal W. *The Agile Mind.* Oxford Univeristy Press; 2013.
133. Fredrickson B. *Love 2.0: How Our Supreme Emotion Affects Everything We Feel, Think, Do and Become.* New York, NY: Penguin Group; 2013.
134. Alloway T., R. Alloway. *The Working Memory Advantage: Train Your Brain to Function Stronger, Smarter, Faster.* New York, NY: Simon & Schuster; 2013.

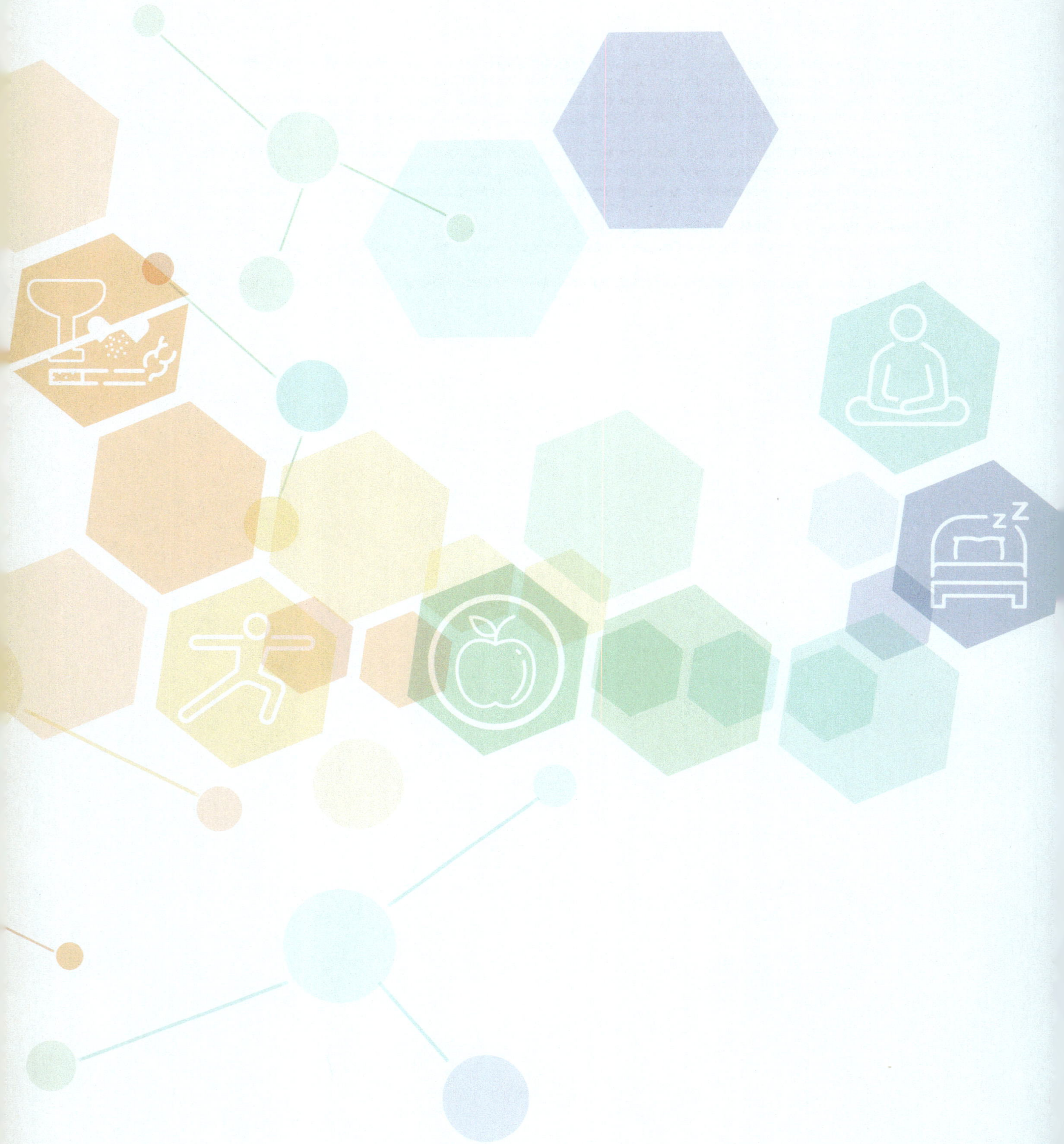

SECTION 8
Sleep Health Science and Interventions

Objective 1 Review the physiology of sleep **268**

Objective 2 Explain the role of light exposure and endogenous melatonin in sleep health **277**

Objective 3 Review sleep's role in health and chronic disease **278**

Objective 4 Identify the lifestyle-based activity and the dietary, environmental, and coping behaviors that can improve sleep health. **282**

Objective 5 Identify at least two lifestyle adjustments related to light exposure and meal composition and timing that support improved sleep. **284**

Objective 6 Identify key factors that differentiate patient subpopulations with insufficient or poor-quality sleep **286**

Section 8 Glossary **289**

Section 8 Review Questions **290**

Section 8 Review Question Answers and Summaries **292**

Section 8 References. **293**

OBJECTIVE 1

Review the physiology of sleep

1) Sleep and culture

a) Previous viewpoint

1. Conscious limiting of sleep; viewing sleep as inconvenient or as "wasted" time
2. Being able to "function" on a small amount of sleep is equated with strength, courage, or productivity.

b) Newer insights

1. Sleep equated to health on all levels: physical, mental and emotional
2. Sleep a key to performance

c) Continued challenge

1. Early morning or late evening may be the only time available for focused, uninterrupted work.
2. 20% of workers are on night shifts.
3. Global economies with a 24-hour and 7-days-a-week expectation.

2) Sleep statistics[1,2,3,4]

a) The average US adult sleeps 6 hours, 57 minutes.

1. 20% sleep less than 6 hours per night.

b) 37% of young adults sleep less than 7 hours per night.

1. This proportion doubled from 1960 to 2002.

c) There has been a significant increase in short sleep duration for all age categories from 1970 to present.

d) 60 million US adults have frequent difficulty sleeping.

1. Only 10% of those with difficulty sleeping seek medical attention.

e) Indirect costs from insomnia are estimated at $60 billion annually and include:

1. Presenteeism (people are at work, but not productive)
2. Increased risk of long-term disability
3. Mistakes, errors, and accidents

3) Amount of sleep[2,3]

a) 1/3 of life is spent sleeping.

b) There is no recognized objective test for how much sleep a person needs.

c) General sleep requirements:

1. 7–9 hours per day for adults, but there's a considerable range of subjective sleep need among individuals
2. Change throughout lifespan (see Figure 8.1)

Figure 8.1 Sleep Duration Recommendations

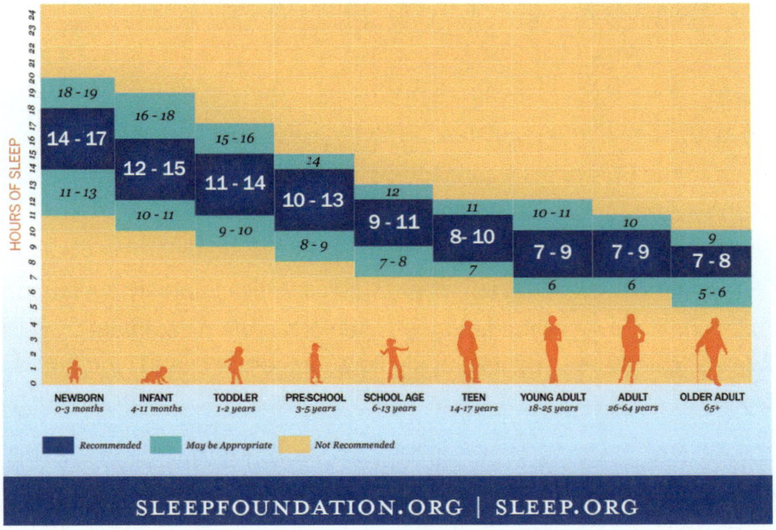

- **d)** Sleep deficiency impairs functional performance, but often individuals are unaware of the level of impairment.

4) Circadian physiology terminology

- **a)** *Circa*: about; *dia*: day
- **b)** Endogenous or internal circadian oscillators: the molecules, cells, and tissues that make up the body's "internal clock." They produce oscillating (alternating) currents through self-regulating positive and negative feedback loops that create the circadian rhythm. Endogenous oscillators include both the central and peripheral oscillators.[5]
- **c)** Central oscillators are found in the suprachiasmic nucleus (SCN), which is the body's main "clock."
- **d)** Peripheral oscillators are present in every major organ in the body (kidney, liver, heart, adrenal glands, and pancreas). They allow for synchrony and alignment between the central and peripheral clocks.
- **e)** Circadian rhythms
  1. Biological process that are regulated by central and peripheral oscillators that are capable of being brought into a rhythm (usually a 24-hour period) in order to help align physiologic functions and behaviors with the solar light-dark cycles.
  2. "Body clocks."
- **f)** Entrainment
  1. The ability to be brought into a rhythm
  2. Synchronization of the internal endogenous oscillators based on external (out of the body) inputs
  3. Sleep propensity is the ability to transition to sleeping, if a person is awake, or to stay asleep, if a person is sleeping.
     - a. The human circadian rhythm is closer to 24.2 hours but is entrained to a 24-hour day.
     - b. For most people, it is easier to stay up later than to go to bed earlier.
     - c. This affects travel as people align to new time zones—it is easier for most people to travel westward, when the person experiences a day being greater than 24 hours.

g) Wakefulness-sleep cycle is entrained by day-night cycle.

h) Awakening cortisol spike

1. Entrained by food anticipation

i) SCN

1. Central "clock"
2. Portion of hypothalamus that regulates melatonin secretion
   a. Nerves from the SCN directly connect to the other tissues and organs allowing for entrainment and control the circadian rhythm (see Figure 8.2).
      (1) Neuronal tract from retina to SCN is used to entrain central oscillators.
      (2) Neuronal tract from SCN to pineal gland controls melatonin secretion.
      (3) Splanchnic nerves of the autonomic nervous system innervate the adrenal glands. Adrenal glands help regulate blood flow, temperature, and food intake through secretion of epinephrine, norepinephrine, glucocorticoids, and aldosterone.

Figure 8.2[6]

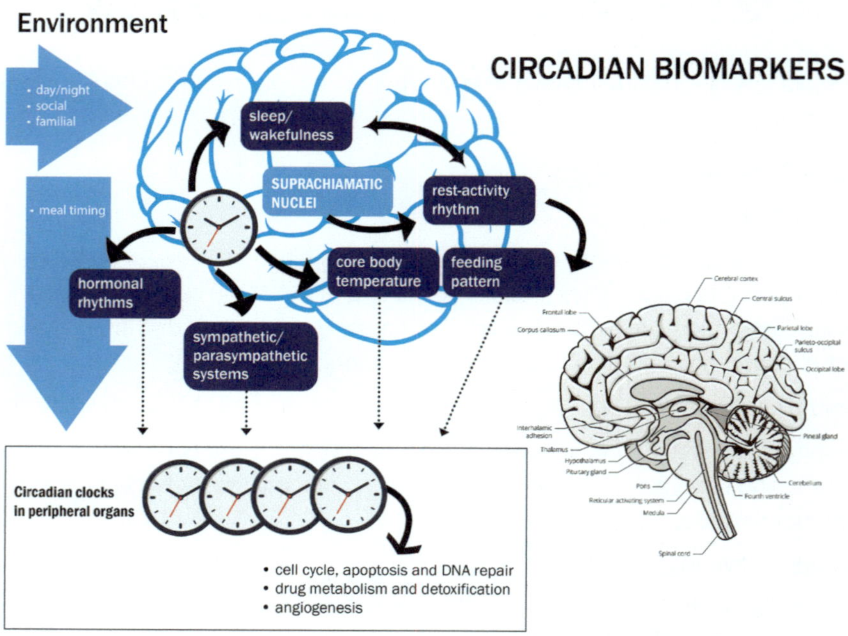

3. Responsible for awakening cortisol spike

j) Retinal ganglion cells (RGC)

1. Nonvisual light-sensitive retinal neurons
2. Relay light intensity/spectra to SCN
3. Melanopsin is the photopigment in the RGC and is the pathway through which the SCN clock is entrained. Melanopsin is maximally sensitive to short wavelengths of light (blue light ~480nm) and stimulates the RGC neurons, which relay light intensity and spectra to the SCN. Based on this signal, melatonin secretion timing may be changed.

5) Circadian system components[7]

a) Circadian system (Figure 8.3)

Figure 8.3 Circadian System

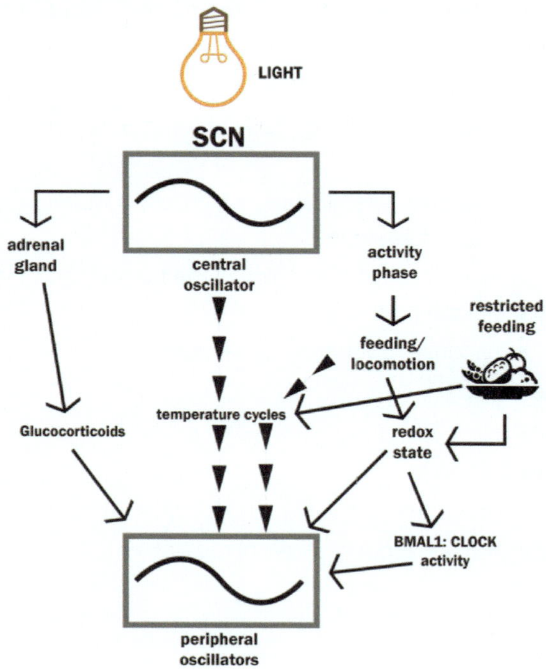

b) Cycle of stimulating the endogenous oscillators (Figure 8.4)[8]

1. Inputs: external and environmental factors that can entrain the circadian rhythm
   a. Light intensity
   b. Light wavelength (frequency, color)
   c. Food (mainly carbohydrates)
   d. Fluid (blood osmolality), which is a measurement of the particles (such as sodium, potassium, and chloride) dissolved in the plasma.[9]
   e. Ambient temperature (temperature of the surrounding environment)
2. Modifiers: change the amount of "input" that gets to the body's operators
   a. Pupillary reflex
      (1) Limits the amount of light getting to retina ganglion cells
   b. Sunglasses or backlight on electronic devices
      (1) Changes the intensity of light reaching retina ganglion cells
   c. Single nucleotide polymorphisms (SNPs)
      (1) SNPs are genetic variations in the DNA. If they occur in the gene-coding portion of DNA, it can lead to an abnormal, enhanced, or nonfunctioning protein.
      (2) PER and CRY proteins are an integral part of the molecular mechanism that controls the circadian rhythm throughout the body in the peripheral oscillators. PER and CRY inhibit function of other proteins (proteins "clock" and "cycle") until they degrade, a process that takes approximately 24 hours. Exposure of retinal ganglion cells to light causes more PER protein to be produced, an important factor for "entrainment" of this molecular cycle.

        (3) If single nucleotide polymorphisms occur in the PER and CRY proteins, these proteins may not be able to function appropriately, and the circadian rhythm in the body may be impaired.

    d. Cutaneous fat stores: these affect core and extremity temperature by accelerating (if there are not enough fat stores) or dampening (if there is too much cutaneous fat) the body's ability to thermoregulate.

    e. Vascular tone

        (1) Affects fluid volume in blood vessels, which modifies core and peripheral temperatures.

            (a) Nitric oxide and estrogen enhance vasodilation, which is the widening of blood vessels, and which lowers blood pressure.

            (b) Sodium causes an acute vasoconstriction, which is the narrowing of blood vessels, and which raises blood pressure.

3. Operators: are the body's reaction or response to the modified inputs

    a. Core body temperature changes

    b. Melatonin suppression or secretion

    c. Cortisol secretion, timing of cortisol spike

    d. Cutaneous blood flow, increase or decrease

4. Outputs: the behavioral and physiological consequences of the operators

    a. Sleep

    b. Functional performance, including:

        (1) Alertness

        (2) Kinetic activity

        (3) Motor skills, including precision

        (4) Strength and stamina

    c. Food-seeking behaviors, including quantity and quality

Figure 8.4 Cycle of Stimulating the Endogenous Oscillators

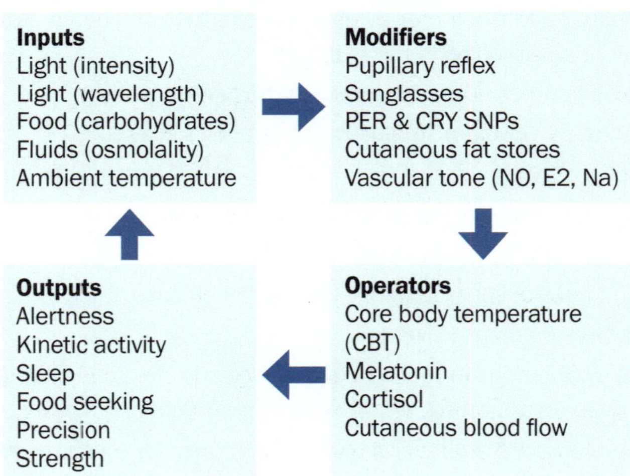

6) Circadian and sleep physiology

a) Sleep onset

1. Darkness triggers pineal melatonin secretion.
2. Melatonin secretion
    a. Cutaneous vasodilation → extremity warming → cooling of core body temperature → sleep initiation

b) Early sleep: sleep onset to mid-sleep

1. Continued rise in melatonin levels
    a. Increase peripheral skin temperature → continued cooling of core body temperature → core body temperature nadir (low point) reached ~2–3 hours before awakening
2. Predominantly slow wave (restorative sleep) on electroencephalogram (EEG)
3. Decreasing core body temperature with increased peripheral skin temperature signals physiologic restorative processes throughout the body.
4. Decreased blood pressure and sympathetic tone

c) Throughout sleep, decreased metabolic demand allows for restoration and repair.

1. DNA remodeling and repair
2. Leptin and ghrelin secretion (control appetite)
3. Increase in growth hormone release
4. Elevated peptide synthesis
5. Gradual increase in cortisol
6. Fatty acid metabolism
7. Regulation of insulin[10]
8. Promotion of ATP synthesis
9. Memory encoding and consolidation
10. Emotional regulation[11]

d) Late sleep: mid-sleep to awakening

1. Declining melatonin levels
    a. Decreasing peripheral skin temperature → increased core body temperature
2. Longer rapid eye movement (REM) periods (important for fear extinguishing and limbic system functioning)
3. Increasing blood pressure, sympathetic tone, and baroreceptor sensitivity as the body prepares to awaken
    a. Baroreceptor sensitivity references the body's ability to change blood pressure rapidly by modifying heart rate, heart contractibility, and peripheral vascular tone.[12]

e) Awakening

1. Cortisol spike (24-hour peak)
    a. Normally the peak cortisol level in a 24-hour period occurs upon awakening. This spike is important in the transition from sleep to wakefulness.

f) Sleep, melatonin, and core temperature[13]

1. Figure 8.5 is a graph of core temperature, sleep propensity, and melatonin levels.

Figure 8.5 The Relationship Between Insomnia and Body Temperatures

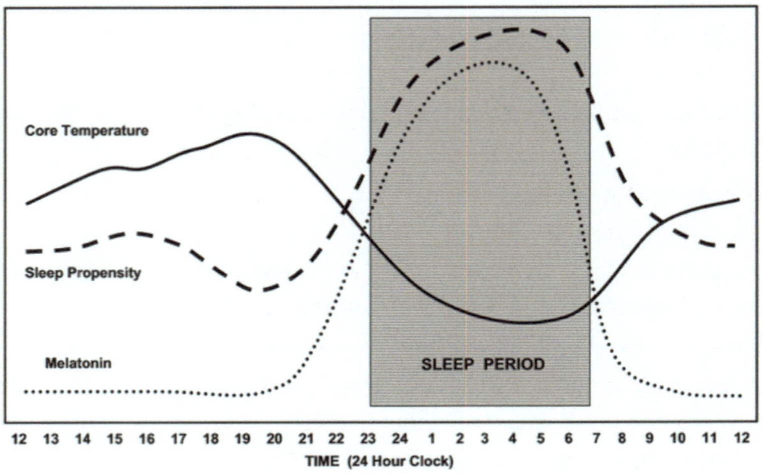

Diagrammatic representation of normally entrained endogenous rhythms of core body temperature (solid curve), plasma melatonin (dotted curve), and objective sleep propensity (dashed curve) placed in the context of the 24-hour clock time and normal sleep period (shaded area).

7) **Circadian physiology and light**

   a) Inputs
      1. Light
      2. Food (carbohydrates)
      3. Exercise
      4. Fluid status (osmolality of blood, temperature)
      5. Ambient temperature

   b) Light is the predominant entraining force of the central SCN clock
      1. Components of light that effect the SCN
         a. Light intensity
         b. Light spectra
         c. Timing of light exposure in a 24-hour cycle
         d. Duration of light exposure

   c) Light intensity
      1. Sunlight is a greater intensity than artificial light
         a. Bright sunlight at noon: 100K lux
         b. Cloudy day: 25K lux
         c. Overcast day: 2–10K lux
         d. Bright industrial lighting: 1–5K lux
         e. Offices and kitchens: 200–500 lux
         f. Household lighting: 50–200 lux
         g. Average nursing home: 50 lux
         h. Street lighting: 20 lux
         i. Full moon: 1 lux

j. Moonless night: 0.001–0.0001 lux (8 orders of magnitude less than bright sunny day). The human eye is extremely sensitive to light and is able to detect light even at this magnitude.

d) Light spectra

1. The visible spectrum of light ranges from violet light (400 nm) to red light (700 nm).
2. Blue light is ~420–480 nm.
3. Blue light is 6500 Kelvin color (blue sky, fluorescent lights) while warm light is 2500 Kelvin color (incandescent light bulbs, light from flames of fire).[14]
   a. Blue light creates greater melatonin suppression at lower intensities and shorter durations.

> **Note:** Kelvin color is a number that describes the dominant color tone produced at a certain temperature in Kelvin. Lower temperatures in Kelvin lead to warmer colors of light (red, orange). Higher Kelvin temperatures lead to cooler lights (blue, violet).

4. Blue light nighttime effects[15]
   a. Increases nighttime heart rate, blood pressure, and core body temperature
   b. Decreases sleepiness
   c. Suppresses melatonin
5. Leads to delayed phase (like eastward travel)
6. Back-lit computers, TV screens, phones, and other screens (which have strong blue spectra components) have powerful melatonin suppressive effects even though the intensity may be low.

e) Timing of light exposure

1. Light during the day
   a. Suppresses melatonin
   b. Supports alertness
2. Blue light at night
   a. Increases cortisol, blood pressure, heart rate, sympathetic tone, alertness, and core body temperature
   b. Suppresses melatonin
   c. Inhibits sleep onset and shifts the sleep cycle later
      (1) Can occur even with typical nighttime household lighting of intensities 50–100 lux
3. Low daylight
   a. Decreases daytime activity, alertness, positive affect, and core body temperature amplitude/max
   b. Increases melatonin suppression with evening light
4. Low daytime light significantly increases the sensitivity of melatonin suppression from light at night.
   a. Daytime exposure to 10K lux of light for 6.5 hours cannot fully eliminate nighttime melatonin suppression from exposure to 90 lux of light.
   b. If low-light exposure has occurred 2–3 days prior, the SCN is more sensitive to light at night, resulting in higher melatonin suppression, possible delayed onset of sleep, and shifting of the sleep cycle.

f) Endogenous SCN clock

1. Ideal SCN clock: 24-hour circadian rhythm with consistent sleep and wake times
   a. Before electricity, solar cycle of day/night provided natural SCN resetting. Now, resetting SCN is more difficult due to inappropriately timed light signals.
2. Phase shifts[16]
   a. Delayed phase shift (delays in the circadian rhythm): SCN clock is longer than 24 hours
      (1) A delay of sleep onset by of 1–3 hours can occur with evening light exposure. This is because light exposure delays melatonin secretion and reduces total melatonin levels. As a result, individuals will get more and more behind in their objective time clocks.
      (2) Can occur with eastward travel
      (3) Can occur with home lighting of 100–1,000K, and home lighting can lead to almost 100% melatonin suppression.
      (4) People who prefer staying up late ("night owls") are more susceptible to melatonin suppression and delay due to evening light.
   b. Advanced phase shift (premature or early resetting of circadian rhythm) SCN clock is shorter than 24 hours.
      (1) Can occur with exposure to light earlier in day; individual will get more and more ahead of objective time (like traveling eastward).
      (2) People who prefer mornings (morning people or "larks") are more susceptible to desynchrony due to morning light, which shifts them to waking earlier.
3. Few people have a SCN clock equal to 24 hours.
   a. Most have 24.2 hours (delayed phase shift)
   b. In general, SCN needs to be reset forward (advanced) or reset backward (delayed) by 5–15 minutes a day.
4. Daily entrainment requirements[7]
   a. Daily adjustments required to maintain entrainment
      (1) If shorter than 24 hours, advancement of ~10 minutes or less is needed
         (a) Example, delaying exposure in light in morning by 10 minutes or ideal wake up time
      (2) If longer than 24 hours, backward setting of ~20 minutes or less is needed
         (a) Example, limiting light 20 minutes earlier in evening so ideal bedtime can be achieved
5. Effects of sleep delay and disruption
   a. Decreased daytime activity/attention, positive affect, sociability, REM sleep, and melatonin
   b. Metabolic effects
      (1) Decreased caloric burn, leptin (appetite control hormone), and core body temperature amplitude/max
      (2) Increased appetite and insulin resistance

g) Food: carbohydrates

1. Skipped, late, or low-carbohydrate breakfast leads to diminished cortisol awakening rise.
2. Eating breakfast shortly after wakening may help shift wake-up time earlier.
3. Eating a high-carbohydrate breakfast may improve sleep-wakefulness transition.

4. Eating dinner too early may contribute to falling asleep too early.
5. Shifting carbohydrates
    (1) If someone is falling asleep too early, they can eat more carbohydrates at dinner.
    (2) If someone is falling asleep too late, they can shift carbohydrates to earlier meals, avoid snacking and carbohydrate-rich dinners, and eat an earlier dinner.

h) Exercise[17,18]

1. Morning and afternoon exercise have been found to have phase-advancing effects.
2. Evening exercise has been shown to have phase-delaying effects.
3. Many hypotheses for exercise having a phase-shifting effect
    a. Relative ATP depletion-leading to higher adenosine levels
    b. Thermoregulation allows for cooling core body temperature in the evening to promote sleep.

i) Fluid status[19]

1. Body temperature is controlled by three main elements: 1) the heat-producing body core, which is generally homeostatic, 2) the heat-losing peripheral body, which varies widely in temperature in response to blood flow, and 3) the ambient temperature of the surrounding environment.
    a. Normally, during the afternoon, core body temperature will rise and peripheral extremities will cool. During the night, the opposite will occur as heat shifts from the core to the peripheral extremities and heart rate and cardiac output are reduced.
2. Higher blood osmolality
    a. In late afternoon, higher blood osmolality leads to higher afternoon peak core body temperature because of an increase in internal temperature threshold, increased blood flow the vital organs, and less output to the peripheral body.[20]
3. Decreased fluid volume
    a. Can reduce amount cutaneous blood flow needed for core cooling at night
    b. Increases cardiac activation, sympathetic tone which shunts blood to core
4. Sleep deficiency
    a. Increases total amount of cortisol secreted during the night.
        (1) Decreases cortisol mineralocorticoid action (salt and fluid regulation), which may exacerbate low fluid effects

j) Ambient temperature

1. Strong determinant of peripheral body temperature
2. If peripheral body is not warm enough during transition to sleep, sleep onset may be inhibited.

k) Impact of timing of sleep on physiology and pathology

1. In addition to quantity of sleep, the timing of sleep also has a discernible influence on health and risk for disorder and disease.

Note: Benzodiazepines, yoga, non-sleep meditation, and autogenic training all produce a similar effect in the body's natural shift of heat to the extremities. With these antecedents, blood is shunted from the core to the extremities as sympathetic activation in the muscles and skin, heart rate, and energy expenditure are all reduced.

OBJECTIVE 2

Explain the role of light exposure and endogenous melatonin in sleep health

1) **Melatonin and sleep health**

   a) Populations that are more sensitive to melatonin suppression include:[21]

      1. Those with behavioral health disorders (see Table 7.1)

         a. Bipolar and seasonal affective disorders

Table 7.1 Decrease in Melatonin Secretion	
Controls	~15%
Major Depressive Disorder	~20%
Seasonal Affective Disorder	~40%
Bipolar Disorder	~45%

      2. Elderly adults

         a. Partially due to cataracts/corneal opacity

         b. Natural trend toward lower production of melatonin with each decade of life

      3. Those with corneal opacity, often due to cataracts

         a. Limits retinal light exposure

            (1) A 45-year-old has 50% lower retinal illuminance than a 10-year-old.

            (2) A 65-year-old has 50% lower retinal illuminance than a 45-year-old.

         b. Retinal illuminance is also reduced as one ages.

            (1) Short light wavelengths are most affected (e.g., blue light), while longer wavelengths are least affected (e.g., red light).

      4. Melatonin suppression correlates with affective disorders.[22]

OBJECTIVE 3

Review sleep's role in health and chronic disease

1) **Sleep disorders**

   a) Behaviorally induced insufficient sleep syndrome (BIISS)[23,24,25]

      1. Inadequate sleep for functional performance

      2. Voluntary restriction of sleep time

      3. Longer sleep duration on weekends

      4. Disparity between sleep needed and obtained

      5. Prevalence: 7.3–20% of general population

      6. Associated with:

         a. Younger age, 30–39 years old

         b. Alcohol abuse

         c. Longer work hours (>40 per week)

         d. Stress

e. Depression

b) Chronic insomnia[24,26]

1. Most common sleep disorder and complaint
2. Difficulty initiating and/or maintaining sleep
3. Daytime consequences
4. Adequate sleep opportunity
5. Ongoing for at least 3 months and occurring at least three times a week
6. Associated with:
   a. Fatigue, malaise, and sleepiness
   b. Concentration/memory impairment
   c. Decreased motivation
   d. Mood disturbances/irritability
   e. Errors or accidents at work/driving
   f. Physical symptoms: headaches, gastrointestinal distress
   g. Persistent worry about sleep
7. Important to appreciate mental as well as physical etiologies towards optimal therapy

c) Obstructive sleep apnea[27,28,29]

1. Recurrent apnea or hypopnea during sleep, lasting 10 seconds or longer, usually quantified as Apnea-Hypopnea Index (AHI) based on polysomnography (in-lab sleep study) or home sleep study
2. AHI Classes
   a. Mild: 5–15, Moderate: 15–30, Severe: 30+
   b. Greatest data on treatment benefits of severe cases
   c. Many treatment modalities; needs to be individualized
3. Prevalence: up to 26% of the general population
   a. 80% undiagnosed
4. Classically associated with one or more of the following:
   a. Overweight or obese
   b. Metabolic syndrome
   c. Hypertension
   d. Atrial fibrillation
   e. Increased neck circumference
   f. Loud snoring

d) Restless Leg Syndrome (RLS)[30]

1. Sensorimotor disorder characterized by feeling an urge to move the limbs or torso, which can occur with an uncomfortable sensation that happens when one rests (sitting or lying down). This most commonly presents in the lower extremities but can also be noted in the upper extremities or torso.
2. These can present as paresthesia or pain.
3. Condition is worse in the evenings than during that day.
4. Movement helps to temporarily relieve the uncomfortable sensation and the urge to move.
5. Symptoms are not due to another primary medical cause.
6. Present in 5–15% of the US population.

7. Associated with:
    a. Periodic movements of sleep (occurs in 85% of patients with restless leg syndrome)
    b. Phase delay of sleep
    c. Disruptions of sleep
    d. Fatigue
    e. Periodic involuntary and jerky movements of limbs while awake or at rest
    f. Both genetic and acquired cases noted
    g. Iron abnormalities
        (1) Low ferritin <75 ng/ml
        (2) Elevated ferritin
    h. Magnesium, yet does not correlate with serum levels
    i. Vitamin D (less robust correlation)

e) Other sleep disorders

1. Short sleep misperception
    a. Mismatch between sleep duration (polysomnography) and interpretation (patient perceives less sleep than actual sleep duration)
2. Secondary insomnia
    a. Possibly due to medications; vascular dysfunction (peripheral hypoperfusion, vasospasm); visual impairment (opacification, retinal degeneration); or renin-angiotensin dysfunction (fluid balance)
3. Narcolepsy
    a. Sudden, uncontrollable onset of sleep
        (1) May occur with or without cataplexy
        (2) Diagnosis of exclusion with corresponding history
        (3) It's appropriate to refer these individuals for a sleep study and a sleep medicine specialist.
4. Periodic limb movements
    a. Limb movements occurring at about a 30-second interval during sleep
    b. Patients are typically unaware of the movements and the resulting brief arousals and do not report abnormal sensations in the extremities.
    c. Increasing frequency with age, especially after 50 years old.
    d. Often associated with restless legs syndrome
    e. Patients may report restless sleep or middle-of-night awakening with increased daytime sleepiness
    f. Diagnosis based on history and polysomnography.

2) Sleep and metabolic disorders[31,32,33,34,35]

a) Healthy sleep duration and quality

1. Lower cortisol and glucose levels
2. Greater insulin sensitivity
3. Higher daytime leptin, reduced food-seeking behaviors

b) Impaired sleep quality and short duration:

1. Higher nighttime cortisol and glucose levels
2. Reduced insulin sensitivity

3. Higher glucose levels
4. Lower daytime leptin levels and higher intake of carbohydrate-dense foods
    a. Men and women who slept 4 hours for 5 nights in a row sought out approximately 300 calories more (and especially calories from saturated fat) during the day.
5. Reduced testosterone levels
6. Reduce growth hormone levels
7. Increased advanced glycation end product (AGE) deposition in to vascular system
8. Dyslipidemia
9. Endothelial dysfunction

c) Short duration and disrupted sleep correlate with:

1. Elevated body mass index (BMI)
2. Obesity (2-fold increased risk)
3. Metabolic syndrome
4. Type 2 diabetes
5. Cardiovascular risk and mortality

3) Sleep and cardiovascular disorders[2,32,36]

a) Healthy sleep duration and quality leads to:

1. Lower sympathetic tone and blood pressure
2. Greater nighttime peripheral perfusion and core body temperature cooling
3. Increased stamina and faster cardiovascular recovery time

b) Impaired sleep quality and/or short duration leads to:

1. Elevated sympathetic tone
2. Endothelial injury
3. Dyslipidemia
4. Elevated blood pressure, especially at night
5. Reduced nighttime peripheral perfusion
6. Increase nighttime core body temperature
7. Refractory and no-reduction of blood pressure in early morning hours
8. Increased heart attacks
9. Increased risk of cardiovascular disease deaths
10. Vasospastic disorders

4) Sleep, mood, and cognition[3,37,38,39,40,41]

a) Healthy sleep duration and quality sleep lead to:

1. Higher proportion of sleep time spent in slow-wave sleep (stage 3, which is the deepest, most restorative stage of non-REM sleep)
2. Higher proportion in REM
    a. Enhanced learning and memory
    b. Faster cognitive processing
    c. Greater anxiety and fear extinguishment

b) Impaired sleep quality and short sleep lead to:

1. Less slow wave and REM sleep

2. Reduced brain-derived neurotrophic factor (BDNF), which is a key substance that triggers repair and regeneration of nerve tissue
3. Impaired learning and memory
4. Emotional distress, impaired moral judgement, and misinterpretation of social cues
5. Decreased alertness and cognitive processing speed
6. Diminished fear extinguishing, as the amygdala is not able to get rid of the memory of fearful events

c) Short sleep duration correlates with:[3,37,38,39,42]

1. Major depression
2. Bipolar disorder
3. Seasonal affective disorder (SAD)
4. Premenstrual syndrome
5. Post-traumatic stress disorder (PTSD) is worsened if sleep deprivation occurs 2 weeks prior to traumatic event.
6. Traumatic brain injury (TBI) is worse if sleep deprivation occurs before and/or follows injury.

5) Sleep health and cancer[43]

a) Healthy sleep duration and quality help with:

1. DNA repair and histone remodeling
2. Apoptosis and anti-cancer cytokines (IL-1, IL-2), TNF-alpha

b) Impaired sleep quality and short duration lead to:

1. Melatonin and immune system suppression
2. Increased cancer-stimulating cytokines (IL-10)
3. Dysfunction in gene transcription and cell cycle
4. Aberrant DNA methylation, meaning DNA expression is not being coded correctly

c) Sleep disruption and short sleep duration correlates with:

1. Breast cancer
2. Endometrial cancer
3. Prostate cancer
4. Colorectal cancer
5. Acute myeloid leukemia

OBJECTIVE 4

Identify the lifestyle-based activity and the dietary, environmental, and coping behaviors that can improve sleep health

1) Lifestyle prescription for sleep[44]

a) Actions and sleep environment

1. Use bed for sleep and sex only
2. Establish regular sleep cycle for bedtime and wake time
3. Increase bedtime peripheral cutaneous vasodilation through:

        a. Bath/shower
        b. Socks or heating pad for cold feet
        c. Non-caffeinated tea/beverages
    4. Allow air temperature to gradually warm extremities using:
        a. Bedding, socks, heating pad, and/or blankets
    5. Minimize/eliminate bedroom noise and lights
        a. Digital displays, charger lights
        b. Alarm clock out of sight
    6. Power naps may be helpful if they're less than 30 minutes

b) Light exposure
    1. Increase daytime exposure to sunlight
        a. Ideally outdoors, open sky
    2. Increase daytime physical activity
    3. Decrease light at night
        a. Turn off or dim unnecessary lights at least 1 hour before bedtime, especially blue light, compact fluorescent, halogen light, and backlit screens.
        b. Use 2,500K color warm spectrum lights.

c) Dietary
    1. Eliminate nighttime caffeinated beverages.
    2. Limit daytime caffeinated beverages.
    3. Avoid alcohol within 3 hours of bed.
    4. Eliminate after-dinner and late-night snacking.
    5. Avoid high-sodium foods, especially at dinner because it affects vascular tone and vasodilation.
    6. Assure adequate daytime fluid intake, especially late afternoon, because it affects vascular tone and vasodilation.
    7. Pursue weight reduction if BMI is elevated.

d) Exercise
    1. Increase daytime physical activity.
        a. Get up and move at least once an hour.
        b. Increase physical activity in the morning or in the late afternoon/early evening.
    2. Daily exercise is helpful to promote circadian regulation and improved quality of sleep.
    3. It is important to personalize prescription of frequency, intensity, type, time, volume, and progression.
    4. With overexertion, pain can disrupt sleep.

e) Minimizing stress
    1. Start settling down 1 hour before bed, including active relaxation.
        a. Bath/shower, meditation, guided imagery, music with 60 bpm
    2. Develop a wind-down routine for the segue from daytime concerns to restfulness.
        a. Stop working or doing stimulating activities 90 minutes before bed.
    3. Mitigate nighttime worrying, planning, and ruminating.
        a. Try mindfulness-based stress reduction (MBSR) and meditation.

4. Practice cognitive behavioral therapy (CBT) techniques for insomnia.

f) Intensive therapies

1. CBT for insomnia (CBT-I)
    a. Recommended as first-line treatment of chronic insomnia over medications[44]
        (1) More likely to produce sustained benefit
        (2) Less risk of tolerance or side effects
        (3) Cognitive therapies combined with behavioral therapies have been shown to facilitate getting off sleep medications and sustaining sleep over time. There is also limited evidence that they reduce daytime fatigue.[45,46]
    b. Behavioral methods[45,47]
        (1) Sleep restriction
            (a) Shown to be effective in moderate to high quality randomized control trials[45,48]
            (b) Meets evidence-based psychological treatment (EBT) criteria for adults >60 years old[49]
        (2) Stimulus control
            (a) Shown to be effective in moderate- to high-quality randomized control trials[49]
            (b) Partially meets evidence-based psychological treatment criteria for adults >60 years old[49]
        3) Relaxation training therapy
            (a) Shown to be effective in moderate- to high-quality randomized control trials[50]
            (b) Did not meet evidence-based psychological treatment criteria for adults >60 years old
        4) Sleep hygiene
            (a) Did not meet evidence-based psychological treatment criteria for adults >60 years old
    c. Cognitive methods
        (1) Cognitive restructuring[47]
            (a) Addressing anxiety-producing or erroneous beliefs about sleep or lack of sleep
2. Supplemental melatonin
    a. Significant inter-individual variation in endogenous melatonin
    b. Efficacious for jetlag mitigation and circadian rhythm disorders
    c. Mixed evidence for insomnia
    d. No evidence for adverse effects at typical doses (1–6 mg), but possible interaction with some cytochrome P-450 drugs
    e. Supplementation does not appear to suppress endogenous melatonin, but there are no long-term studies
    f. Sublingual preparation may have better bioavailability
    g. Sustained preparation may be more helpful for westward jetlag, but may cause morning drowsiness
    h. Supplements with vitamin B6 may cause an acute altering effect in some individuals
3. Hypnotic or sedative medication use and mortality[49]
    a. Medications that are used to induce and/or maintain sleep can be prescription-strength (benzodiazepines) or over-the-counter (Benadryl, doxylamine).
    b. Prescription-strength hypnotic medications are associated with:

(1) A significant increase in death rates in adults aged 18–55[51]

(2) An increased risk of all-cause mortality in all age groups that used hypnotics from overdose, car accidents, falls, depression, cancer, and suicide[52]

OBJECTIVE 5

Identify at least two lifestyle adjustments related to light exposure and meal composition and timing that support improved sleep

1) Sleep disruptions

a) Delayed sleep onset or difficulty with sleep initiation

1. Environment: use bed only for sleep and sex, minimize noise and lights, allow natural cooling of temperature through night, and warm extremities at ideal bedtime (clothing, bathing, or warm beverage).
2. Light exposure: increase early morning sunlight, increase afternoon physical activity (outdoors preferred), and decrease light at night.
3. Diet: reduce/eliminate nighttime caffeine, alcohol, and high sodium foods; eat a carbohydrate-rich breakfast and a low carbohydrate dinner.
4. Exercise: seek to exercise in the morning or afternoon, if possible.
5. Stress: start winding down at least 1 hour before bed and include active relaxation.
    a. Bath/shower, meditation, guided imagery

b) Sleep fragmentation and difficulty maintaining sleep

1. Environment: darken bedroom, allow bedroom to cool gradually through night, and keep a glass of cool water at bedside.
2. Light: increase morning and mid-afternoon sunlight exposure, increase physical activity (preferably outdoors), use red-toned nightlights if light is necessary, and avoid turning on the lights if one wakes up.
3. Diet: increase late-afternoon hydration, and avoid evening diuretic beverages (soda, caffeine, and alcohol).
4. Exercise: seek an exercise program without creating a burden of pain.
5. Stress: mitigate nighttime worrying, planning, and ruminating.

c) Sleep deficiency from waking up too early

1. Environment: assure sufficient bedcovers to be warm in early morning.
2. Light
    a. Avoid bright lights until ideal wake-up time.
    b. Increase late-afternoon and evening sunlight to increase melatonin production (usually morning people, or "larks," naturally gravitate to more early morning light).
    c. Increase evening physical activity.
    d. Use blue spectrum 6,500K lights until 1 hour before bedtime.
3. Diet: Avoid eating or drinking caffeine until 30–60 minutes after ideal wakeup time, and shift carbohydrates from breakfast to dinner.

d) Jet lag traveling east

1. Environment

a. Get exposure to bright light, preferably outdoors, close to new ideal wake-up time.
b. Get only dim-light exposure starting 1 hour before new ideal sleep time.

2. Diet: Eat a hearty breakfast within 30–45 minutes of new ideal wake-up time.
3. Take melatonin 1 mg sublingual 1 hour before new ideal sleep time.

e) Jet lag traveling west

1. Environment
   a. Get late-afternoon and early evening bright light, preferably outdoors.
   b. Avoid dim-light exposure until 1 hour before new ideal sleep time.
2. Diet
   a. Eat a hearty breakfast within 30–45 minutes after new ideal wake-up time.
   b. Eat a complex carbohydrate–rich dinner 2–3 hours before new ideal sleep time.
3. Take melatonin 1 mg sublingual 1 hour before new ideal sleep time.

OBJECTIVE 6

Identify key factors that differentiate patient subpopulations with insufficient or poor-quality sleep

1) Sleep assessments[44,53,54]

a) Mini sleep assessment

1. Typical weekday hours of sleep
2. Typical weekend hours of sleep
3. Perceived sleep quality
4. Red flags
   a. Less than 7 hours duration
   b. 1 or more hours weekday-weekend difference
   c. Irregular sleep timing, or duration (especially shiftwork)
   d. Poor sleep quality despite 7 or more hours in bed
   e. More than 9 hours
5. Frequency of daytime fatigue (fatigue inhibiting daily activities), sleepiness, and/ or difficulty waking up
6. Frequency and type of sleep disturbance
   a. Fall asleep more than 8 hours before ideal wakeup time
   b. Sleep onset more than 15–20 minutes after lights out
   c. Prolonged wakefulness after initial sleep onset
   d. Awaking less than 7–9 hours after bedtime
7. Attitude toward sleep, misunderstanding about healthy sleep, and sleep barriers. Extremes include:
   a. Cavalier about sleep need: "I don't have time for sleep."
   b. Highly distressed by any sleep disturbance
   c. Belief about sleep not needed or I can sleep anywhere

2) **STOP-BANG: Brief obstructive sleep apnea (OSA) assessment 30 screens for OSA, not for central sleep apnea[29]**

   a) Snoring (loud)
   b) Tired often, fatigued, and sleepiness during daytime that inhibits functioning
   c) Observed patient apnea episodes
   d) Pressure: elevated blood pressure or taking hypertension medications
   e) BMI >35
   f) Age greater than 50
   g) Neck Size ≥17 inches (43 cm) in a male, ≥16 inches (41 cm) in a female
   h) Gender: male
   i) Scoring
      1. 0–2 Yes = low risk for OSA
      2. 3–4 Yes = intermediate risk for OSA
      3. 5–8 Yes = high risk for OSA: refer for sleep study
         a. Additional scoring criteria for high risk of OSA
            (1) Yes to 2 or more of 4 STOP questions + male gender
            (2) Yes to 2 or more of 4 STOP questions + BMI >35 kg/m^2
            (3) Yes to 2 or more of 4 STOP questions + neck circumference

3) **Sleep hygiene assessment[31,44]**

   a) Daytime naps of more than 30 minutes
   b) Poor daytime hydration
   c) Variations in sleep onset/offset
   d) Prolonged non-sleep periods in bed
   e) Stimulating activities pre-bedtime
   f) Going to bed stressed, angry, or upset
   g) Reading, watching TV, or eating in bed
   h) Uncomfortable bed and/or bedroom
   i) Think, plan, or worry in bed
   j) Caffeine or alcohol within 3 hours of bedtime

4) **Epworth Sleepiness Scale (ESS)[55] to assist healthcare providers in their recognition of daytime sleepiness**

   a) Scoring the ESS[56]
      1. Patients with scores of 8 or above would benefit from a thorough review of their sleep pattern and possible sleep disorders.
      2. In contrast to just feeling tired, how likely are you to doze off or fall asleep in the following situations? (Even if you have not done some of these things recently, try to work out how they would have affected you.) Use the following scale to choose the most appropriate number for each situation:
         a. 0 – Would never doze
         b. 1 – Slight chance of dozing

c. 2 – Moderate chance of dozing
d. 3 – High chance of dozing

3. Score the following situations
    a. Sitting and reading
    b. Watching TV
    c. Sitting inactive in a public place (i.e., theater)
    d. As a car passenger for an hour without a break
    e. Lying down to rest in the afternoon
    f. Sitting and talking to someone
    g. Sitting quietly after lunch without alcohol
    h. In a car, while stopping for a few minutes in traffic

5) Pittsburgh Sleep Quality Index (PSQI)[57]

a) A self-rated questionnaire that assesses sleep quality and disturbances over a 1-month time interval.

b) 19 individual items generate seven "component" scores
1. Subjective sleep quality
2. Sleep latency
3. Sleep duration
4. Habitual sleep efficiency
5. Sleep disturbances
6. Use of sleeping medication
7. Daytime dysfunction

c) Sum of scores for these seven components yields one global score.

d) The client self-rates each of these seven areas of sleep.

e) Scoring of the answers is based on a 0–3 scale, whereby 3 reflects the negative extreme on the Likert Scale.

f) A global sum of 5 or greater indicates a "poor" sleeper.

SECTION 8 GLOSSARY

Blood osmolality: a measurement of the particles (such as sodium, potassium, and chloride) dissolved in the plasma.

Blue light: a specific range within the spectrum of light. Blue light creates greater melatonin suppression at lower intensities and shorter durations and has disruptive nighttime effects.

Central oscillators: these are found in the suprachiasmic nucleus (SCN), which is the main internal "clock."

Circadian rhythm: a biological process that regulates physiologic functions and behaviors over a 24-hour period that aligns with the light-dark cycles. It's also known as the "internal clock." The circadian rhythm is regulated by endogenous oscillators.

Endogenous or internal circadian oscillators: the molecules, cells, and tissues that make up the body's "internal clock." They produce oscillating (alternating) currents through self-regulating positive and negative feedback loops that produce the circadian rhythm. Endogenous oscillators include both the central and peripheral oscillators.

Entrainment: the ability to be brought into a rhythm.

Inputs: the external and environmental factors that can entrain the circadian rhythm. Modifiers: things that change the amount of "input" that gets to the body's operators. Operators: the body's reaction or response to the modified inputs.

Melatonin: a natural hormone that is made in the pineal gland and helps regulate sleep and wake cycles.

Outputs: the behavioral and physiological consequences of the operators. Ambient temperature: temperature of the surrounding environment.

Peripheral oscillators: these are present in many major organs in the body (kidneys, liver, heart, adrenal glands, and pancreas). They allow for synchrony and alignment between the central and peripheral clocks.

Retinal Ganglion Cells (RGC): are non-visual light-sensitive retinal neurons that relay light intensity/ spectra to the suprachiasmic nuclieus.

Suprachiasmic nucleus (SCN): the main body "clock" or central "clock." This is a portion of the hypothalamus that regulates melatonin secretion and creates the circadian rhythm in the body.

SECTION 8 REVIEW QUESTIONS

1. **In order to readjust the circadian rhythm after traveling several time zones to the east, the process of entrainment is best accomplished by:**
   - **A.** Sleeping an extra hour a day for the next few days
   - **B.** Eating a large, carbohydrate-based meal immediately before the new ideal sleep time
   - **C.** Exposing oneself to blue light prior to the new ideal sleep time
   - **D.** Taking melatonin (1 mg sublingual) 1 hour before the new ideal sleep time

2. **Unhealthy sleep is best characterized as:**
   - **A.** A rise in melatonin during the first 4 hours of sleep.
   - **B.** A cortisol spike during the first 4 hours of sleep.
   - **C.** Slow waves on the EEG during the first 4 hours of sleep.
   - **D.** Decreased blood pressure during the first 4 hours of sleep.

3. **A patient with a sleep disorder who snores loudly, is obese, has hypertension, and is not responding well to first-line medication most likely has a diagnosis of:**
   - **A.** Behaviorally induced insufficient sleep syndrome (BIISS)
   - **B.** Chronic insomnia
   - **C.** Obstructive sleep apnea
   - **D.** Secondary insomnia

4. **Which of the following actions would most likely disrupt sleep?**
   - **A.** Drinking three cups of coffee every morning
   - **B.** Drinking a glass of red wine with dinner each evening
   - **C.** Consuming a low-carbohydrate dinner each evening
   - **D.** Watching television in bed while falling asleep each night

5. **An overweight medical student presents with anxiety, depression and difficulty sleeping. He consumes caffeine and snacks to stay alert so that he can study late at night. He tries to catch up on sleep during the weekend. This patient most likely has a diagnosis of:**
   - **A.** Behaviorally induced insufficient sleep syndrome (BIISS)
   - **B.** Chronic insomnia
   - **C.** Obstructive sleep apnea
   - **D.** Secondary insomnia

6. **A 50-year-old office worker comes to you complaining of fatigue. She has trouble getting up in the morning, so she drinks two cups of coffee to start her day. Then she has difficulty staying alert in the afternoon, so she has another cup of coffee. She gets home late, so she has a late dinner with a glass of wine to relax. She then has trouble getting to sleep, so she stays up watching TV and falls asleep in her chair. She comes to you for advice. You would be correct to recommend which of the following?**
   - **A.** Eliminate daytime caffeine and eliminate evening alcohol within 3 hours of bedtime.
   - **B.** Shift meals that have a higher concentration of carbohydrates to later in the day.
   - **C.** Eat higher sodium foods in the evening to help promote vasodilation.
   - **D.** Continue to have a glass of wine within 2 hours of bedtime in order to relax.

7. **A 60-year-old woman complains to you that she is waking up two hours early most days and can't get back to sleep. She also feels tired later in the day. You suggest:**
   - **A.** Shifting breakfast and any caffeine to 15 minutes after her ideal wakeup time
   - **B.** Avoiding any bright lights until 30 minutes before her ideal wakeup time
   - **C.** Going outside for a walk in the sunshine in the late afternoon
   - **D.** Understanding that she is getting older, and this is a common problem with age

8. **A 30-year-old male comes in complaining of decreased concentration at work and wonders if a stimulant would help. He stays up late or gets up early to get work done and gets about 6 hours of sleep during the week. On the weekend he gets 10 hours of sleep to try and catch up. He doesn't feel rested during the week or on the weekend. You advise him that his sleep patterns may be more the issue. "Red flags" on the Mini Sleep Assessment you take include:**
   - **A.** Getting less than 6 hours of sleep at a time
   - **B.** One or more hours sleep duration differentiation between the weekday and weekend
   - **C.** Regular sleep timing
   - **D.** More than 8 hours of sleep at a time

9. **Describe the correct circadian physiology during the sleep cycle.**
   - **A.** The steps of sleep initiation include: 1) darkness triggering the pineal gland to secrete melatonin, 2) cutaneous vasodilation, 3) extremity warming, and 4) cooling of core body temperature.
   - **B.** With a continued rise in melatonin, there is a decrease in peripheral skin temperature and continued cooling of core body temperature. The nadir of core body temperature occurs about 4 hours after sleep onset.
   - **C.** Between mid-sleep and awakening, melatonin starts to increase as peripheral skin temperature increases. This is followed by decreased core body temperature.
   - **D.** In the awakening phase, melatonin and cortisol levels decrease, initiating the transition from sleep to wakefulness.

10. **Which is a correct statement about blue light spectra?**
    - **A.** Melatonin suppression is less with higher light intensities and increased duration of light exposure.
    - **B.** Decreases nighttime heart rate, blood pressure, and core body temperature
    - **C.** Increases sleepiness
    - **D.** Leads to delayed phase sleep similar to westward travel

11. **Which of the following statements about sleep duration and quality is true?**
    - **A.** Healthy sleep duration and quality are associated with a lower proportion of slow wave sleep and higher proportion of REM sleep.
    - **B.** Healthy sleep duration and quality is associated with higher daytime leptin and reduced food-seeking behaviors.
    - **C.** Impaired sleep quality leads to increased fear extinguishing and preserved memory of fearful events.
    - **D.** PTSD is worse if a person is sleep deprived for the 2 days after the event.

SECTION 8 REVIEW QUESTION ANSWERS AND SUMMARIES

1. **Answer: D.** Melatonin may help with entrainment. The other responses would all contribute to a delay of sleep onset at the new ideal time.

2. **Answer: B.** With healthy sleep, cortisol spikes upon awakening, not during the first 4 hours of sleep. The remaining answers characterize normal sleep during the initial hours of sleep.

3. **Answer: C.** The patient profile best fits obstructive sleep apnea (OSA).

4. **Answer: D.** Watching television exposes people to blue light, which contributes to a delayed sleep onset.

5. **Answer: A.** The patient profile best fits BIISS: A chronic, voluntary sleep restriction that commonly causes excessive daytime sleepiness and daytime fatigue.

6. **Answer: A.** Eliminate daytime caffeine and eliminate alcohol within 3 hours of bedtime. Avoid high sodium foods as they restrict vasodilation. Dim lights 30–60 minutes prior to bedtime.

7. **Answer: C.** Shift breakfast and any caffeine until 45 minutes after her ideal wakeup time. Avoid any bright lights until her ideal wakeup time. Light in the late afternoon increases melatonin production and will help her sleep cycle. While D is true, patient may be able to change her lifestyle to help improve her sleep.

8. **Answer: B.** A Mini Sleep Assessment includes asking about typical weekday hours of sleep, typical weekend hours of sleep, and perceived sleep quality. In addition to the above, other "red flags" include poor sleep quality despite 7 or more hours in bed and getting more than 9 hours of sleep.

9. **Answer: A.** Melatonin and peripheral skin temperature are directly related. B is incorrect because as melatonin increases, so does the peripheral skin temperature. In mid-sleep and awakening, melatonin starts to decrease and peripheral skin temperature decreases. This is followed by increased core body temperature. In the awakening phase, melatonin decreases and cortisol levels increase, initiating the transition from sleep to wakeful.

10. **Answer: D.** Blue light creates greater melatonin suppression at higher intensities and higher durations. It increases nighttime heart rate, blood pressure, and core body temperature. Blue light decreases sleepiness. It also leads to delayed phase sleep that is similar to westward travel (e.g., it postpones sleep onset by making the body think it's earlier than it is).

11. **Answer: B.** Healthy sleep duration and quality is associated with higher daytime leptin and reduced food-seeking behaviors. Healthy sleep duration and quality are associated with a higher proportion of slow wave sleep and REM sleep. Impaired sleep quality leads to decreased fear extinguishing and memory preservation of fearful events. PTSD is worse if a person is sleep deprived for the 2 weeks prior to the event.

SECTION 8 REFERENCES

1. National Sleep Foundation . Sleepiness and low levels of action. 2020. https://www.sleepfoundation.org/professionals/sleep-america-polls/2020-sleepiness-and-low-action
2. Banks S., Dinges D. F. Behavioral and physiological consequences of sleep restriction. *J Clin Sleep Med.* 2007;3(5):519-528.
3. Egger G., Binns A., Rossner S. *Lifestyle Medicine: Managing Diseases of Lifestyle in the 21st Century.* New York, NY: McGraw-Hill; 2010.
4. Hirshkowitz M., Whiton K., Albert S. M., et al. National Sleep Foundation's sleep time duration recommendations: methodology and results summary. *Sleep Health.* 2015;1(1):40-43.
5. Bell-Pedersen D., Cassone V. M., Earnest D. J., et al. Circadian rhythms from multiple oscillators: lessons from diverse organisms. *Nat Rev Genet.* 2005;6(7):544-556.
6. Scully C. G., Karaboué A., Liu W. M., et al. Skin surface temperature rhythms as potential circadian biomarkers for personalized chronotherapeutics in cancer patients. *Interface Focus.* 2011;1(1):48-60. https://doi.org/10.1098/rsfs.2019.0098
7. Stratmann M., Schibler U. Properties, entrainment, and physiological functions of mammalian peripheral oscillators. *J Biol Rhythms.* 2006;21(6):494-506.
8. Weaver D. R. Introduction to circadian rhythms and mechanisms of circadian oscillations. In: Gumz M. L., ed., *Circadian Clocks: Role in Health and Disease; Physiology in Health and Disease.* New York, NY: Springer; 2016.
9. Tuazon S. A., Cardona R., Tuazon J. A. Serum osmolality. November 20, 2019. https://emedicine.medscape.com/article/2099042-overview. Accessed July 18, 2019.
10. Mesarwi O., Polak J., Jun J., Polotsky V. Y. Sleep disorders and the development of insulin resistance and obesity. *Endocrinol Metab Clin North Am.* 2013;42(3):617-634.
11. Anderson K. N., Bradley A. J. Sleep disturbance in mental health problems and neurodegenerative disease. *Nat Sci Sleep.* 2013;5:61-75.
12. DSI, a Division of Harvard Bioscience. Baroreceptor sensitivity (BRS). https://www.datasci.com/solutions/cardiovascular/baroreceptor-sensitivity-(brs). Accessed March 21, 2018.
13. Lack L. C., Gradisar M., Van Someren E. J., Wright H. R., Lushington K. The relationship between insomnia and body temperatures. *Sleep Med Rev.* 2008;12(4):307-317.
14. NLPIP. Introduction: light sources and color. 2004. https://www.lrc.rpi.edu/programs/nlpip/lightinganswers/lightsources/abstract.asp. Accessed March 21, 2018.
15. Cajochen C., Münch M., Kobialka S., et al. High sensitivity of human melatonin, alertness, thermoregulation, and heart rate to short wavelength light. *J Clin Endocrinol Metab.* 2005;90(3):1311-1316.
16. Zeitzer J. M., Dijk D. J., Kronauer R., Brown E., Czeisler C. Sensitivity of the human circadian pacemaker to nocturnal light: melatonin phase resetting and suppression. *J Physiol.* 2000;526 Pt 3(Pt 3):695-702.
17. Youngstedt S. D., Kline C. E., Elliott J. A., Zielinski M. R., Devlin T. M., Moore T. A. Circadian phase-shifting effects of bright light, exercise, and bright light + exercise. *J Circadian Rhythms.* 2016;14:2.
18. Wang C. Y. Circadian rhythm, exercise, and heart. *Acta Cardiol Sin.* 2017;33(5):539-541.
19. Krauchi K., Deboer T. The interrelationship between sleep regulation and thermoregulation. *Front Biosci (Landmark Ed).* 2010;15:604-625.
20. Shibasaki M., Aoki K., Morimoto K., Johnson J. M., Takamata A. Plasma hyperosmolality elevates the internal temperature threshold for active thermoregulatory vasodilation during heat stress in humans. *Am J Physiol Regul Integr Comp Physiol.* 2009;297(6):R1706-1712.
21. Turner P. L., Mainster M. A. Circadian photoreception: ageing and the eye's important role in systemic health. *Br J Ophthalmol.* 2008;92(11):1439-1444.
22. Nathan P. J., Burrows G. D., Norman T. R. Melatonin sensitivity to dim white light in affective disorders. *Neuropsychopharmacology.* 1999;21(3):408-413.
23. American Academy of Sleep Medicine. *International Classification of Sleep Disorders,* 3rd ed. Darien, IL: American Academy of Sleep Medicine; 2014.
24. Chattu V. K., Manzar M. D., Kumary S., Burman D., Spence D. W., Pandi-Perumal S. R. The global problem of insufficient sleep and its serious public health implications. *Healthcare (Basel).* 2018;7(1).
25. Van Cauter E., Spiegel K., Tasali E., Leproult R. Metabolic consequences of sleep and sleep loss. *Sleep Med.* 2008;9 Suppl 1(0 1):S23-28.
26. Sateia M. J. International classification of sleep disorders-third edition: highlights and modifications. *Chest.* 2014;146(5):1387-1394.
27. Vgontzas A. N., Bixler E. O., Chrousos G. P. Sleep apnea is a manifestation of the metabolic syndrome. *Sleep Med Rev.* 2005;9(3):211-224.
28. Wolf J., Lewicka J., Narkiewicz K. Obstructive sleep apnea: an update on mechanisms and cardiovascular consequences. *Nutr Metab Cardiovasc Dis.* 2007;17(3):233-240.
29. Chung F., Subramanyam R., Liao P., Sasaki E., Shapiro C., Sun Y. High STOP-Bang score indicates a high probability of obstructive sleep apnoea. *Br J Anaesth.* 2012;108(5):768-775.
30. Winkelman J. W., Armstrong M. J., Allen R. P., et al. Practice guideline summary: treatment of restless legs syndrome in adults: report of the Guideline Development, Dissemination, and Implementation Subcommittee of the American Academy of Neurology. *Neurology.* 2016;87(24):2585-2593.

31. Carmelli D., Swan G. E., Bliwise D. L. Relationship of 30-year changes in obesity to sleep-disordered breathing in the Western Collaborative Group Study. *Obes Res.* 2000;8(9):632-637.
32. Spiegel K., Knutson K., Leproult R., Tasali E., Van Cauter E. Sleep loss: a novel risk factor for insulin resistance and type 2 diabetes. *J Appl Physiol (1985).* 2005;99(5):2008-2019.
33. Cappuccio F. P., Taggart F. M., Kandala N. B., et al. Meta-analysis of short sleep duration and obesity in children and adults. *Sleep.* 2008;31(5):619-626.
34. Van Cauter E., Knutson K. L. Sleep and the epidemic of obesity in children and adults. *Eur J Endocrinol.* 2008;159 Suppl 1(S1):S59-66.
35. Spiegel K., Leproult R., L'Hermite-Balériaux M., Copinschi G., Penev P. D., Van Cauter E. Leptin levels are dependent on sleep duration: relationships with sympathovagal balance, carbohydrate regulation, cortisol, and thyrotropin. *J Clin Endocrinol Metab.* 2004;89(11):5762-5771.
36. Martino T. A., Sole M. J. Molecular time: an often overlooked dimension to cardiovascular disease. *Circ Res.* 2009;105(11):1047-1061.
37. Ferrie J. E., Shipley M. J., Cappuccio F. P., et al. A prospective study of change in sleep duration: associations with mortality in the Whitehall II cohort. *Sleep.* 2007;30(12):1659-1666. https://pubmed.ncbi.nlm.nih.gov/18246975.
38. Vgontzas A. N., Fernandez-Mendoza J., Bixler E. O., et al. Persistent insomnia: the role of objective short sleep duration and mental health. *Sleep.* 2012;35(1):61-68.
39. Pace-Schott E. F., Milad M. R., Orr S. P., Rauch S. L., Stickgold R., Pitman R. K. Sleep promotes generalization of extinction of conditioned fear. *Sleep.* 2009;32(1):19-26. https://pubmed.ncbi.nlm.nih.gov/19189775.
40. Fernandez-Mendoza J., Calhoun S., Bixler E. O., et al. Insomnia with objective short sleep duration is associated with deficits in neuropsychological performance: a general population study. *Sleep.* 2010;33(4):459-465. https://pubmed.ncbi.nlm.nih.gov/20394314.
41. van der Helm E., Gujar N., Walker M. P. Sleep deprivation impairs the accurate recognition of human emotions. *Sleep.* 2010;33(3):335-342. https://pubmed.ncbi.nlm.nih.gov/20337191.
42. Szklo-Coxe M., Young T., Peppard P. E., Finn L. A., Benca R. M. Prospective associations of insomnia markers and symptoms with depression. *Am J Epidemiol.* 2010;171(6):709-720.
43. Blask D. E. Melatonin, sleep disturbance and cancer risk. *Sleep Med Rev.* 2009;13(4):257-264.
44. Mastin D. F., Bryson J., Corwyn R. Assessment of sleep hygiene using the Sleep Hygiene Index. *J Behav Med.* 2006;29(3):223-227.
45. Qaseem A., Kansagara D., Forciea M. A., Cooke M., Denberg T. D., Clinical Guidelines Committee of the American College of Physicians. Management of Chronic Insomnia Disorder in Adults: A Clinical Practice Guideline From the American College of Physicians. *Ann Intern Med.* 2016;165(2):125-133. http://europepmc.org/abstract/MED/27136449.
46. Irwin M. R., Cole J. C., Nicassio P. M. Comparative meta-analysis of behavioral interventions for insomnia and their efficacy in middle-aged adults and in older adults 55+ years of age. *Health Psychol.* 2006;25(1):3-14.
47. Sharma M. P., Andrade C. Behavioral interventions for insomnia: theory and practice. *Indian J Psychiatry.* 2012;54(4):359-366.
48. Falloon K., Elley C. R., Fernando A. 3rd, Lee A. C., Arroll B. Simplified sleep restriction for insomnia in general practice: a randomised controlled trial. *Br J Gen Pract.* 2015;65(637):e508-515.
49. McCurry S. M., Logsdon R. G., Teri L., Vitiello M. V. Evidence-based psychological treatments for insomnia in older adults. *Psychol Aging.* 2007;22(1):18-27.
50. Trauer J. M., Qian M. Y., Doyle J. S., Rajaratnam S. M., Cunnington D. Cognitive behavioral therapy for chronic insomnia: a systematic review and meta-analysis. *Ann Intern Med.* 2015;163(3):191-204.
51. Kripke D. F., Langer R. D., Kline L. E. Hypnotics' association with mortality or cancer: a matched cohort study. *BMJ Open.* 2012;2(1):e000850.
52. Basta M., Chrousos G. P., Vela-Bueno A., Vgontzas A. N. Chronic insomnia and stress system. *Sleep Med Clin.* 2007;2(2):279-291.
53. Pagel J. F. *Pharmacological Treatment of Insomnia in Primary Care Sleep Medicine: A Practical Guide,* 2nd ed. New York, NY: Springer; 2014.
54. Youngstedt S. D., Kripke D. F. Long sleep and mortality: rationale for sleep restriction. *Sleep Med Rev.* 2004;8(3):159-174.
55. Johns M. W. A new method for measuring daytime sleepiness: the Epworth sleepiness scale. *Sleep.* 1991;14(6):540-545.
56. Rosenthal L. D., Dolan D. C. The Epworth sleepiness scale in the identification of obstructive sleep apnea. *J Nerv Ment Dis.* 2008;196(5):429-431.
57. Buysse D. J., Reynolds C. F. 3rd, Monk T. H., Berman S. R., Kupfer D. J. The Pittsburgh Sleep Quality Index: a new instrument for psychiatric practice and research. *Psychiatry Res.* 1989;28(2):193-213.

SECTION 9
Fundamentals of Tobacco Cessation and Managing Risky Alcohol Use

Objective 1 Describe the societal and health effects of tobacco use **296**

Objective 2 Explain the role of tobacco cessation in preventing and treating chronic disease **297**

Objective 3 List at least five recommendations on tobacco cessation from the US Public Health Service.......... **298**

Objective 4 Summarize the evidence-based literature on tobacco cessation interventions.......... **299**

Objective 5 Demonstrate the ability to assist patients in developing and implementing plans for tobacco cessation.......... **303**

Objective 6 Summarize coverage for tobacco cessation counseling **307**

Objective 7 Describe the role of moderating alcohol use in preventing and treating chronic diseases.......... **308**

Objective 8 Describe the clinical process for screening for alcohol misuse...... **311**

Objective 9 Summarize the evidence-based literature on alcohol misuse interventions, and develop and implement plans for avoiding risky alcohol use... **312**

Section 9 Glossary.......... **316**

Section 9 Review Questions **317**

Section 9 Review Questions Answers and Explanations **319**

Section 9 References.......... **320**

OBJECTIVE 1

Describe the societal and health effects of tobacco use

1) Tobacco use and exposure[1]

- **a)** Economic costs of tobacco
    1. ~$300 billion annually
        - a. $170 billion in direct medical costs[2]
        - b. $150 billion in lost productivity
- **b)** Human costs of tobacco
    1. Tobacco is the single largest preventable cause of morbidity and mortality in the US.[3]
        - a. In 2017, preliminary research by Cleveland Clinic and the New York School of Medicine presented that obesity has become the leading preventable cause of disease and death. The Centers for Disease Control and Prevention still states that smoking is the number one cause of preventable death.[4]
    2. ~50 million Americans die prematurely every year.
    3. ~16 million suffer from diseases caused by smoking.
    4. Compared to people who have never smoked, smokers:
        - a. Suffer more health problems and disability
        - b. Lose ~10 years of life

2) Health effects of modern cigarettes[1]

- **a)** Today's smokers smoke fewer cigarettes but have a greater risk of lung cancer.
    1. Changes in cigarette design and composition have led to an increased risk of lung adenocarcinoma, the most common type of lung cancer. These changes include:
        - a. Ventilated filters, which allow more vigorous inhalation, thereby drawing cancer-causing chemicals deeper into lung tissue
        - b. Chemical additives: 70 chemicals in cigarette smoke are known carcinogens (cancer-causing chemicals), and the levels of some chemicals in cigarettes have increased through changes in the manufacturing process.
- **b)** Smoking-related deaths in the US
    1. 480,000 die each year in the US (approximately one of five deaths).
    2. Tobacco products kill one of every two people who use them.
    3. Smoking causes:
        - a. 87% of lung cancer deaths
        - b. 32% of coronary heart disease deaths
        - c. 80% of all deaths from chronic obstructive pulmonary disease (COPD)
- **c)** Smoking and cancer[3,5]
    1. 40+ cancers are related to tobacco use, and these cancers occur in almost any part of the body.
    2. If no one smoked or used tobacco products, one in three cancer deaths would not happen.
- **d)** Smoking leads to or worsens:
    1. Diabetes (risk of developing diabetes is 30–40% for current smokers)[6]
    2. Rheumatoid arthritis

3. Impaired immune system/immune function, in part because of high levels of tar and other chemicals that damage the immune system[3]
4. Reduced quality of life
5. Problems with reproduction in men and women
6. Poorer-quality, slower wound healing
7. Tuberculosis disease
8. Ectopic pregnancy, preterm delivery stillbirth, or low birth weight, and sudden infant death syndrome (SIDS)
9. Cleft lip and cleft palate (if mothers smoke while the child is in utero)
10. Erectile dysfunction
11. Age-related macular degeneration
12. Failure rate of treatment for all cancers
13. Risk of bone fractures
14. Muscle aches and pains

3) Nicotine dependence[7]

a) Nicotine is the most common form of chemical dependence in the US.
1. Nicotine is the key drug in the addiction cycle of tobacco products.
2. It may be as addictive as heroin, cocaine, or alcohol.

b) Effective treatment exists but often requires repeated treatment.

OBJECTIVE 2

Explain the role of tobacco cessation in preventing and treating chronic disease

1) Health benefits of quitting[7,8]

a) Reduces the risk of disease, including lung cancer, coronary heart disease, stroke, peripheral vascular disease, chronic obstructive pulmonary disease, and infertility

b) Timeline of smoking cessation benefits
1. Immediate: people who quit smoking cut their risk of having a heart attack by 50% compared to someone who continues to smoke[8]
2. 1 year: the risk of heart disease is 50% of a non-smoker.
3. 2–5 years: the risk of stroke is approximately that of a non-smoker.
4. 10 years: the risk of lung cancer is reduced by 50%.

c) Reduces the risk of premature death and lowers rates of heart attacks, strokes, and lethal cancers

d) Quitting is beneficial at any age, but there are more benefits to quitting the younger someone quits.
1. Quitting at 30 years of age gains 10 years of life expectancy.
2. Quitting at 60 years of age gains 3 years of life expectancy.

2) Tobacco cessation[7,9]

a) Smokers can and do quit.

b) Today there are more former smokers in the world than current smokers.

c) Most tobacco users want to quit.

1. 68.8% of current US smoking adults want to quit completely.
2. Only 5% of those who want to stop will be able to quit without assistance.

d) By absolute numbers, most people who quit smoking have quit without using evidence-based treatments; however, quitting "cold turkey," or abrupt complete cessation, is the least effective long-term treatment.[9]

1. 50% will resume smoking within 14 days of quitting smoking.
2. 75% will resume within 30 days.

e) Physicians using evidence-based programs can double quitting success rates.

1. Among patients in treatment programs under medical guidance, 40–50% will be tobacco-free 3 months after their "quit date."[9]

f) Effective evidence-based treatments include:

1. Counseling
    a. Brief clinical interventions
    b. Individual, group, or telephone counseling
    c. Behavioral therapies
    d. Intensive treatments with a high amount of person-to-person contact
    e. Program treatments using mobile phones
2. Medication
    a. Over-the-counter or prescription nicotine replacement therapy
    b. Prescription non-nicotine medications
3. Counseling and medication are more potent than either alone.

g) Providers and tobacco users must both be persistent.

h) Slips and relapses are normal and considered part of the change process.

3) Lung Cancer Screening[10]

a) US Preventive Services Task Force recommends yearly low-dose computed tomography screening for those who meet the following criteria:

1. Greater or equal to 30 pack-year smoking history
2. Current smoker or quit within the past 15 years
3. Between the ages of 55–80 years of age

OBJECTIVE 3

List at least five recommendations on tobacco cessation from the US Public Health Service

1) US Public Health Service (USPHS) Clinical Practice Guidelines are for clinicians using evidence-based treatments for tobacco cessation and their effectiveness and guidelines for system changes that can increase tobacco assessment, intervention, and cessation rates.[11]

a) The 10 key recommendations from USPHS' guidelines

1. Clinicians need to recognize that tobacco dependence is a chronic disease and should be treated and appropriately followed up.
    a. Effective treatments and medications exist for tobacco dependence.

b. Often, quitting requires repeated interventions and attempts.

2. Clinicians and healthcare workers should consistently assess and document tobacco use.
3. Tobacco use treatments are effective across a broad range of populations.
   a. Clinicians should encourage everyone willing to change to use effective treatments.
4. Brief tobacco dependence treatment is effective.
   a. Minimal interventions (lasting less than 3 minutes) still increase overall tobacco abstinence rates.
5. Individual, group, and telephone counseling is effective.
   a. There is a dose-response relationship
      (1) The more intense the intervention, the more effective it is.
      (2) Person-to-person treatment (more than four sessions) appears to be especially effective.
   b. The most effective counseling includes:
      (1) Practical counseling, which includes problem-solving and skills training
      (2) Social support that is delivered as part of the treatment
6. Numerous effective medications exist.
   a. Medication use should be encouraged by clinicians, unless the medication is medically contraindicated and for specific populations (pregnant women, smokeless tobacco users, light smokers, and adolescents).
   b. Certain combinations are more effective.
7. A combination of counseling and medication is more effective than either alone.
   a. Interventions offered in multiple formats increase abstinence rates.
   b. Tailored materials (web-based or in print) are also effective in helping people quit.
8. Telephone "quitline" counseling is effective.
   a. Clinicians and counselors should make sure patients have access to quitline use.
9. If a tobacco user is not ready to quit, clinicians should use motivational interviewing skills that can increase future quit attempts.
10. Tobacco dependence treatments are clinically effective and very cost-effective compared to interventions for other disorders.

OBJECTIVE 4

Summarize the evidence-based literature on tobacco cessation interventions

1) Pharmacotherapy guidelines for patients wanting to quit[11]

a) The US Department of Health and Human Services (HHS) recommends that clinicians encourage all patients to use effective medications except:

1. Those where treatment is contraindicated
2. Special populations where there is insufficient evidence (pregnant women, smokeless tobacco users, light smokers, and adolescents)

b) There are seven US Food and Drug Administration (FDA) approved first-line medications including:[9,12]

1. Five nicotine replacement therapies (NRTs)
   a. Mechanism of action (see Figure 9.1): direct stimulation of nicotinic receptors in the ventral tegmental area of the brain, which leads to dopamine release.[13]

Figure 9.1

Brain reward (dopamine) pathways

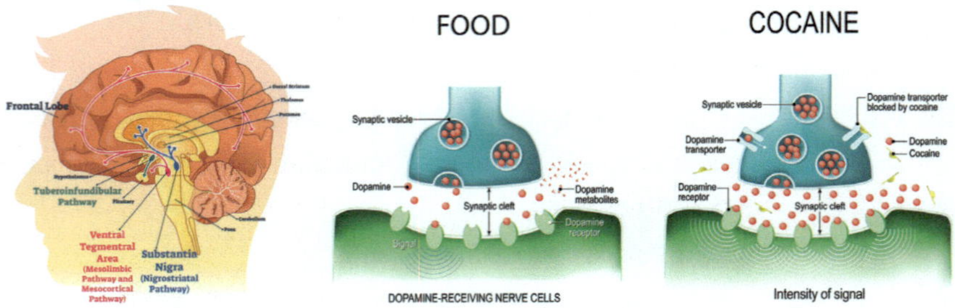

These brain circuits are important for natural rewards such as food, music, and sex.

Typically, dopamine increases in response to natural rewards such as food.
When cocaine is taken, dopamine increases are exaggerated, and communication is altered.

   b. Nicotine patch, gum, and lozenge (over-the-counter)
      (1) Patch alone: 45% tobacco-free at 8 weeks (placebo 30%)
      (2) Lozenge alone: 40% tobacco-free at 8 weeks (placebo 30%)
   c. Nicotine replacement inhaler or nasal spray (prescription only)
2. Two non-nicotine medications
   a. Vareniclin
      (1) Varenicline is the most effective monotherapy.
         (a) 51% tobacco-free at the end of the 12-week program (21% smoke-free with placebo)
         (b) 35% tobacco-free at 6 months (17% smoke-free with placebo)
      (2) Mechanism of action: varenicline acts as a nicotinic receptor partial agonist, meaning the medication binds to the same receptors as nicotine, but less strongly. Therefore, it causes some of the effect of nicotine (thereby preventing withdrawals) while blocking nicotine from attaching to the receptor (thereby stopping nicotine highs).
   b. Bupropion
      (1) 40% tobacco-free at 8 weeks (placebo 30%)
      (2) Mechanism of action: bupropion inhibits the reuptake of norepinephrine and dopamine at the nerve synapse so that more norepinephrine and dopamine are available to attach to the corresponding receptors and stimulate the postsynaptic neuron.[14]

c) Treatment combinations are more effective than monotherapies (data is based on treatment of individuals without chronic disease or psychiatric illness)

1. The combination of varenicline and bupropion is the most effective treatment.
   a. 71% tobacco-free at the end of a 12-week program
   b. 58% tobacco-free at 6 months
2. The combination of bupropion, patch, and lozenge
   a. 54% tobacco-free at eight weeks
3. The combination of bupropion and lozenge

        a. 50% tobacco-free at 8 weeks
   4. Recent studies show nicotine replacement therapies plus varenicline may be an effective treatment without worsening medication side effects.
   5. The combination of varenicline, bupropion, and nicotine replacement therapies may be even more effective, but only preliminary data is currently available.

d) For those with one or more chronic disease(s) or mental illness
   1. A triple medication regime is recommended (bupropion, patch, and one nicotine replacement therapy).
      a. 62% tobacco-free at 8 weeks, versus 37% with the patch alone
      b. 35% at 6 months, versus 19% with the patch alone

e) Two second-line medications for tobacco cessation (off-label use):
   1. Clonidine and nortriptyline
   2. The use of these medications is on a case-by-case basis. They may be used if first-line medications have not worked or are contraindicated.

f) Factors to consider when prescribing
   1. Clinician's familiarity with medications
   2. Contraindications
   3. Patient preference
   4. Previous patient experience with medications or treatments (successes/failures)
   5. Patient characteristics: history of depression, suicide attempt, weight gain concerns, or recent myocardial infarction (MI)
      a. Concerns about weight gain
         (1) Average weight gain <10 lbs (4.5 kg) (this gain is more common in women)
         (2) Bupropion and nicotine replacement therapy may delay but not prevent weight gain
   6. Frequency of tobacco use and level of dependence
      a. Light smokers (<10 cigarettes per day) show no significant benefit from nicotine replacement therapy.

g) Patients with mental illness[15]
   1. Most require medication to be successful
   2. May need higher doses, longer duration of treatment, and a combination of medications
   3. Bipolar patients
      a. Do not use bupropion.
      b. Patch is recommended treatment.
   4. Schizophrenia
      a. Patch is recommended.

h) Patients with cardiovascular disease[12]
   1. There is no association between the nicotine patch and acute cardiovascular events, even among those who continued to smoke while on patch.
   2. Nicotine replacement therapy packaging recommends caution for patients with acute cardiovascular disease.

i) Pregnant smokers[12]
   1. Counseling is best.
      a. The benefits of over-the-counter nicotine replacement (patches, lozenge, and gum) outweigh the risk. No harm is expected, but this is based on limited studies.[16,17]

b. Bupropion and varenicline: FDA category C for use during pregnancy
c. Prescription nicotine replacement therapy: category D with a potential risk of birth defects

2. Continuing to smoke
   a. Increases risk of premature or stillbirth, intrauterine growth restriction
   b. Likely has a higher risk of harm than birth defects from nicotine replacement therapy

j) Adolescents[12]

1. Nicotine replacement therapy is safe, but there is very little research on adolescents who smoke and on adolescents who are trying to quit.

k) Long-term pharmacotherapy[12]

1. Helpful for tobacco users with persistent withdrawal symptoms
2. Long-term nicotine replacement therapy has no known health risks.
3. Bupropion is approved for up to 6 months.
4. Varenicline is recommended for 12 weeks and may be repeated for 12 more weeks (6 months total).

2) Other treatment modalities that are not evidence-based[11]

a) Treatments that have not demonstrated effectiveness

1. Acupuncture
2. Hypnosis
3. Prior unsuccessful quit attempts with conventional therapies do not justify the use of unproven alternative cessation methods. Multiple attempts with evidence-based methods may be necessary to achieve abstinence.

b) Treatments that have insufficient evidence

1. Physiological feedback or biofeedback
2. Restricted environmental stimulation therapy
3. Use of incentives
4. Cigarette fading (cutting down slowly or reduce to quit)

c) Electronic nicotine delivery systems (e-cigarettes, e-hookahs, vaping, "Juuling")[18]

1. These are not FDA regulated or approved for tobacco cessation treatments and even some canisters labeled "no nicotine" have been found to contain nicotine.
2. Made of three main parts: 1) a chamber to hold liquid (the liquid contains nicotine but can be used for marijuana or other drugs), 2) a heating device, and 3) a battery (defective batteries have led to fires and explosions).
3. The heated liquid becomes an aerosol that can be inhaled into the lungs by primary and secondhand exposure.
4. Nicotine liquid can cause poisoning to children and adults if swallowed or absorbed through the skin or eyes.
5. Aerosol has less harmful chemicals than tobacco smoke, which as more than 7,000 chemicals. Still, it contains heavy metals such as nickel, tin, and lead, as well as other cancer-causing and lung- damaging chemicals.
6. Lack of definitive data regarding associated benefits and harms.
7. E-cigarette use is recently associated with an e-cigarette or vaping product use-associated lung injury (EVALI). Most, but not all EVALI cases involved vaping THC (the active ingredient in marijuana), and is likely caused by vitamin E acetate in the vaping oil. The investigation is ongoing, but providers should be aware of the latest recommendations from the Centers for Disease Control and Prevention.[19]

8. More youths are using e-cigarettes than adults (10.5% of middle schoolers and 27.5% of high schoolers). Nicotine can harm the developing adolescent brain. E-cigarettes are associated with higher use of other tobacco products.[20]
9. Most adult users are purchasing e-cigarettes to quit. However, studies find that these adults are not quitting smoking, but rather, continuing to use both e-cigarettes and cigarettes (dual use).

3) Effective counseling in helping people quit

a) Practical counseling (which includes problem-solving skills and skills training):

1. Help patients recognize and avoid high-risk situations.
2. Identify triggers.
3. Address specific barriers to behavior change.
4. Develop physical and mental coping skills.
5. Provide basic information about smoking and successful quitting.
6. Provide support and encouragement (intra-treatment support), and communicate care and concern.
7. Engage patient in discussions about the quitting process.

OBJECTIVE 5

Demonstrate the ability to assist patients in developing and implementing plans for tobacco cessation

1) Facilitating behavior change with those willing to quit with the 5A's model (see Table 9.1)[11]

a) Tobacco Cessation: 5A's Model

Table 9.1

5A's of Behavior Change	5A's in Tobacco Cessation
1. Assess practices in the context of health risks.	**1. Ask:** Identify tobacco use and document for every patient.
2. Advise change to practices with clear, specific, and personalized advice for behavior change.	**2. Advise:** Use a clear, strong, and personalized manner when advising quitting.
3. Agree on the focus of counseling and treatment based the patient's interest and willingness to change.	**3. Assess:** Is the tobacco user ready and willing to make a quit attempt?
4. Assist the patient in setting and achieving goals to change practices. a. Address motivational barriers via counseling and self-help techniques. b. Determine whether the patient needs additional information or help. c. Refer the patient to a dietitian or other resources as needed.	**4. Assist:** Provide counseling and/or pharmacotherapy for those who are ready to make a quit attempt.
5. Arrange regular follow-up and support.	**5. Arrange:** Schedule follow-up and accountability appointment, preferentially 1 week prior to quit date and 3 days following quit date.

Note: This is similar, but different from other 5A's utilized in behavior change. Be aware of the differences.

1. Alternative model (when time constraints are present)
    a. Ask, Advise, Refer
    b. Ask: identify tobacco use and document for every patient.
    c. Advise: use a clear, strong, and personalized manner when advising quitting.
    d. Refer: connect the patient with behavioral support and intensive treatment.
        (1) Many quitlines have fax or electronic referral programs for quick and easy use.

b) Ask: identify all tobacco users every visit.
1. Action: implement an office-wide system to ensure that tobacco use status is queried and documented for every patient and every visit.
2. Implementation strategies: expand vital signs to include tobacco use or use an alternate universal identification system (like stickers, electronic notice).

c) Advise to quit
1. Action: advise quitting in a clear, strong, and personalized manner.
2. Implementation strategies
    a. Be clear: "There is no safe level of smoking. Occasional and light smoking are still dangerous."
    b. Be strong: "This is the most important thing you can do for your long-term health."
    c. Personalize the message: "Continuing to smoke will continue to worsen your asthma. Quitting may improve your breathing."

d) Assess the patient's willingness to make a quit attempt.
1. Action: assess every tobacco user's willingness to quit.
2. Implementation strategies
    a. If they are willing, provide assistance
    b. If they are willing to participate in an intensive program, refer them
    c. If they are unwilling, provide motivational intervention to increase future quit attempts

e) Assist the patient in quitting.
1. Action:
    a. Help the patient develop a quit plan
    b. Recommend and prescribe medication if it's not contraindicated and the patient is not in a special population.
    c. Provide or refer for counseling (especially that includes problem-solving and skills training).
    d. Provide intra-treatment support.
2. Implementation (patient preparations)
    a. Set a quit date, ideally within 2 weeks of the agreement to quit smoking.
    b. Encourage the patient to tell family and friends about the quit attempt.
    c. Prescribe medications, and explain how to use them to increase success and reduce withdrawal symptoms.
    d. Counseling

(1) Refer if necessary

(2) Discuss

(a) Striving for total abstinence from smoking after the quit date

(b) Past quit experiences

(c) Removing tobacco from the environment (home, work, car, etc.)

(3) Anticipate triggers or challenges patient will face.

(a) Alcohol (which is often a strong trigger)

(b) Other smokers in the home

(c) Withdrawal symptoms

(d) High-risk times (stress, parties, etc.)

e. Intra-treatment support

(1) Encourage patients in their quit attempt

f. Supplementary materials

(1) Connect the patient with resources for further support, including:

(a) Federal agencies

(b) Nonprofit agencies

(c) National quitline network (1-800-Quit-Now)

(d) Local/state/tribal health departments and quitlines

f) Arrange follow-up contact

1. Action:

a. Establish follow-up in person, telephone, or electronically.

2. Implementation strategies

a. Arranging follow-up

(1) First, follow up around quit date, ideally 3 days after quit date.

(2) Second, follow up within first month after quit day.

(3) Schedule additional follow-ups as needed.

b. Actions to discuss during follow-up appointments

(1) Problems encountered

(2) Anticipating challenges

(3) Assess medication use and problems

(4) Discuss quitline support

(5) Address tobacco use at each following visit

(6) Congratulate if successful on quit attempt

2) Motivational interviewing[11]

a) Motivational interviewing can increase future quit attempts (see Table 9.2 and Table 9.3).

Table 9.2 Motivational Interviewing Principles	
Express empathy	a. Use open-ended questions (explore)
	b. Use reflective listening (gain shared understanding)
	c. Normalize feelings and concerns
	d. Support autonomy and right to choose or reject change
Develop discrepancy	a. Highlight discrepancy between the patient's values, goals, priorities, and present behavior
	b. Reinforce and support "change talk" and "commitment language"
	c. Build and deepen commitment to change
Roll with resistance	a. Back off and use reflection when the patient expresses resistance
	b. Express empathy
	c. Ask permission to provide information
Support self-efficacy	a. Help the patient identify and build on past successes
	b. Offer options for achievable small steps toward change (for example, call the quitline, read handouts, or change smoking pattern)

Table 9.3 Five R's of Motivational Interviewing[11]	
Relevance	a. Ask the patient to identify the negative consequences of smoking
	b. The provider may highlight those pertinent to the patient
Risks of smoking	a. Acute risks: shortness of breath, asthma exacerbations, respiratory infections, impotence, pregnancy complications, fetal harm, and infertility
	b. Long-term risks: heart attacks, strokes, lung cancers, other cancers, chronic obstructive pulmonary disease (COPD), osteoporosis, long-term disability, and need for extended care
	c. Environmental risks of secondhand smoke: In spouses: increased risk of heart disease and lung cancer. In children: increased risk of low birth weight, sudden infant death syndrome (SIDS), asthma, middle ear infections, and respiratory infections.
Rewards of quitting	a. Have the patient list potential benefits (the clinician can highlight those that are most relevant)
	b. Examples: lower risk of the diseases above, a better sense of smell, setting a good example for family, improved appearance of skin, and whiter teeth
Roadblocks to quitting	a. Patient's identified barriers
	b. Frequent barriers include withdrawal symptoms, fear of failure, weight gain, change of relationships and friendships, lack of support, depression, enjoyment of tobacco, limited knowledge of effective treatment options, and being around others who smoke
Repetition	a. Repeat the steps above at every visit if the patient is unmotivated
	b. Encourage patients who have failed attempts that most people must try multiple times before succeeding

OBJECTIVE 6

Summarize coverage for tobacco cessation counseling

Summarize coverage for tobacco cessation counseling in the US

1) Medicaid[21]
   a) 47 states cover individual counseling for nicotine dependence.
   b) 29 states cover group counseling.
   c) There is variable state coverage for phone counseling.
   d) Telephone counseling through the state quitlines is available free to callers in all 50 states and the District of Columbia. National Quitline portal: 1-800-QUIT-NOW.[23]
2) Medicare[22]
   a) Coverage is available for outpatient and hospitalized beneficiaries who use tobacco, whether or not the person has symptoms of tobacco-related illnesses.
   b) Coverage includes:
      1. Four cessation counseling sessions for one attempt to quit
      2. Eight counseling sessions (two cessation attempts) every 12 months
   c) Counseling session
      1. Refers to face-to-face patient contact at one of two levels
         a) Intermediate: 3–10 minutes (CPT code 99406)
         b) Intensive: more than 10 minutes (CPT code 99407)
      2. May be performed by a qualified practitioner
         a) Prescription drug benefit covers smoking cessation treatments prescribed by a physician.
         b) Over-the-counter medicines are not covered.
3) Private insurers[12]
   a) Most insurers provide coverage for:
      1. One or more type of behavioral intervention
      2. One or more pharmacotherapy treatments
   b) ICD-10 (international classification of diseases) billing codes
      1. Preventive medicine treatments
      2. Tobacco dependence treatment
         a. Part of initial or periodic comprehensive preventive medicine exam
         b. As specific counseling and/or risk factor reduction
   c) Coverage varies

OBJECTIVE 7

Describe the role of moderating alcohol use in preventing and treating chronic diseases

1) **Background and rationale of screening for alcohol use disorder (AUD), which refers to disorders related to drinking**
   - **a)** 15 million adults in the US have some form of alcohol use disorder.[25]
   - **b)** 30% of US adults exceed the National Institutes of Health (NIH) daily limits at least once per year.
     1. 26% are at-risk drinkers or have mild AUD
     2. 3% have moderate AUD
     3. 1% have severe AUD
   - **c)** Alcohol misuse is hazardous alcohol consumption.[26,27]
     1. Excessive alcohol use associated with:
        - a. 10% of all cancers
        - b. 20% of all intentional injuries
        - c. 7% of all deaths, including:
          - (1) Road crash injury
          - (2) Cancer
          - (3) Suicide
        - d. 88,000 attributable deaths per year[24]
        - e. 2.5 million years of life lost per year among US adults
     2. Heavy drinking increases the risk of:
        - a. High blood pressure
        - b. Stroke
        - c. Unintentional injuries
        - d. Cancer
     3. Moderate alcohol consumption may have possible health benefits. Note, the health benefits appear to be due to the health properties of red grapes, and the same benefits may be acquired directly from just eating the grapes.
   - **d)** Regions and groups at higher risk of alcohol misuse
     1. Northeast, upper Midwest, Alaska, and Hawaii
        - a. People in these areas are more likely to binge drink at least once a year
        - b. Individuals in the southern US are least likely
     2. Higher prevalence groups[27]
        - a. Ages: 18–34 (28%)
        - b. Prevalence increases with income
        - c. Whites > blacks or Asians
        - d. Men (23%) >Women (11%)
        - e. Smokers
        - f. Psychiatric patients
        - g. Trauma patients
        - h. Positive family history of alcohol abuse

e) People with AUD only received appropriate assessment and treatment from primary care providers 10% of the time.[28]

f) AUD can be treated with anti-relapse medications (ARMs).

   1. Anti-relapse medications can be prescribed by non-specialist physicians.

g) Anti-relapse medications plus medical management

   1. Is as effective as addiction counseling for mild to moderate AUD

h) Chronic care management

   1. Effective for patients with AUD and alcohol-related serious medical illness

i) Identification and brief advice by a healthcare provider (Grade B US Preventitive Services Task Force recommendation) is an effective way to reduce drinking and its associated risks.

2) **Definitions**

a) Standard alcoholic drink in the US

   1. 12 oz (340 g) regular beer
   2. 5 oz (142 g) table wine
   3. 1.5 oz (43 g) of 80-proof spirits (shot)

b) Typical containers

   1. 750 ml (25 oz) wine bottle = 5 drinks
   2. 750 ml (25 oz) "fifth" of spirits = 18 drinks
   3. 1 L (34 oz) spirits = 24 drinks

c) US Dietary Guidelines for Alcohol Consumption (DGAC)[29]

   1. The DGAC recommends that when consuming alcohol, it should be consumed in moderation, and only by adults of legal drinking age.
   2. Moderate alcohol consumption is defined as:
      a. daily consumption of up to one drink per day for women
      b. daily consumption of up to two drinks per day for men

d) "Binge" drinking

   1. Drinking enough that blood alcohol level increases to 0.08 mg/L
   2. Five drinks in 2 hours for men, four drinks in 2 hours for women

e) Heavy alcohol use

   1. Binge drinking on more than 5 days in the past month
   2. The National Institute on Alcohol Abuse and Alcoholism (NIAAA) defines heavy alcohol use as more than four drinks on any day for men or more than three drinks for women.

f) At-risk drinking

   1. Exceeds the levels above for any day or week
   2. Binge drinking at least once a month
   3. Drinking that increases the risk of future problems, even though there are no current symptoms

g) AUD

   1. DSM-5 term for disorders related to drinking
      a. Previously, in DSM-4, AUD was referred to as "alcohol abuse and dependence."
      b. "Alcohol use disorder" is a more appropriate term because this disorder is a continuous spectrum.

c. The terms "alcoholism" and "alcoholic" are imprecise and stigmatizing, and no longer used.

2. The most common symptoms of AUD include:
   a. Significant distress or impairment
   b. Impaired control over use
   c. Cravings and preoccupations
   d. Persistent but unsuccessful desire to quit or cut down
   e. Use despite adverse consequences, such as hangover, nausea, heartburn, depression, and other health problems
   f. 10% of people with AUD develop serious adverse consequences, including job, legal, and role-failure problems.
   g. The most severe 10% are over-represented in rehabs, jails, and hospitals.

3) DSM-5 Diagnostic Criteria for AUD[30,31]

a) Eleven questions to ask that demonstrate signs or symptoms over the past 12 months

1. "Did you have times when you ended up drinking more, or longer, than you intended?"
2. "More than once did you want to cut down or stop drinking, or tried to, but couldn't?
3. "Did you spend a great deal of time in activities necessary to obtain alcohol, use alcohol, or recover from its effects?"
4. "Do you spend a lot of time drinking? Or being sick or getting over other aftereffects of drinking too much?"
5. "Do you find that drinking—or being sick from drinking—often interferes with taking care of your home or family? Or causes job troubles? Or school problems?"
6. "Do you continue to drink even though it causes trouble with your family or friends?"
7. "Have you given up or cut back on activities that were important or interesting to you, or gave you pleasure, in order to drink?"
8. "More than once have you gotten into situations while or after drinking that increased your chances of getting hurt such as driving, swimming, using machinery, walking in a dangerous area, or having unsafe sex?"
9. "Have you continued to drink even though it was making you feel depressed, anxious, or added to another health problem? Or continued to drink after having a memory blackout?"
10. "Do you have to drink much more than you once did to get the effect you want? Or found that your usual number of drinks had much less effect than before?"
11. "Have you found that when the effects of alcohol were wearing off, you had withdrawal symptoms, such as trouble sleeping, shakiness, restlessness, nausea, sweating, a racing heart, or a seizure? Or have you had delusions, such as sensing things that were not there?"

b) AUD diagnostic criteria (≥2 of the above signs and symptoms during the past 12 months)

1. 0–1: criteria met; no AUD
2. 2–3: mild (similar to DSM-4 alcohol abuse)
3. 4–5: moderate (similar to DSM-4 alcohol dependence)
4. 6+: severe

c) 12-month prevalence of DSM-5 AUD[32]

1. Mild
   a. Men ~10%
   b. Women ~5%

2. Moderate to Severe
    a. Men ~6%
    b. Women ~2%

OBJECTIVE 8

Describe the clinical process for screening for alcohol misuse

1) Timing of screening

- **a)** Annual prevention examination or "physical"
- **b)** High-risk groups
    1. Younger people
    2. High-risk regions and groups
    3. Trauma/sexually transmitted diseases
    4. Family history
    5. Pregnant or planning to be pregnant
    6. Heavy smokers
    7. Clinical suspicion

2) Oral survey

- **a)** All patients should be asked about drinking.
    1. "How many times in the past year have you had greater than four drinks (women), five (men) in a day?"
        a. If screening outcomes on 1 or more days is positive, then the following should be documented:
            (1) Number of drinking days per week
            (2) Number of drinks per day
            (3) Advice should be given to reduce or stop if:
                (a) Women: >3 drinks per day, >7 drinks per week
                (b) Men: >4 drinks per day, >14 drinks per week
            (4) Additional written screening should be completed

3) Written screening[33]

- **a)** Alcohol Use Disorder Identification Test (AUDIT)
    1. The AUDIT screening test is 10 self-reported items (available at https://www.drugabuse.gov/sites/default/files/audit.pdf)[29,34]
        a. AUDIT is the recommended screening test, as it provides meaningful information with a low burden to patients and staff.
        b. Questions are rated 0 (never, low number of occurrences) to 4 (daily, high number of occurrences)
            (1) How often do you have a drink containing alcohol?

> **Note:** AUDIT screens for six or more drinks, but NIH states high risk drinking is five or more drinks.

(2) How many drinks containing alcohol do you have on a typical day when you are drinking?
(3) How often do you have six or more drinks on one occasion?
(4) During the last year, how often have you found that you were not able to stop drinking once you started?
(5) How often during the last year have you failed to do what was normally expected of you because of drinking?
(6) During the last year, how often have you needed a first drink in the morning to get yourself going after a heavy drinking session?
(7) How often during the last year have you had a feeling of guilt or remorse after drinking?
(8) How often during the last year have you been unable to remember what happened the night before because of your drinking?
(9) Have you or someone else been injured because of your drinking?
(10) Has a relative, friend, doctor, or other healthcare worker been concerned about your drinking or suggested you cut down?

2. AUDIT Scores help guide therapy
   a. 5–10: at-risk drinker (20% will have AUD)
   b. 11–15: more at risk (40% have AUD)
   c. 16+: high probability of moderate or severe AUD (90%)
   d. Higher scores have higher sensitivity
3. AUDIT-C (consumption) has three items
   a. Questions are rated 0 (never, low number of occurrences) to 4 (daily, high number of occurrences).
      (1) How many drinks containing alcohol do you have on a typical day when you are drinking?
      (2) How many drinks containing alcohol do you have on a typical day when you are drinking?
      (3) How often do you have six or more drinks on one occasion?
4. AUDIT-C Scores
   a. A score of more than 5 on the AUDIT-C may indicate hazardous or harmful drinking.

OBJECTIVE 9

Summarize the evidence-based literature on alcohol misuse interventions, and develop and implement plans for avoiding risky alcohol use

1) At-risk drinkers with mild AUD

a) Signs and symptoms[34,35,36,37,38]

1. Exceed five or more drinks per drinking occasion at least monthly
2. One to three symptoms of AUD
3. Risk increases with intensity and frequency of drinking

4. Primary risks: AUD development, liver disease, and marital problems

b) Risk reduction by clinicians or medical staff[30,39]

1. Brief advice to reduce
2. Naltrexone 25–50mg by mouth, used as needed at time of drinking occasion
3. Follow-up booster sessions to improve effectiveness

c) Behavioral intervention

1. Listen and reflect to ensure understanding.
2. Be non-judgmental and accepting.
3. Give matter of fact, clear opinions and recommendations.
4. Roll with resistance.
5. Use optimism, confidence, and acceptance.
6. Accept setbacks as expected, and know that change may be slow.

d) Resource

1. "Rethinking Drinking," developed by the NIH, is available online at https://www.rethinkingdrinking.niaaa.nih.gov

2) Mild to moderate AUD

a) Symptoms of impaired control include:

1. Going over limits
2. Desire to cut down
3. Use despite adverse consequences
4. Tolerance

b) Usually occurs as an isolated episode, possibly lasting 3–4 years, then resolves.

c) Few receive treatment

d) Similar to functional depression

e) Management[40]

1. Primary care setting, not an addiction clinic
2. Behavioral health
3. Anti-relapse medication
   a. As effective as addiction counseling
   b. Similar effect size as SSRI antidepressants

> "Antidepressants help about 27 people out of 100 not relapse within 2 years of a major depressive episode when compared to placebo pills (RR 0.46). You would need to treat four depressed people with an antidepressant to help one not have a relapse within 2 years."[39,41]

3) Severe recurrent AUD

a) Risk factors include:

1. Family history
2. Early childhood neglect
3. Behavior problems in childhood
4. Early-onset (mid-teens)
5. Chronic or recurrent course
6. Other substance abuse and psychiatric disorders

b) Treatment[42]

1. Counseling

2. Consider anti-relapse medications (ARMs)
    a. Due to the level of impairment, lifestyle intervention may be difficult
    b. Medications are comparable to Alcoholics Anonymous and counseling
    c. Medications are at least as good as SSRI's for depression treatment
    d. ARMs improve the proportion of patients who enter long-term recovery
3. Provide medical management for withdrawal symptoms.
4. Recruit assistance from family members when appropriate.
5. Relate medical disorders to drinking if applicable.
6. Encourage attempts to stop or reduce use.

c) Refer to an addiction specialist.

1. Especially if there is life impairment and the patient is not compliant with lifestyle changes or the initial interventions are not effective

4) Tracking outcomes

a) Use quantitative measures, not just abstinent versus not abstinent.

1. Valid measure (incorporate to electronic medical record if possible)
2. Number of heavy drinking days (more than five drinks in the past month)
3. AUDIT or AUDIT-C

b) Gamma-glutamyl transferase (GGT)

1. Helpful to track if initially elevated

5) Available ARMs[43]

a) Naltrexone 50 mg by mouth daily or twice a day[44]

1. Blocks mu-opioid receptor
2. Compared to placebo, reduced risk of heavy drinking by 83% and reduced drinking days by 4%

b) Acamprosate

1. Modulates glutamate neurotransmission
2. Compared to placebo, reduced rate of any drinking (RR 0.86, NNT = 9) and increased abstinence duration by 11 days, but not found to have an effect on heavy drinking

c) Second-line medications

1. Disulfiram 250 mg by mouth daily
    a. An aversion agent that inhibits aldehyde dehydrogenase, therefore, acetaldehyde (a metabolite of alcohol) builds up and leads to unpleasant side effects (nausea, vomiting, headache, sweating, etc.)
    b. Has high rates of non-compliance and is not found to be more effective than a placebo
2. Gabapentin 300–600 mg by mouth two to three times a day
    a. Abstinent rates were higher in 900 and 1800 mg/day gabapentin groups (11%, 17%) than placebo (4%) over a 12-week treatment course.
    b. Well tolerated, but there's a concern for possible abuse potential
3. Topiramate, starting at 100–150 mg by mouth twice a day
    a. Off-label use for AUD treatment
    b. Decreased percentage of heavy drinking days versus placebo over 14 weeks (43.8% versus 51.8%)

SECTION 9 GLOSSARY

Alcohol use disorders (AUD): refer to disorders related to drinking alcoholic beverages.

Anti-relapse medications (ARMs): treatments that help prevent relapse in people with alcohol use disorder.

E-cigarette or vaping associated lung injury (EVALI): lung disease associated with the use of vaping products that can be severe and life-threatening. Symptoms can initially mimic common pulmonary diagnoses like pneumonia, but individuals typically do not respond to antibiotic therapy. Individuals usually seek care within a few days to several weeks when symptoms first arise. EVALI remains a diagnosis of exclusion because, at present, no specific test or marker exists for its diagnosis, and evaluation should be guided by clinical judgment.

NIAAA: National Institute on Alcohol Abuse and Alcoholism

Nicotine: a highly addictive chemical used in tobacco products. Nicotine dependence is the most common form of chemical dependence in the US.

Nicotine replacement therapy (NRT): medications that are used to help people quit smoking by providing some small doses of nicotine to the user.

SECTION 9 REVIEW QUESTIONS

1. **Which behavior is the single largest preventable cause of morbidity and mortality in the US?**
   - **A.** Alcohol use
   - **B.** Unprotected sexual intercourse
   - **C.** Tobacco use
   - **D.** Intravenous drug use
2. **Which of the following is most effective when counseling a patient about smoking cessation?**
   - **A.** Tell them quitting is a simple and easy task.
   - **B.** Stress that one cessation attempt is their only chance for success.
   - **C.** Encourage them to quit smoking "cold turkey" or all at once.
   - **D.** Use open ended questions and reinforce change talk.
3. **Which is true about smoking cessation?**
   - **A.** It leads to a 20% reduction in the risk of heart disease after a year of smoking cessation.
   - **B.** Quitting at age 30 leads to the same gain in life expectancy as quitting at age 60.
   - **C.** It leads to a reduction in the risk of premature death.
   - **D.** Most smokers do not want to quit.
4. **Which treatment for smoking cessation is most effective?**
   - **A.** Counseling
   - **B.** Medication
   - **C.** Hypnosis
   - **D.** Counseling and medication
5. **Which of the following includes a list of all FDA-approved first-line medication options for smoking cessation?**
   - **A.** Varenicline, clonidine, nicotine patches
   - **B.** Bupropion, nicotine gum, nortriptyline
   - **C.** Nicotine patches, varenicline, bupropion SR
   - **D.** Naltrexone, nicotine lozenges, nicotine patches
6. **Which statement is true about smoking cessation for the following special populations?**
   - **A.** First-line for bipolar patients is bupropion.
   - **B.** Counseling is the best option for smoking cessation in pregnant smokers.
   - **C.** Nicotine replacement therapy is not an option for adolescents.
   - **D.** Patients with cardiovascular disease are at higher risk of acute coronary syndrome if using nicotine replacement therapy (NRT).
7. **Which of the following represents the 5A's model for smoking cessation?**
   - **A.** Assist, Argue, Allow, Assist, Advise
   - **B.** Admit, Assess, Agree, Assist, Arrange
   - **C.** Address, Arrange, Allow, Agree, Assist
   - **D.** Ask, Advise, Assess, Assist, Arrange

8. **"At-risk drinking" is defined as:**

   A. Drinking to avoid alcohol withdrawal symptoms

   B. Drinking that increases the risk of future problems, but with no current symptoms

   C. Getting a DUI

   D. Alcohol dependence

9. **Which patient would be characterized as having moderate alcohol use disorder (AUD)?**

   A. A woman who has 1–2 drinks, 5 nights per week over 12 months.

   B. A male who has no more than 4 drinks on any single day and no more than 14 drinks per week over 12 months.

   C. A male who does not like to go to a party if there is not going to be alcohol there, has developed tolerance to alcohol use, wakes up craving vodka, and has experienced alcohol withdrawal over a 12-month period.

   D. A woman who has lost custody of her children because of her drinking, does not like to go to a party if there is not going to be alcohol there, has developed tolerance to alcohol use, wakes up craving vodka, has experienced alcohol withdrawal, drives drunk, and has tried to quit five times without success, all over 12 months.

10. **Which of the following includes a list of all anti-relapse medications (ARMs) for alcohol use disorder?**

   A. Nortriptyline, topiramate, clonidine

   B. Acamprosate, varenicline, disulfaram

   C. Gabapentin, clonidine, buproprion

   D. Naltrexone, acamprosate, gabapentin

SECTION 9 REVIEW QUESTIONS ANSWERS AND EXPLANATIONS

1. **Answer: C.** According to the Centers for Disease Control and Prevention, tobacco use is the leading cause of preventable death in the US. Physical inactivity is the fourth leading risk factor for global mortality.

2. **Answer: D.** Motivational interviewing techniques are key to helping drive health behavior change. Expressing empathy, developing discrepancy, rolling with resistance, and supporting self-efficacy are the main principles of mastering motivational interviewing.

3. **Answer: C.** Quitting smoking has many significant health benefits that lead to the reduction of risk for premature death. Smoking cessation leads to a 50% reduction in the risk of heart disease after a year of smoking cessation. Quitting at age 30 adds 10 years of life expectancy versus quitting at age 60 adds only three years of life expectancy. Lastly, more than two-thirds of current smokers want to quit completely.

4. **Answer: D.** The combination of counseling and medication is more effective than either alone, and hypnosis is less effective than either counseling or medication.

5. **Answer C.** Nicotine patches, varenicline, and bupropion are first-line medications for tobacco cessation. Clonidine and nortriptyline are currently second-line medications for tobacco cessation. They should be prescribed on a case-by-case basis when first-line medications are contraindicated or have not been effective.

6. **Answer: B.** Counseling is the best option for pregnant smokers, as there could be a potential risk of congenital disabilities with nicotine replacement therapies (NRT). Bipolar patients should not use bupropion but can use the patch. NRT is safe for adolescents. There is no association between nicotine patch use and acute coronary syndrome.

7. **Answer: D.** The 5A's model for tobacco cessation helps to facilitate behavior change. It is comprised of Ask, Advise, Assess, Assist, Arrange.

8. **Answer: B.** At-risk drinking is drinking that increases the risk for future problems, but with no current symptoms, binge drinking ≥1 time a month, or exceeding the low-risk drinking guidelines at any time. Getting a DUI is considered a sign of alcohol use disorder (AUD) as it is continued use despite adverse consequences. Drinking to avoid withdrawal symptoms is not part of the definition of at-risk drinking or AUD. "Alcohol abuse and dependence" was the DSM-4 terminology for AUD.

9. **Answer: C.** Alcohol use disorder (AUD) is diagnosed by the presence of at least 2 out of 11 possible signs or symptoms of DSM-5 AUD criteria during a 12-month period. Moderate AUD is categorized by the presence of 4–5 signs or symptoms that occur over a 12-month period.

10. **Answer: D.** Anti-relapse medications include naltrexone, acamprosate, disulfiram, gabapentin, and topiramate.

SECTION 9 REFERENCES

1. Centers for Disease Control and Prevention. The health consequences of smoking. 2014. https://www.ncbi.nlm.nih.gov/books/NBK179276/pdf/Bookshelf_NBK179276.pdf. Accessed December 2, 2020.
2. Centers for Disease Control and Prevention. Tobacco use. March 18, 2019. https://www.cdc.gov/chronicdisease/resources/publications/factsheets/tobacco.htm. Accessed December 2, 2020.
3. Centers for Disease Control and Prevention. Fact sheet: health effects of smoking. April 28 2020. https://www.cdc.gov/tobacco/data_statistics/fact_sheets/health_effects/effects_cig_smoking/index.htm. Accessed December 2, 2020.
4. Caffrey M. Obesity tops list of causes for lost years of life beating tobacco. The American Journal of Managed Care. April 24, 2017. http://www.ajmc.com/newsroom/obesity-tops-list-of-causes-for-lost-years-of-life-beating-tobacco. Accessed 2018.
5. National Institutes of Health. Health effects. https://smokefree.gov/quitting-smoking/reasons-quit/health-effects. Accessed September, 2017.
6. Centers for Disease Control and Prevention. Smoking and diabetes. March 23, 2020. https://www.cdc.gov/tobacco/campaign/tips/diseases/diabetes.html. Accessed May 27, 2020.
7. Centers for Disease Control and Prevention. Quitting smoking: smoking and tobacco use 2017. February 1, 2017. https://www.cdc.gov/tobacco/data_statistics/fact_sheets/cessation/quitting/index.htm. Accessed September 10, 2017.
8. World Health Organization. Fact sheet about health benefits of smoking cessation. http://www.who.int/tobacco/quitting/en_tfi_quitting_fact_sheet.pdf. Accessed September 10, 2017.
9. Sachs DPL, Leone FT, Farber HJ, et al. Smoking and tobacco use. In: *American College of Chest Physicians Tobacco-Dependence Treatment Tool Kit*, 3rd ed. Northbrook, IL: American College of Chest Physicians; 2009.
10. Centers for Disease Control and Prevention. Smoking and cancer. March 23, 2020. https://www.cdc.gov/tobacco/campaign/tips/diseases/cancer.html. Accessed September 4, 2020.
11. Fiore M. C., Jaén C. R., Baker T. B., et al. *Treating Tobacco Use and Dependence: 2008 Update.* Rockville, MD: US Department of Health and Human Services. Public Health Service; 2008.
12. American Academy of Family Physicians. Treating tobacco dependence. http://www.aafp.org/dam/AAFP/documents/patient_care/tobacco/ask-act-clinician-presentation.pdf. Accessed September 10, 2020.
13. Molyneux A. Nicotine replacement therapy. *BMJ.* 2004;328(7437):454-456.
14. Stahl S. M., Pradko J. F., Haight B. R., Modell J. G., Rockett C. B., Learned-Coughlin S. A review of the neuropharmacology of bupropion, a dual norepinephrine and dopamine reuptake inhibitor. *Prim Care Companion J Clin Psychiatry.* 2004;6(4):159-166.
15. Missouri Department of Mental Health. Toolkits and clinical guidelines for tobacco cessation. https://dmh.mo.gov/mental-illness/tobacco/toolkits-and-guides. Accessed December 3, 2020.
16. Epocrates. Nicotine transdermal. https://online.epocrates.com/drugs/102313/nicotine-transdermal/Pregnancy-Lactation. Accessed December 3, 2020.
17. Epocrates. Nicotine transmucosal. https://online.epocrates.com/drugs/3580/nicotine-transmucosal. Accessed December 2, 2020.
18. Centers for Disease Control and Prevention. Electronic cigarettes. September 9, 2020. https://www.cdc.gov/tobacco/basic_information/e-cigarettes/. Accessed December 3, 2020.
19. Blount B. C., Karwowski M. P., Shields P. G., et al. Vitamin e acetate in bronchoalveolar-lavage fluid associated with EVALI. *N Engl J Med.* 2020;382(8):697-705.
20. Centers for Disease Control and Prevention. Youth and tobacco use. https://www.cdc.gov/tobacco/data_statistics/fact_sheets/youth_data/tobacco_use/index.htm. Accessed December 2, 2020.
21. Kaiser Family Foundation. State medicaid program coverage of tobacco dependence treatments by type of coverage. 2018. https://www.kff.org/medicaid/state-indicator/cessation-treatment-under-medicaid/?currentTimeframe=0&sortModel=%7B%22colId%22:%22Location%22,%22sort%22:%22asc%22%7D. Accessed December 2, 2020.
22. Medical Learning Network. Counseling to prevent tobacco use; MM7133. Center for Medicare and Medicaid Service. 2009. https://www.cms.gov/Outreach-and-Education/Medicare-Learning-Network-MLN/MLNMattersArticles/Downloads/MM7133.pdf. Accessed March 16, 2021
23. Centers for Disease Control and Prevention. STATE system Medicaid coverage of tobacco cessation treatments fact sheet. March 18, 2020; https://www.cdc.gov/statesystem/factsheets/medicaid/Cessation.html. June 29, 2020.
24. CDC WONDER: Underlying Cause of Death, 1999–2018. Centers for Disease Control and Prevention; 2018. Updated December 3, 2020. https://wonder.cdc.gov/. Accessed March 12, 2020.
25. National Institute on Alcohol Abuse and Alcoholism. Understanding alcohol use disorder. https://www.niaaa.nih.gov/alcohol-health/overview-alcohol-consumption/alcohol-use-disorders. Accessed Dec 2, 2020.
26. Egger G., Binns A., Rossner S. *Lifestyle Medicine: Managing Diseases of Lifestyle in the 21st Century.* New York, NY: mcGraw-Hill; 2010.
27. Centers for Disease Control and Prevention. Binge drinking prevalence frequency, and intensity among adults – United States, 2010; morbidity and mortality weekly report. January 2012. https://www.cdc.gov/mmwr/preview/mmwrhtml/mm6101a4.htm. Accessed 2017.
28. National Institute on Alcohol Abuse and Alcoholism. Helping patients who drink too much: a clinician's guide. January 2007. https://pubs.niaaa.nih.gov/publications/Practitioner/CliniciansGuide2005/clinicians_guide.htm. Accessed Septermber 10, 2017.
29. Centers for Disease Control and Prevention. Dietary guidelines for alcohol. December 30, 2019; https://www.cdc.gov/alcohol/fact-sheets/moderate-drinking.htm.

30. American Psychiatric Association. *Diagnostic and Statistical Manual of Mental Disorders (DSM-5)*. 5th ed. Arlington, VA: American Psychiatric Publishing; 2013.
31. National Institute of Alcohol Abuse and Alcoholism. Alcohol use disorder: a comparison between DSM–IV and DSM–5. 2016. https://pubs.niaaa.nih.gov/publications/dsmfactsheet/dsmfact.htm.
32. Agrawal A., Heath A. C., Lynskey M. T. DSM-IV to DSM-5: the impact of proposed revisions on diagnosis of alcohol use disorders. *Addiction (Abingdon, England)*. 2011;106(11):1935-1943.
33. Rubinsky A. D., Kivlahan D. R., Volk R. J., Maynard C., Bradley K. A. Estimating risk of alcohol dependence using alcohol screening scores. *Drug Alcohol Depend*. 2010;108(1-2):29-36.
34. World Health Organization. *AUDIT: The Alcohol Use Disorders Identification Test*. Geneva, Switzerland; World Health Organization; 2001. https://www.drugabuse.gov/sites/default/files/files/AUDIT.pdf.
35. Dawson D. A., Li T. K., Grant B. F. A prospective study of risk drinking: at risk for what? *Drug Alcohol Depend.* 2008;95(1-2):62-72.
36. Saha T. D., Chou S. P., Grant B. F. Toward an alcohol use disorder continuum using item response theory: results from the National Epidemiologic Survey on Alcohol and Related Conditions. *Psychol Med.* 2006;36(7):931-941.
37. Moss H. B., Chen C. M., Yi H. Y. Subtypes of alcohol dependence in a nationally representative sample. *Drug Alcohol Depend.* 2007;91(2-3):149-158.
38. Gould J. F., Treyvaud K., Yelland L. N., et al. Does n-3 LCPUFA supplementation during pregnancy increase the IQ of children at school age? Follow-up of a randomised controlled trial. *BMJ Open.* 2016;6(5):e011465.
39. Whitlock E. P., Polen M. R., Green C. A., Orleans T., Klein J. Behavioral counseling interventions in primary care to reduce risky/harmful alcohol use by adults: a summary of the evidence for the US Preventive Services Task Force. *Ann Intern Med.* 2004;140(7):557-568.
40. O'Malley S. S., Rounsaville B. J., Farren C., et al. Initial and maintenance naltrexone treatment for alcohol dependence using primary care vs specialty care: a nested sequence of 3 randomized trials. *Arch Intern Med.* 2003;163(14):1695-1704.
41. Institute for Quality and Efficiency in Health Care. Depression: How effective are antidepressants? InformedHealth.org. https://www.ncbi.nlm.nih.gov/books/NBK361016/. Updated June 18 2020. Accessed 12/1/2020.
42. Jonas D. E., Amick H. R., Feltner C., et al. Pharmacotherapy for adults with alcohol use disorders in outpatient settings: a systematic review and meta-analysis. *JAMA.* 2014;311(18):1889-1900.
43. Jung Y. C., Namkoong K. Pharmacotherapy for alcohol dependence: anticraving medications for relapse prevention. *Yonsei Med J.* 2006;47(2):167-178.
44. Seneviratne C., Johnson B. A. Advances in medications and tailoring treatment for alcohol use disorder. *Alcohol Res.* 2015;37(1):15-28.

SECTION 10
The Role of Connectedness and Positive Psychology

Objective 1 Identify lifestyle interventions that promote emotional well-being **322**

Objective 2 Explain how physical activity affects emotional well-being **322**

Objective 3 Describe the role sleep plays in emotional well-being **323**

Objective 4 Describe the science of how a plant-based diet impacts emotional well-being **323**

Objective 5 Apply positive psychology in motivational interviewing and health behavior change counseling. **325**

Objective 6 Describe how positive psychology and emotional well-being support achieving and sustaining healthy behaviors **326**

Objective 7 Compare and contrast eudaimonia and hedonia.................. **327**

Objective 8 Explain how eudaimonia relates to physical health and longevity **327**

Objective 9 Describe how connectedness and social networks affect emotional well-being, physical health, and longevity **328**

Objective 10 State the effect social media has on one's emotional well-being. **328**

Section 10 Glossary... **329**

Section 10 Review Questions **330**

Section 10 Review Question Answers and Summaries **331**

Section 10 References... **332**

OBJECTIVE 1

Identify lifestyle interventions that promote emotional well-being

1) **A healthy lifestyle should promote mental and emotional well-being as well as physical health.**

2) **Therapeutic lifestyle change (TLC) to address mental health and emotional well-being**

   a) TLC can be as effective as psychotherapy and pharmacotherapy.[1]

      1. TLC can help treat and control multiple mental disorders; preserve and improve cognitive processing; and cultivate personal and social well-being, including in adolescents.[2,3]
      2. Diet, sleep, and physical activity play an especially important role in the prevention, progression, and treatment of major depression and anxiety.[4,5]
      3. TLC interventions include:
         a. Exercise and physical activity
         b. Nutrition and diet
         c. Time in nature
         d. Supportive relationships
         e. Recreation, relaxation, and stress management
         f. Religious or spiritual involvement
         g. Service to others
         h. Modification of sleeping patterns

OBJECTIVE 2

Explain how physical activity affects emotional well-being[6,7,8,9,10]

1) **Physical activity can improve mood and reduce symptoms of depression and anxiety.[11]**

2) **Exercise has shown a small positive effect on treatment of depression compared to no treatment or control treatment (pharmacology and psychology interventions). However, exercise alone has not yet been shown to be better than psychotherapy or pharmacotherapy.**

3) **Exercise is as effective as pharmacotherapy for mild to moderate depression. Further longitudinal studies are needed to examine the dose-response relationship for exercise and depression.[12]**

4) **Some studies show a synergistic effect of exercise in combination with antidepressant medications.**

5) **Exercise may be an effective treatment for depression in the elderly.**

6) **Routine physical activity in childhood may be protective against depression as a young adult.**

OBJECTIVE 3

Describe the role sleep plays in emotional well-being

1) **Among ~100,000 Japanese young adults, those who slept 7–9 hours a night had improved mental health compared to those who slept less than 7 or more than 9. There was also a linear relationship between sleep quality and mental health.[13]**

2) **A sleep intervention directed at a sample of the UK student population led to a reduction in symptoms of depression, anxiety, and psychosis following improved sleep.[14] A sample of 3,755 students from 26 UK universities were assigned to digital cognitive behavioral therapy (CBT) intervention or usual practice. Measures of insomnia, paranoia, and hallucinations were all lower in the treatment group at the end of a 10-week intervention.**

OBJECTIVE 4

Describe the science of how a plant-based diet impacts emotional well-being

1) **Mood disorders and an unhealthy diet**
   - **a)** Depression was more likely to develop in adults who frequently ate fast food compared to those who avoided it, HR 1.36 (CI 95% CI 1.02, 1.81; P trend = 0.003).[15]
   - **b)** An increased rate of depression occurs in a linear dose-response curve with higher *trans*-fat intake, whereas depression is negatively associated with intake of mono- and poly-unsaturated fats.[16]
   - **c)** Fried foods, refined grains, sugary products, and beer were associated with higher rates of anxiety and depression in adult Australian and Norwegian women, whereas a "traditional" diet of fruit, vegetables, whole grains, fish, and meat was associated with lower rates.[17,18]
   - **d)** Preliminary randomized control trial evidence now exists for a link between improved diet and relief of major depressive episodes.[19] In this study "improved diet" consisted mostly of whole grains, vegetables, fruits, legumes, and nuts, with small allowances for fish, lean meats, eggs, and olive oil. "Extras" foods, such as sweets, refined cereals, fried food, fast-food, processed meats, sugary drinks, and alcohol were also reduced.
   - **e)** Dietary patterns, rather than nutrient deficiencies, are likely to account for the incidence of depression, according to a meta-analysis of 21 studies from 10 countries.[20] A dietary pattern characterized by high intakes of fruit, vegetables, whole grain, fish, olive oil, low-fat dairy, and antioxidants, and low intakes of animal foods, was associated with a decreased risk of depression. A dietary pattern characterized by a high consumption of red and/or processed meat, refined grains, sweets, high-fat dairy products, butter, potatoes, and high-fat gravy, and low intakes of fruits and vegetables, is associated with an increased risk of depression.

2) **Mood disorders and nutrients**
   - **a)** Higher rates of mood disorders are seen with deficiencies in folate, vitamin B12, calcium, iron, selenium, zinc, and omega-3 fatty acids.[21,22]
   - **b)** Some studies show fish oil may help reduce symptoms of depression. However, other studies show little benefit of treating depression with fatty acids.[22]

c) Treatment with omega-3 fatty acids does appear beneficial among some populations, such as those with depression or bipolar disorder. A short 4-month trial among patients with bipolar disorder showed longer periods of remission when they were treated with omega-3 fatty acids. Fatty acids were well-tolerated.[23,24]

d) The data suggest that some nutritional supplements may be useful as adjunctive therapies in the treatment of mental disorders.[25]

3) Diets high in plant foods and emotional well-being

a) Fruit and vegetable consumption have been associated with:

1. Increased eudemonic feelings (engagement, meaning, and purpose) and behaviors (curiosity and creativity) among young adults[26]
2. Improvement in depression, anxiety, and productivity[27]
3. Lower scores for mood disturbance among men and women, lower anxiety scores among men, and lower stress scores among women[28]
4. Significant improvement in mood scores in 2 weeks for omnivores placed on a vegetarian diet (no fish or meat intake)[29]
5. Significantly, there are fewer negative emotions among vegetarians than omnivores, despite the lower intake of long-chain omega-3 fatty acids.[30]
6. Higher optimism[31]
7. Improved health, quality of life, and productivity in the workplace[32]
8. Lower risk of depression in adults[33]
9. More positive attitudes on the day foods are eaten and on the following day among healthy young adults. This suggests that fruit and vegetable intake is the cause of a more positive attitude and not the reverse.[34]
10. Increases in scores for vitality, flourishing, and motivation in 14 days in young adults who were provided with two additional servings of fruits and vegetables a day on top of their normal diets. This suggests fruit and vegetable intake is important for psychological benefits.[35]

b) Studies have shown improvement in mood with intake of saffron, turmeric, probiotics, flaxseeds, walnuts, and carbohydrate-rich evening meals.[1,4,36,37] While long term efficacy (beyond 8 weeks) is not yet established, the results are promising for curcumin, an active ingredient in turmeric, in particular.[38]

4) A plant-based diet and the potential mechanisms of action for improved mental health and emotional well-being[1,27,28,29,30,32,33]

a) While the current evidence does not support causation, there is evidence of association between some nutrients and mood. For example, arachidonic acid, which is found in chicken and eggs, is associated with increased depression rates. A reduction in suicide risk in pregnant women may also be associated with avoidance of arachidonic acid.[39]

b) Vitamin C is a co-factor for the neurotransmitter dopamine production. This may support improvement and/or stability of mood.[26]

5) Mood and eating patterns

a) A positive mood helps one resist the temptation of unhealthy snacks through activating the centers of the brain that control long-term goals, such as health.[40,41]

b) In adolescent girls, 11–19 years old, happiness was significantly associated with lower body mass index (BMI), fruit and vegetable consumption, physical activity, meaningful time with family, and no exposure to second-hand smoke.[42]

c) In Chilean college students, being "very happy" was associated with eating fruits and vegetables daily, being physically active daily, having a favorable view of stress, and being younger and female.[43]

6) **A brief overview of meditation, mindfulness, and emotional well-being**

a) The field of mindfulness currently requires more research and more rigorous study design. In particular, a uniform definition of mindfulness is needed.[44]

1. Mindfulness can mildly lower stress scores even in people who have mental health disorders, such as depression or anxiety.[45]
2. College students who practiced mindfulness reported lower stress levels, less use of avoidance, and greater use of assertive coping skills like addressing the situation.[46]

b) Meditation can result in mild to moderate reductions in the negative dimensions of mental stress.[47]

7) **The provider's role in promoting emotional well-being activities for patients is to:**

a) Be mindful that all the major elements of a lifestyle medicine approach (involving attention to diet, exercise, sleep, social support, substance avoidance, and stress management) potentiate emotional well-being and mental health.

b) Prescribe dosed therapeutic lifestyle change as part of a treatment plan for mental and emotional wellness.

OBJECTIVE 5

Apply positive psychology in motivational interviewing and health behavior change counseling

1) **Positive psychology**

a) Positive psychology is the study of that which allows individuals and communities to thrive. It does not minimize misery or even the experience of negative emotional states, but focuses on amplifying well-being through positive affect, engagement, and meaning.[48]

b) Consider this definition: A scientific approach to studying human thoughts, feelings, and behavior, with a focus on strengths instead of weaknesses, building the good in life instead of repairing the bad, and taking the lives of average people up to "great" instead of focusing solely on moving those who are struggling up to "normal."[49]

c) Positive affect is defined as the experience of pleasurable emotions arising from engagement in one's environment, contentment with the past, happiness in the present, and hope for the future.

2) **Pillars of positive psychology (PERMA)[50]**

a) Positive emotion: the ability to be optimistic and the ability to view the past, present, and future in a positive fashion.

b) Engagement: being fully absorbed into the present moment with a "blissful immersion" that stretches intelligence, skill, and emotional capacity.

c) Relationship: one of the most important aspects of life is the development of positive social connections with other humans emotionally and physically. From a neuro-imaging perspective, social isolation looks neurologically like physical pain.[51]

d) Meaning: having a purpose for why one is on the Earth is important to living a life of fulfillment and happiness. Meaning also encompasses the value one places upon activities, one's views, and one's attitudes.

e) Accomplishments: having ambition and accomplishing realistic goals produces a sense of satisfaction, pride, and fulfillment.

3) Individual virtues and strengths are used to increase our experience of engagement

1. Character strengths include: appreciation of beauty and excellence, bravery, creativity, curiosity, fairness, forgiveness, gratitude, honesty, hope, humility, humor, judgement, kindness, leadership, love, love of learning, perseverance, perspective, prudence, self-regulation, social intelligence, spirituality, and teamwork.
2. See a free online inventory at https://www.viacharacter.org.

4) Positive emotions and chronic disease

a) The use of positive psychology activities in patients with chronic disease increases positive emotions and produces emotional well-being. It also lowers the risk of distressing thoughts and lowers the risk of suicidal ideation in those patients.[52]

5) Health promotion and positive psychology

a) The direct impact of positive psychology on physical diseases needs further research. Links between positive psychological assets (optimism, life satisfaction, positive emotions, purpose, and social support) have been prospectively associated with better health. However, it is not yet known if positive psychology is an effective treatment for chronic illnesses such as diabetes, heart disease, or cancer.[53] Impacts of positive psychology interventions on well-being and depression show small, but significant, impact.[54]

OBJECTIVE 6

Describe how positive psychology and emotional well-being support achieving and sustaining healthy behaviors

1) Positive psychology is a key framework for intervention in behavior change therapy.

2) Health providers should:

a) Continue screening, diagnosing, and referring to mental health providers (as appropriate).

b) In addition to the above they should:

1. Prescribe positive psychology activities, such as those listed below.
2. Leverage positive psychology in behavior change conversations.

3) Positive psychology practical techniques and specific actions[55,56]

a) Habits for emotional well-being

1. Finding and improving signature strengths[57]
2. Counting blessings[57,58]
3. Expressing appreciation[57,58,59]
4. Savoring the pleasing things in life[57,59]
5. Writing down how one wants to be remembered[57]
6. Regularly practicing acts of kindness[57,58,59]

7. Thinking of one's happiest days frequently[57]
8. Doing activities that feel meaningful[57,59,60]
9. Connecting and interacting with others regularly in person and not solely or mainly through social media[57,60]

OBJECTIVE 7

Compare and contrast eudaimonia and hedonia

1) **The authors Deci and Ryan define eudaimonia as, "concerned with living well or actualizing one's human potentials. This conceptualization maintains that well-being is not so much an outcome or end state as it is a process of fulfilling or realizing one's 'daimon' or true nature—that is, of fulfilling one's virtuous potentials and living as one was inherently intended to live."[61]**

2) **Eudaimonia may contain aspects of meaningful goal-directedness unique from hedonia.[62]**

3) **Hedonia is well-being created by maximizing one's happiness and characterized by the presence of positive emotions and expressions, the absence of negative emotions and expressions, and the satisfaction of desires.[61,62]**

OBJECTIVE 8

Explain how eudaimonia relates to physical health and longevity[63]

1) **Having a purpose in life is important in mitigating disease risk and promoting longevity.**

- **a)** A high purpose in life was associated with a reduction in mortality among elderly people in the community (HR 0.60).
- **b)** Those with a high score for life purpose were less likely to be diagnosed with Alzheimer's disease or mild cognitive impairment and had a slower rate of cognitive decline.[64]
- **c)** The Health and Retirement Study showed older individuals with higher levels of life purpose were less likely to have strokes and heart attacks and were more likely to participate in preventive labs and screening exams.[65,66]
- **d)** Individuals with chronic conditions who responded with higher levels of purpose in life, positive relationships, and positive affect had lower levels of inflammatory markers Interleukin-6 (IL-6) and C-reactive protein (CRP).[67]
- **e)** Eudaimonia is associated with gene regulation: pro-inflammatory genes are downregulated while antibody synthesis genes are upregulated. Hedonia is associated with the opposite pattern.[68,69]
- **f)** Neuroscience shows higher psychological well-being is associated with less activation of the amygdala, more engagement of higher cortical function with negative stimuli, and sustained activation of the reward circuit with positive stimuli.[70]
- **g)** Having a purpose in life appears to aid adaptive and protective functions, such as quicker recovery from negative events.[71]
- **h)** Eudaimonia well-being was positively associated with greater insular cortex grey matter volume.[72]

OBJECTIVE 9

Describe how connectedness and social networks affect emotional well-being, physical health, and longevity[73]

1) **Connection is the "quality, state, or capability to be connected," as defined by Merriam-Webster.[74]**
   a) Longevity, health, and physiologic measures, such as heart rate, are improved with positive resonance and micro-moments of connection.[73,75]
      1. Positive resonance means social interactions characterized by shared positivity, mutual care, and concern.[75]
      2. Micro-moments of connection are brief authentic social interactions.
2) **Connection mechanism**
   a) Connection and nurturing activate the parasympathetic nervous system, in contrast to experiences of unmanaged stress, which activate the sympathetic nervous system.
3) **Social connection and longevity**
   a) A 75-year cohort study on adult development looked at 268 male Harvard students from graduating years 1939–1944 and 456 men from inner city Boston and concluded that the single most important predictor of happiness and longevity is having social connections.[76,77]

OBJECTIVE 10

State the effect social media has on one's emotional well-being

1) **Social media use and mood**
   a) A sample of 1,787 young adults, aged 19–32, were asked about their social media use. Those in the highest quartile for social media use had significantly higher rates of depression (adjusted odds ratio = 2.74, 95% CI = 1.86–4.04) than those in the lowest quartile. Causation could not be assessed from this trial. Results were linear in a dose dependent trend.[78]
   b) 44% of a sample of young adults in the US reported problematic social media use (PSMU). PSMU is strongly and independently associated with depressive symptoms. Frequency of social media use may be a distinct behavioral component of PSMU.[79]
   c) A study of media use, sleep quality, and well-being in 467 adolescents, which examined emotional investment in social media and overall versus nighttime-specific use found social media use is associated with poor sleep, anxiety, depression, and low self-esteem; poor sleep is most strongly associated with nighttime-specific social media use; anxiety and depression are most strongly associated with emotional investment in sites.[80]
   d) Patterns of social media use (SMU), rather than single aspects of SMU (e.g., quantity, frequency) appear to relate more strongly to mental health outcomes.[81]

SECTION 10 GLOSSARY

Connection: developing and maintaining a relationship with another person, such that emotional experiences can be shared.

Eudaimonia: is concerned with living well or actualizing one's human potential. This conceptualization maintains that well-being is not so much an outcome or end state as it is a process of fulfilling or realizing one's "daimon" or true nature—that is, of fulfilling one's virtuous potentials and living as one was inherently intended to live.

Hedonia: happiness is characterized by the presence of positive emotions and expressions, the absence of negative emotions and expressions, and the satisfaction of desires.

Micro-moment of connection: brief and authentic social interaction.

Positive affect: the experience of pleasurable emotions arising from engagement in one's environment.

Positive psychology: the study of human thoughts, feelings, and behavior, with a focus on strengths and virtues that allow individuals and communities to thrive. It does not minimize misery, but focuses on amplifying happiness through positive affect and building the good in life instead of repairing the bad.

Positive resonance: positive social interaction characterized by shared positivity, mutual care, and concern.

Therapeutic lifestyle changes: using positive lifestyle changes, such as improving diet, activity, sleep, relationships, substance use and spirituality, to address and support mental health and emotional well-being. Dosing is considered relevant.

SECTION 10 REVIEW QUESTIONS

1. **Which is the best example of a recommended intervention for a patient with mild depression?**
   - **A.** Low-carb diet combined with resistance exercise
   - **B.** Focus on relationships and religious community involvement
   - **C.** High protein, low-fat diet combined with service to others
   - **D.** A diet high in fruits and vegetables, low in saturated fat, regular physical activity, combined with cognitive behavioral therapy

2. **Which of the following statements is the most accurate with respect to a plant-based diet and mental health?**
   - **A.** Depression is no more likely to develop in adults who frequently eat fast food compared to those who avoided it.
   - **B.** An increased rate of depression occurs in a linear dose-response curve with higher monosaturated-fat intake.
   - **C.** A plant-based diet has been shown to alleviate depression symptoms in those changing from a Western diet pattern.
   - **D.** Fish oil is the most effective therapeutic nutraceutical to treat depression.

3. **Which of the following is a demonstrated effect of a plant-based diet on emotional well-being?**
   - **A.** Increased eudemonic feelings (engagement, meaning, and purpose) and behaviors (curiosity and creativity) in young adults
   - **B.** Young adults receive little to no benefit from increased fruit and vegetable intake
   - **C.** Decreased productivity in the workplace
   - **D.** Higher scores for mood disturbance among men and women, lower anxiety scores among men, and higher stress scores among women

4. **Which of the following combinations of habits is least likely to support emotional well-being?**
   - **A.** Finding and improving signature strengths and regularly practicing acts of kindness.
   - **B.** Doing activities that feel pleasurable and interacting with others regularly through social media.
   - **C.** Expressing appreciation and writing down how one wants to be remembered.
   - **D.** Savoring the pleasing things in life, counting blessings, and thinking of one's happiest days frequently.

5. **Which of the following is the best example of "M" in the PERMA model of positive psychology?**
   - **A.** Appreciation of beauty, excellence, gratitude, and love
   - **B.** Evaluation of an activity one completes as a significant contribution to something much larger
   - **C.** Being fully absorbed into the present moment with a "blissful immersion" that stretches intelligence, skill, or emotional capacity
   - **D.** The ability to be optimistic and the ability to view the past, present, and future in a positive fashion

6. **Which of the following is an aspect of a hedonic approach to health and well-being?**
   - **A.** Seeking experiences in which meaning and purpose can be discovered or inferred.
   - **B.** Less activation of the amygdala, more engagement of higher cortical function with negative stimuli, and sustained activation of the reward circuit with positive stimuli.
   - **C.** Seeking experiences of pleasure and joy for their own sake.
   - **D.** Pro-inflammatory genes are down-regulated while antibody synthesis genes are upregulated.

SECTION 10 REVIEW QUESTION ANSWERS AND SUMMARIES

1. **Answer: D.** Of the options listed, counseling sessions with behavioral health providers combined with eating a diet high in fruits and vegetables (not necessarily a low-carbohydrate or high-protein diet), regular physical activity, and avoiding saturated fat would be most effective for mild depression. Recreation and social support could be helpful as an adjunct to other interventions.

2. **Answer: C.** The SMILES trial, conducted in Australia[19] showed a marked improvement in depressive symptomatology in adults who followed a plant-based diet, in contrast to their regular Western pattern diet. Depression is more likely to occur in those who eat fast food (HR 1.36).[15] Mono and polyunsaturated fats were associated with decreased depression whereas *trans*-fats increased rates.[16,22] Young adults reported high vitality, flourishing, and motivation within 14 days of two additional servings of fruits and vegetables to their typical diet.[35] Studies of fish oil benefits are mixed.[22]

3. **Answer: A.** A plant-based diet has been associated with increased eudemonic feelings (engagement, meaning, and purpose) and behaviors (curiosity and creativity) in young adults; lower scores for mood disturbance among men and women, lower anxiety scores among men, and lower stress scores among women; and increased productivity in the work place. There is an absence of demonstrated research to marital and relational impact.

4. **Answer: B.** Connecting and interacting with others is important. However, it is most important to regularly connect and interact with others in person and not solely or mainly through social media. The use of social media has been connected to higher rates of depression.

5. **Answer: B.** The "M" in PERMA represents "meaning." This is experienced when one perceives an activity as part of something much bigger or more purposeful.

6. **Answer: C.** Hedonia represents the experience of pleasure-seeking, largely for its own sake. Eudaimonia represents the ideas of discovering meaning and purpose in order to find what nourishes the capacity to live life in a full, purposeful, and deeply satisfying manner.

SECTION 10 REFERENCES

1. Walsh R. Lifestyle and mental health. *Am Psychol.* 2011;66(7):579-592.
2. Zaman R., Hankir A., Jemni M. Lifestyle factors and mental health. *Psychiatri Danub.* 2019;31(Suppl 3):217-220.
3. Loewen O. K., Maximova K., Ekwaru J. P., et al. Lifestyle behavior and mental health in early adolescence. *Pediatrics.* 2019;143(5).
4. Lopresti A. L., Hood S. D., Drummond P. D. A review of lifestyle factors that contribute to important pathways associated with major depression: diet, sleep and exercise. *J Affect Disord.* 2013;148(1):12-27.
5. Cheung T., Wong S. Y., Wong K. Y., et al. Depression, anxiety and symptoms of stress among baccalaureate nursing students in Hong Kong: a cross-sectional study. *Int J Environ Res Public Health.* 2016;13(8).
6. Eriksson S., Gard G. Physical exercise and depression. *Physical Therapy Reviews.* 2011;16(4):261-268. https://doi.org/10.1179/1743288X11Y.0000000026.
7. Eriksson M., Holmgren L., Janlert U., et al. Large improvements in major cardiovascular risk factors in the population of northern Sweden: the MONICA study 1986–2009. *J Intern Med.* 2011;269. http://dx.doi.org/10.1111/j.1365-2796.2010.02312.x.
8. Cooney G. M., Dwan K., Greig C. A., et al. Exercise for depression. *Cochrane Database Syst Rev.* 2013(9):Cd004366.
9. Mura G., Carta M. G. Physical activity in depressed elderly. A systematic review. *Clin Pract Epidemiol Ment Health.* 2013;9:125-135.
10. McKercher C., Sanderson K., Schmidt M. D., et al. Physical activity patterns and risk of depression in young adulthood: a 20-year cohort study since childhood. *Soc Psychiatry Psychiatr Epidemiol.* 2014;49(11):1823-1834.
11. Kandola A., Vancampfort D., Herring M., et al. Moving to beat anxiety: epidemiology and therapeutic issues with physical activity for anxiety. *Curr Psychiatry Rep.* 2018;20(8):63.
12. Netz Y. Is the comparison between exercise and pharmacologic treatment of depression in the clinical practice guideline of the american college of physicians evidence-based? *Front Pharmacol.* 2017;8:257-257. https://pubmed.ncbi.nlm.nih.gov/28555108.
13. Kaneita Y., Ohida T., Osaki Y., et al. Association between mental health status and sleep status among adolescents in Japan: a nationwide cross-sectional survey. *J Clin Psychiatry.* 2007;68(9):1426-1435.
14. Freeman D., Sheaves B., Goodwin G. M., et al. The effects of improving sleep on mental health (OASIS): a randomised controlled trial with mediation analysis. *Lancet Psychiatry.* 2017;4(10):749-758.
15. Sánchez-Villegas A., Toledo E., de Irala J., Ruiz-Canela M., Pla-Vidal J., Martínez-González M. A. Fast-food and commercial baked goods consumption and the risk of depression. *Public Health Nutr.* 2012;15(3):424-432.
16. Sánchez-Villegas A., Verberne L., De Irala J., et al. Dietary fat intake and the risk of depression: the SUN Project. *PLoS One.* 2011;6(1):e16268.
17. Jacka F. N., Pasco J. A., Mykletun A., et al. Association of Western and traditional diets with depression and anxiety in women. *Am J Psychiatry.* 2010;167(3):305-311.
18. Jacka F. N., Mykletun A., Berk M., Bjelland I., Tell G. S. The association between habitual diet quality and the common mental disorders in community-dwelling adults: the Hordaland Health study. *Psychosomat Med.* 2011;73(6):483-490.
19. Jacka F. N., O'Neil A., Opie R., et al. A randomised controlled trial of dietary improvement for adults with major depression (the 'SMILES' trial). *BMC Med.* 2017;15(1):23.
20. Li Y., Lv M. R., Wei Y. J., et al. Dietary patterns and depression risk: a meta-analysis. *Psychiatry Res.* 2017;253:373-382.
21. Leung B. M., Kaplan B. J. Perinatal depression: prevalence, risks, and the nutrition link–a review of the literature. *J Am Diet Assoc.* 2009;109(9):1566-1575.
22. Bodnar L. M., Wisner K. L. Nutrition and depression: implications for improving mental health among childbearing-aged women. *Biol Psychiatry.* 2005;58(9):679-685.
23. Bloch M. H., Hannestad J. Omega-3 fatty acids for the treatment of depression: systematic review and meta-analysis. *Mol Psychiatry.* 2012;17(12):1272-1282.
24. Stoll A. L., Severus W. E., Freeman M. P., et al. Omega 3 fatty acids in bipolar disorder: a preliminary double-blind, placebo-controlled trial. *Arch Gen Psychiatry.* 1999;56(5):407-412.
25. Sarris J., Murphy J., Mischoulon D., et al. Adjunctive nutraceuticals for depression: a systematic review and meta-analyses. *Am J Psychiatry.* 2016;173(6):575-587.
26. Conner T. S., Brookie K. L., Richardson A. C., Polak M. A. On carrots and curiosity: eating fruit and vegetables is associated with greater flourishing in daily life. *Br J Health Psychol.* 2015;20(2):413-427.
27. Agarwal U., Mishra S., Xu J., Levin S., Gonzales J., Barnard N. D. A multicenter randomized controlled trial of a nutrition intervention program in a multiethnic adult population in the corporate setting reduces depression and anxiety and improves quality of life: the GEICO study. *Am J Health Promot.* 2015;29(4):245-254. https://journals.sagepub.com/doi/10.4278/ajhp.130218-QUAN-72?url_ver=Z39.88-2003&rfr_id=ori:rid:crossref.org&rfr_dat=cr_pub%3dpubmed.
28. Beezhold B., Radnitz C., Rinne A., DiMatteo J. Vegans report less stress and anxiety than omnivores. *Nutr Neurosci.* 2015;18(7):289-296.
29. Beezhold B. L., Johnston C. S. Restriction of meat, fish, and poultry in omnivores improves mood: a pilot randomized controlled trial. *Nutr J.* 2012;11:9. https://www.ncbi.nlm.nih.gov/pmc/articles/PMC3293760/pdf/1475-2891-11-9.pdf.
30. Beezhold B. L., Johnston C. S., Daigle D. R. Vegetarian diets are associated with healthy mood states: a cross-sectional study in seventh day adventist adults. *Nutr J.* 2010;9:26.

31. Boehm J. K., Williams D. R., Rimm E. B., Ryff C., Kubzansky L. D. Association between optimism and serum antioxidants in the midlife in the United States study. *Psychosomat Med.* 2013;75(1):2-10.
32. Katcher H. I., Ferdowsian H. R., Hoover V. J., Cohen J. L., Barnard N. D. A worksite vegan nutrition program is well-accepted and improves health-related quality of life and work productivity. *Ann Nutr Metab.* 2010;56(4):245-252.
33. Lai J. S., Hiles S., Bisquera A., Hure A. J., McEvoy M., Attia J. A systematic review and meta-analysis of dietary patterns and depression in community-dwelling adults. *Am J Clin Nutr.* 2014;99(1):181-197.
34. White B. A., Horwath C. C., Conner T. S. Many apples a day keep the blues away–daily experiences of negative and positive affect and food consumption in young adults. *Br J Health Psychol.* 2013;18(4):782-798.
35. Conner T. S., Brookie K. L., Carr A. C., Mainvil L. A., Vissers M. C. Let them eat fruit! The effect of fruit and vegetable consumption on psychological well-being in young adults: a randomized controlled trial. *PLoS One.* 2017;12(2):e0171206.
36. Noorbala A. A., Akhondzadeh S., Tahmacebi-Pour N., Jamshidi A. H. Hydro-alcoholic extract of Crocus sativus L. versus fluoxetine in the treatment of mild to moderate depression: a double-blind, randomized pilot trial. *J Ethnopharmacol.* 2005;97(2):281-284.
37. Wurtman R. J., Wurtman J. J., Regan M. M., McDermott J. M., Tsay R. H., Breu J. J. Effects of normal meals rich in carbohydrates or proteins on plasma tryptophan and tyrosine ratios. *Am J Clin Nutr.* 2003;77(1):128-132.
38. Ng Q. X., Koh S. S. H., Chan H. W., Ho C. Y. X. Clinical use of curcumin in depression: a meta-analysis. *J Am Med Dir Assoc.* 2017;18(6):503-508.
39. Vaz J. S., Kac G., Nardi A. E., Hibbeln J. R. Corrigendum to "Omega-6 fatty acids and greater likelihood of suicide risk and major depression in early pregnancy" [*J Affect Disord.* 152-154 (2014) 76-82]. *J Affect Disord.* 2016;190:893.
40. Fedorikhin A., Patrick V. Positive mood and resistance to temptation: the interfering influence of elevated arousal. *J Consum Res.* 2010;37:698-711.
41. Gardner M. P., Wansink B., Kim J., Park S. Better moods for better eating? How mood influences food choice. *J Consum Psychol.* 2014;24(3):320-335. https://onlinelibrary.wiley.com/doi/abs/10.1016/j.jcps.2014.01.002.
42. Fararouei M., Brown I. J., Akbartabar T. M., Estakhrian H. R., Jafari J. Happiness and health behaviour in Iranian adolescent girls. *J Adolesc.* 2013;36(6):1187-1192.
43. Piqueras J. A., Kuhne W., Vera-Villarroel P., van Straten A., Cuijpers P. Happiness and health behaviours in Chilean college students: a cross-sectional survey. *BMC Public Health.* 2011;11:443.
44. Davidson R. J., Kaszniak A. W. Conceptual and methodological issues in research on mindfulness and meditation. *Am Psychol.* 2015;70(7):581-592.
45. Bohlmeijer E., Prenger R., Taal E., Cuijpers P. The effects of mindfulness-based stress reduction therapy on mental health of adults with a chronic medical disease: a meta-analysis. *J Psychosom Res.* 2010;68(6):539-544.
46. Weinstein N., Brown K., Ryan R. A multi-method examination of the effects of mindfulness on stress attribution, coping, and emotional well-being. *J Res Pers.* 2009;43:374-385.
47. Goyal M., Singh S., Sibinga E. M., et al. Meditation programs for psychological stress and well-being: a systematic review and meta-analysis. *JAMA Intern Med.* 2014;174(3):357-368.
48. Ackerman C. What is positive psychology & why is it important? June 12, 2020; https://positivepsychology.com/team/courtney-ackerman/.
49. Peterson C. What is positive psychology, and what is it not? May 16, 2008. https://www.psychologytoday.com/us/blog/the-good-life/200805/what-is-positive-psychology-and-what-is-it-not.
50. Pascha M. The PERMA model: your scientific theory of happiness. May 22, 2018. https://positivepsychologyprogram.com/perma-model/.
51. Eisenberger N. I. The neural bases of social pain: evidence for shared representations with physical pain. *Psychosomat Med.* 2012;74(2):126-135.
52. Hirsch J. K., Duberstein P. R., Unützer J. Chronic medical problems and distressful thoughts of suicide in primary care patients: mitigating role of happiness. *Int J Geriatr Psychiatry.* 2009;24(7):671-679.
53. Park N., Peterson C., Szvarca D., Vander Molen R. J., Kim E. S., Collon K. Positive psychology and physical health: research and applications. *Am J Lifestyle Med.* 2016;10(3):200-206.
54. White C. A., Uttl B., Holder M. D. Meta-analyses of positive psychology interventions: the effects are much smaller than previously reported. *PLoS One.* 2019;14(5):e0216588.
55. Pursuit of Happiness. The science of happiness and positive psychology. https://www.pursuit-of-happiness.org/science-of-happiness/.
56. Seligman M. *History of happiness: happiness is understandable, obtainable, and teachable.* https://www.pursuit-of-happiness.org/history-of-happiness/martin-seligman-psychology/.
57. Seligman M. *Flourish: A Visionary New Understanding of Happiness and Well-Being.* New York, NY: Atria Books; 2011.
58. Fredrickson B. *Positivity: Groundbreaking Research Reveals How to Embrace the Hidden Strength of Positive Emotions, Overcome Negativity, and Thrive.* New York, NY: Random House; 2009.
59. Lyubomirsky S. *The How of Happiness: A Scientific Approach to Getting the Life You Want.* New York: Penguin Press; 2007.
60. Csikszentmihalyi M. *Flow: The Psychology of Optimal Experience.* New York, NY: Harper & Row; 1990.
61. Deci E. L., Ryan R. M. Hedonia, eudaimonia, and well-being: an introduction. *J Happiness Stud.* 2008;9(1):1-11. https://doi.org/10.1007/s10902-006-9018-1.
62. Disabato D. J., Goodman F. R., Kashdan T. B., Short J. L., Jarden A. Different types of well-being? A cross-cultural examination of hedonic and eudaimonic well-being. *Psychol Assess.* 2016;28(5):471-482.
63. Ryff C. D. Psychological well-being revisited: advances in the science and practice of eudaimonia. *Psychother Psychosom.* 2014;83(1):10-28.

64. Boyle P. A., Buchman A. S., Barnes L. L., Bennett D. A. Effect of a purpose in life on risk of incident Alzheimer disease and mild cognitive impairment in community-dwelling older persons. *Arch Gen Psychiatry.* 2010;67(3):304-310.
65. Kim E. S., Sun J. K., Park N., Kubzansky L. D., Peterson C. Purpose in life and reduced risk of myocardial infarction among older US adults with coronary heart disease: a two-year follow-up. *J Behav Med.* 2013;36(2):124-133.
66. Kim E. S., Sun J. K., Park N., Peterson C. Purpose in life and reduced incidence of stroke in older adults: 'The Health and Retirement Study'. *J Psychosomat Res.* 2013;74(5):427-432.
67. Friedman E. M., Ryff C. D. Living well with medical comorbidities: a biopsychosocial perspective. *J Gerontol B Psychol Sci Soc Sci.* 2012;67(5):535-544.
68. Fredrickson B. L., Grewen K. M., Coffey K. A., et al. A functional genomic perspective on human well-being. *Proc Natl Acad Sci U S A.* 2013;110(33):13684-13689.
69. Fredrickson B. L., Grewen K. M., Algoe S. B., et al. Psychological well-being and the human conserved transcriptional response to adversity. *PLoS One.* 2015;10(3):e0121839. https://doi.org/10.1371/journal.pone.0121839.
70. van Reekum C. M., Urry H. L., Johnstone T., et al. Individual differences in amygdala and ventromedial prefrontal cortex activity are associated with evaluation speed and psychological well-being. *J Cogn Neurosci.* 2007;19(2):237-248.
71. Schaefer S. M., Morozink Boylan J., van Reekum C. M., et al. Purpose in life predicts better emotional recovery from negative stimuli. *PLoS One.* 2013;8(11):e80329.
72. Lewis G. J., Kanai R., Rees G., Bates T. C. Neural correlates of the 'good life': eudaimonic well-being is associated with insular cortex volume. *Soc Cogn Affect Neurosci.* 2014;9(5):615-618.
73. Fredrickson B. *Love 2.0: How Our Supreme Emotion Affects Everything We Feel, Think, Do and Become.* New York, NY: Penguin Group; 2013.
74. Meriam-Webster. Connection. https://www.merriam-webster.com/dictionary/connection. Accessed 2021.
75. Major B. C., Le Nguyen K. D., Lundberg K. B., Fredrickson B. L. Well-being correlates of perceived positivity resonance: evidence from trait and episode-level assessments. *Pers Soc Psychol Bull.* 2018;44(12):1631-1647. https://doi.org/10.1177/0146167218771324.
76. Grant W. T. Study of adult development. Harvard Second Generation Study. 2015. https://www.adultdevelopmentstudy.org/grantandglueckstudy. Accessed 2018.
77. Mineo L. Good genes are nice, but joy is better. *The Harvard Gazette.* April 11, 2017. https://news.harvard.edu/gazette/story/2017/04/over-nearly-80-years-harvard-study-has-been-showing-how-to-live-a-healthy-and-happy-life/.
78. Lin L. Y., Sidani J. E., Shensa A., et al. Association between social media use and depression among us young adults. *Depression Anxiety.* 2016;33(4):323-331.
79. Shensa A., Escobar-Viera C. G., Sidani J. E., Bowman N. D., Marshal M. P., Primack B. A. Problematic social media use and depressive symptoms among US young adults: a nationally-representative study. *Soc Sci Med.* 2017;182:150-157.
80. Woods H. C., Scott H. #Sleepyteens: social media use in adolescence is associated with poor sleep quality, anxiety, depression and low self-esteem. *J Adolescence.* 2016;51:41-49.
81. Shensa A., Sidani J. E., Dew M. A., Escobar-Viera C. G., Primack B. A. Social media use and depression and anxiety symptoms: a cluster analysis. *Am J Health Behav.* 2018;42(2):116-128.

KEY ARTICLES

Lifestyle Heart Trial 336

Percutaneous Coronary Angioplasty Compared with Exercise Training in Patients with Stable Coronary Artery Disease 338

Comparison of the Atkins, Ornish, Weight Watchers, and Zone Diets for Weight Loss and Heart Disease Risk Reduction 342

The GEMINAL Study: Gene Expression Modulation by Intervention with Nutrition and Lifestyle 345

Reversal of Type 2 Diabetes: Normalisation of Beta Cell Function in Association with Decreased Pancreas and Liver Triacylglycerol 347

The DIETFITS Randomized Clinical Trial 350

DiRECT 352

Fasting-Mimicking Diet Promotes Ngn3-Driven β-Cell Regeneration to Reverse Diabetes 355

From Diabetes Care to Diabetes Cure—The Integration of Systems Biology, eHealth, and Behavioral Change 358

Lifestyle Heart Trial

Citation: Ornish D., Scherwitz L. W., Billings J. H., et al. Intensive lifestyle changes for reversal of coronary heart disease. *JAMA.* 1998;280(23):2001-2007.

Objective

To determine the feasibility of patients to sustain intensive lifestyle changes for a total of 5 years, and their effects on coronary heart disease (CHD) without lipid-lowering drugs.

Study design

Randomized controlled trial (parallel, not double-blind, though radiologists evaluating angiograms were blinded)

Sample population

N = 48 adults with moderate to severe CHD

Location/venue

Two tertiary care university medical centers

Intervention

Intensive lifestyle changes included a low-fat (10% of calories) vegetarian diet, aerobic exercise, smoking cessation, stress management, and group psychosocial support. No lipid-lowering medications were used.

Control

Usual-care control group instructed to follow their doctor's lifestyle recommendations. They received written information about the American Heart Association (AHA) Step 2 diet.

Outcome(s) of interest

- Continued reduction in stenoses with lifestyle changes at 1 year and 5 years
- Association between adherence and regression of stenoses in the experimental group
- Reduction in cardiac events

Summary of methods

N = 48 men and women with moderate to severe CHD were recruited from two medical centers and randomized into either an intensive lifestyle change group or a usual-care control group. The active intervention lasted one year. N = 35 completed a 5-year follow-up. Quantitative coronary arteriograms were assessed with blinding after 1 and 5 years. Results are based on N = 35 subjects (N = 20 experimental and N = 15 control) who had both baseline and 5-year angiograms.

Key results

- Mean relative reduction in stenoses of 7.9% (41.3 to 37.3 absolute % stenosis) for experimental group and increase in stenoses of 27.7% (40.7 to 51.9 absolute % stenosis) for control (P = 0.001; 95% CI, 1.48–4.20).
- 46.7% relative increase in stenoses in the controls who were not taking lipid-lowering medications (40.7–59.7 absolute % stenosis). Note: these controls may provide a better comparison to the experimental group, who took no lipid-lowering medications. (95% CI, 1.48–4.20)
- 45 cardiac events (e.g., angioplasty, bypass surgery, hospitalization, myocardial infarction, or death) in control group versus 25 cardiac events in the experimental group (risk ratio 2.47; 95% CI, 1.48–4.20). More regression of CAD occurred after 5 years than after 1 year in the experimental

group, meaning the intervention continued to reverse CAD, whereas the control group had continued progression and >2x rate of cardiac events.

- Low-density lipoprotein (LDL) reductions of the experimental group compare to those achieved with lipid-lowering drugs in an ambulatory population, (40% at 1 year [P = 0.003], and 20% after 5 years [P = 0.76]). In contrast, the Step 2 diet reduces LDL cholesterol by only 5% or less.
- There was dose-response association between adherence and regression of stenoses in the experimental group, with 82% of the experimental group showing regression versus continued progression in the control group, (P = 0.001; 95% CI, 1.48–4.20).
- Experimental group after 1 year
    - 37.2% reduction in LDL cholesterol levels
    - 91% reduction in the frequency of anginal episodes
    - Reduced LDL cholesterol levels by 37.2%, compared to 6% in the control group
- Control group after 1 year
    - 165% increase in the frequency of reported anginal episodes
    - Average percent diameter stenosis progressed from 42.7% to 46.1%
    - >2x as many cardiac events per patient compared to experimental group

Limitations

- Small number of subjects
- Half the patients invited declined to participate
- 35 of 48 completed 5-year follow-up = 27% loss to follow-up (mostly due to unwillingness to undergo a 3rd angiogram; original study was only 1 year with two angiograms.)

Strengths

- Differences were highly significant, both clinically and statistically
- Significantly fewer cardiac events among the experimental group
- No evidence of bias in the dropout rate; same between experiment and controls
- One of few intensive lifestyle studies to follow subjects for that many years

Key conclusions

Comprehensive lifestyle changes in ambulatory patients with moderate to severe CHD resulted in significant reductions in both LDL cholesterol and anginal episodes after one year and showed even more regression of coronary atherosclerosis after 5 years. In contrast, patients following usual care showed even more progression of coronary atherosclerosis after 5 years than after 1 year, with more than twice as many cardiac events.

Significance for lifestyle medicine

It is possible for patients with mild to severe CHD to significantly reduce stenoses and risk of cardiac events using aggressive lifestyle changes, and without lipid-lowering medications. In fact, the LDL reductions of the experimental group compare to those achieved with lipid-lowering drugs in an ambulatory population.

A strong dose-response relationship between self-reported adherence and angiographic changes was found, with "excellent" adherence during the first year in maintaining the dietary and lifestyle changes, and "good" adherence after 5 years, as measured by percent diameter stenosis. In contrast, patients following conventional lifestyle recommendations showed continued progression of coronary atherosclerosis after 5 years with more than twice as many cardiac events as patients making comprehensive lifestyle changes. Overall, self-reported adherence was highly correlated with % stenosis.

Questions

1. **Which of the following statements about the Lifestyle Heart Trial is true?**
   - **A.** It used a pre vs post design with each subject serving as their own control.
   - **B.** It compared a low-fat diet to a low-carb diet in the secondary prevention of CHD.
   - **C.** The treatment group had a relative difference in progression of -35.6% at 5 years compared to all controls, and a difference of -54.6% compared to controls not taking lipid-lowering medications.
   - **D.** There was no association between adherence and change in stenoses or risk factors.
2. **Which of the following statements about the Lifestyle Heart Trial is true?**
   - **A.** It used a randomized, double-blind, parallel cohort design.
   - **B.** It compared a low-fat diet and smoking cessation to usual care.
   - **C.** It compared intensive lifestyle interventions to no lifestyle interventions.
   - **D.** In spite of its small sample size, the trial found both statistically significant and clinically significant differences between optimal usual care and intensive lifestyle treatment.

Answers to questions

1. **Answer: C.** The study used a randomized parallel design, not pre vs post. It compared a low-fat diet to usual care, which typically recommends the American Heart Association (AHA) Step 2 diet (not a low-carb diet) for patients with diagnosed CHD. There was a strong dose-response relationship between self-reported adherence and angiographic changes. The treatment group had a 7.9% reduction in stenoses at 5 years, while all controls had a progression of 27.7%, for a net difference of -35.6%. Those controls who were not taking lipid-lowering medications had a progression of 46.7%, for a net difference of -54.6%.
2. **Answer: D.** The study was randomized parallel but not double-blind. It compared a multifactorial lifestyle intervention, (a low-fat vegetarian diet, aerobic exercise, stress management, smoking cessation, and group psychosocial support) to optimized usual care, not merely low-fat diet and smoking cessation. The study compared intensive lifestyle changes to non-intensive lifestyle changes, because the control group was instructed to follow their doctor's lifestyle recommendations and received written information about the AHA Step 2 diet. The study had a small number of subjects, but the differences were highly significant, both clinically and statistically, as there were far fewer cardiac events among the experimental group, and most differences had P-values <0.05.

Percutaneous Coronary Angioplasty Compared with Exercise Training in Patients with Stable Coronary Artery Disease

Citation: Hambrecht R., Walther C., Möbius-Winkler S., et al. Percutaneous coronary angioplasty compared with exercise training in patients with stable coronary artery disease: a randomized trial. *Circulation*. 2004;109(11):1371-1378.

Objective

To determine if patients with stable coronary artery disease (CAD) can improve myocardial perfusion and reduce disease progression, and to compare the effects of exercise training to standard percutaneous coronary intervention (PCI) with stenting on:

1. Clinical symptoms

2. Angina-free exercise capacity
3. Myocardial perfusion
4. Cost-effectiveness
5. Frequency of a combined clinical end point (end point = death of cardiac cause: stroke, coronary artery bypass grafting, angioplasty, acute myocardial infarction, and worsening angina with objective evidence resulting in hospitalization)

Study design

Randomized control trial in a 12-month period

Sample population

N = 101 male patients aged ≤70 years with stable CAD and one native coronary artery stenosis of ≥75% by visual assessment, and amenable to PCI

Location/venue

Medical institution in Leipzig, Germany

Intervention

20 minutes of bicycle ergometry per day

Control

Percutaneous coronary angioplasty

Outcome(s) of interest

Compared with PCI, a 12-month program of regular physical exercise in selected patients with stable CAD resulted in:

- Superior event-free survival and improved exercise capacity at lower costs
- Reduced re-hospitalizations
- Fewer repeated revascularizations

Summary of methods

N = 101 male patients aged ≤70 years recruited after routine coronary angiography, randomized to either 12 months of exercise training (N = 51), or to PCI (N = 50). 47 patients in both groups completed the initial as well as follow-up coronary angiograms.

Cost efficiency was calculated based on the average expense (in US dollars) needed to improve the Canadian Cardiovascular Society (CCS) class by 1 class.

Key results

- Exercise training was associated with:
  - Higher event-free survival (88% vs 70% in the PCI group; 0.33, 95% CI 0.12 to 0.90, P = 0.023)
  - Increased maximal oxygen uptake (+16%, from 22.7 ± 0.7 to 26.2 ± 0.8 ml 02/kg, P <0.001 as compared to baseline, P<0.001 as compared to PCI group after 12 months)
  - Increased exercise tolerance by 20% (from 133 ± 5 to 159 ± 5 W, P <0.001 as compared to baseline and as compared to PCI group)
  - Elevated ischemic threshold by 30% (from 98 ± 6 to 127 ± 8 W, P = 0.03 as compared to baseline)
  - Significantly increased HDL serum levels after 12 months (from 1.3 ± 0.1 to 1.4 ± 0.1 mmol/L, P <0.01 vs PCI group for change), whereas high-density lipoprotein (HDL) dropped in the control group (from 1.4 ± 0.1 to 1.2 ± 0.1 mmol/L, P <0.05 as compared to baseline). LDL cholesterol levels remained unchanged during the study period.

- To gain 1 CCS class, $6,956 was spent in the PCI group versus $3,429 in the training group.
- Clinical symptoms significantly improved in both groups during the study period, though the training group's average CCS class decreased from 1.5 ± 0.1 at baseline to 0.4 ± 0.1 after 12 months (P <0.001 vs baseline), compared to the PCI group of mean CCS score reduction from 1.7 ± 0.1 to 0.7 ± 0.1 (P <0.001 vs baseline)
- In the PCI group, only the ischemic threshold showed a significant increase after 12 months. Maximal exercise tolerance was increased significantly along with the ischemic threshold was elevated by 30% (from 98 ± 6 to 127 ± 8 W, P = 0.03 vs baseline).

Limitations

Two patients in each group terminated before the final examinations were completed. One patient in the training group declined repeat coronary angiography. In total, 47 training patients and 47 PCI patients completed both the initial and follow-up coronary angiograms. Of these, the angiograms of 10 patients in the PCI group and 4 in the training group were excluded from quantitative coronary angiography owing to hard clinical events (stroke, target-vessel revascularization.)

Strengths

Consistent with previous clinical trials and strategies in stable CAD, supporting the notion that the interventional approach yields more rapid relief from the symptoms of exercise-induced angina pectoris.

Key conclusions

- After 12 months of exercise training, maximal exercise tolerance was increased significantly along with the ischemic threshold.
- Exercise training was associated with a 16% increase in maximal oxygen uptake.
- Expenses for 1 year of exercise training averaged $3,708, compared with $6,086 per PCI patient.
- In both groups, clinical symptoms improved significantly during the study period.

Significance for lifestyle medicine

Compared with PCI, a 12-month program of regular physical exercise in selected patients with stable CAD resulted in superior event-free survival and improved exercise capacity at lower costs, as well as reduced re-hospitalizations and fewer repeated revascularizations (Figure K.1 and Table K.2).

More than double US dollars were spent to lessen angina, ($6,956 spent in the PCI group vs $3,429 in the exercise group).

Figure K.1 Event-Free Survival After 12 Months

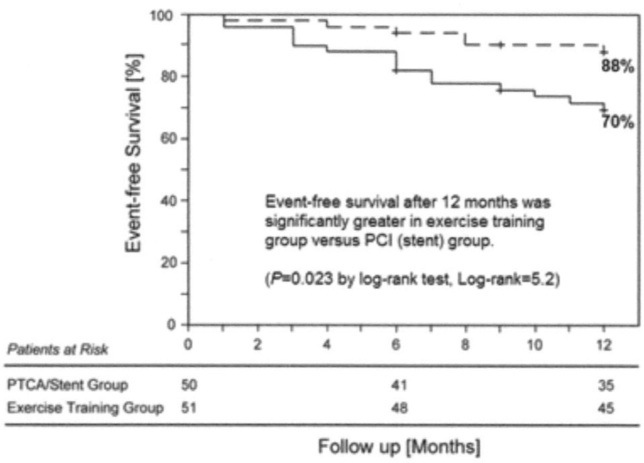

Table K.1 Ergospirometry Results				
	Exercise Training Group (N = 43)		**PCI Group (N = 33)**	
	Baseline	**End of Study**	**Baseline**	**End of Study**
Resting heart rate, bpm	71±2	65±1*†	70±2	70±1
Ischemic threshold, W	98±6	127±8‡	99±5	119±7‡
Maximal heart rate, bpm	131±3	137±3*	132±3	133±3
Physical work capacity, W	133±5	159±5§	130±5	130±5
Vo_2 max, mL - kg^{-1} - min^{-1}	22.6±0.7	26.2±0†	22.3±0.6	22.8±0.9

Vo_2 max indicates oxygen uptake at peak exercise; ischemic threshold, first occurrence of angina pectoris and/or ST-segment depression during stress test.

In the training group of 51 patients, 6 patients with clinical events and 2 dropouts were excluded; in the PCI group of 50 patients, 15 patients with clinical events and 2 dropouts were excluded. Data are mean ±SEM.

*P <0.01, significantly different, 12 months vs baseline, †P <0.01, significantly different, exercise training vs PCI

‡P <0.05, significantly different, 12 months vs baseline, §P <0.001, significantly different, exercise training vs PCI

Questions

1. **Based on results in the figure and the table above, which of the following is the most appropriate conclusion?**
   - **A.** As compared to the PCI group, resting heart rate was statistically significantly higher in the exercise training group at the end of the study.
   - **B.** As compared to the PCI group, maximal heart rate was statistically significantly lower in the exercise training group at the end of the study.
   - **C.** As compared to the PCI group, physical work capacity was statistically significantly higher in the exercise training group at the end of the study.
   - **D.** As compared to the PCI group, VO_2 max was statistically significantly lower in the exercise training group at the end of the study.
2. **Which of the following statements is true?**
   - **A.** Exercise training was equally cost effective as compared to PCI with respect to changing the CCS risk class.
   - **B.** Exercise training was less cost effective as compared to PCI with respect to changing the CCS risk class.
   - **C.** Exercise training was more cost effective as compared to PCI with respect to both changing the CCS risk class and improving exercise capacity.
   - **D.** Exercise training was less cost effective as compared to PCI with respect to improving exercise capacity.

Answers to questions

1. **Answer: C.** In the exercise training group, physical work capacity increased from 133w at baseline to 159w at the end of the study. This change was statistically significant as compared to almost no change observed in the PCI group. The resting heart rate was lower in the exercise-training group, and the maximal heart rate and VO_2 max were higher in the exercise-training group at the end of the study as compared to the PCI group. The exercise group was 88% event free after 12 months, compared to only 70% of the PCI group, resulting in a 26% lower risk in the exercise group than the PCI group.

2. **Answer: C.** Exercise training cost $3,429 to change by one class of the CCS as compared to PCI which cost $6,956. Exercise training was superior to PCI, in improved exercise capacity at lower costs, largely due to lower repeat hospitalizations and revascularizations. Therefore, exercise training was more cost effective as compared to PCI for both CCS and exercise capacity.

Comparison of the Atkins, Ornish, Weight Watchers, and Zone Diets for Weight Loss and Heart Disease Risk Reduction

Citation: Dansinger M. L., Gleason J. A., Griffith J. L., Selker H. P., Schaefer E. J. Comparison of the Atkins, Ornish, Weight Watchers, and Zone diets for weight loss and heart disease risk reduction: a randomized trial. *JAMA.* 2005;293(1):43-53.

Objective

This study sought to provide a valuable comparison of the popular diets—Atkins, Zone, Weight Watchers and Ornish—for both patients and clinicians.

Study design

Randomized control trial for 1 year

Sample population

N = 160 overweight or obese participants between the ages of 22 and 72 years who had diagnosed hypertension, dyslipidemia, or fasting hyperglycemia.

Location/venue

Academic medical center in Boston, MA

Outcome(s) of interest

- Each diet significantly reduced the low-density lipoprotein (LDL) to high-density lipoprotein (HDL) cholesterol ratio by approximately 10% (all $P < 0.05$), with no significant effects on blood pressure or glucose at 1 year.
- The amount of weight loss was associated with self-reported dietary adherence levels ($R = 0.60$; $P < 0.001$), but not with diet type ($R = 0.07$; $P = 0.40$). The association was a nonlinear quadratic association exhibiting a threshold effect.
- For each diet, weight loss was significantly associated with decreasing levels of total to HDL cholesterol ratios, C-reactive protein and insulin (mean R = 0.36, 0.37, and 0.39, respectively), with no significant difference between diets (P = 0.48, P = 0.57, P =0 .31, respectively).
- Overall adherence rates were low (<25%).

Summary of methods and intervention

N = 160 randomized into four dietary groups

1. Atkins (low carbohydrate, N = 40)
2. Zone (macronutrient balance, N = 40),
3. Weight Watchers (calorie restriction, N = 40)
4. Ornish (low-fat, N = 40)

Key results

- Each of the various dietary approaches can be used to reduce weight and improve markers of cardiovascular risk. All four diets resulted in modest weight loss at 1 year, with no statistically significant differences between diets ($P = 0.40$)

- As adherence scores increased, weight loss increased, regardless of the dietary program the participants followed.
- After 1 year of follow-up, weight loss (mean ±SD) for each of the above diets was:
    1. 4.6 ± 10.6 lbs (2.1 ± 4.8 kg) for Atkins
    2. 7.1 ± 13.2 lbs (3.2 ± 6.0 kg) for Zone
    3. 6.6 ± 10.8 lbs (3.0 ± 4.9 kg) for Weight Watchers
    4. 7.2 ± 16.1 lbs (3.3 ± 7.3 kg) for Ornish
- Greater changes were observed in subjects who completed the study.
- Each diet significantly reduced the LDL to HDL cholesterol ratio by approximately 10% (all $P < 0.05$), with no significant effects on blood pressure or glucose at 1 year.
- The amount of weight loss was associated with self-reported dietary adherence levels ($R = 0.60$; $P < 0.001$) but not with diet type ($R = 0.07$; $P = 0.40$).
- For each diet, weight loss was significantly associated with decreasing levels of total to HDL cholesterol ratios, C-reactive protein, and insulin (mean $R = 0.36$, 0.37, and 0.39, respectively), with no significant difference between diets ($P = 0.48$, $P = 0.57$, $P = 0.31$, respectively).
- No significant caloric or macronutrient differences between diet groups at baseline were found, nor any short-term safety risks.
- Measurements of dietary intake and adherence relied on self-reporting and are therefore subjective.

Limitations

- This trial did not test the treatment effects of the individual diets because it did not provide the lifestyle medicine interventions needed to produce and maintain adherence. Instead, it tested the effect of instructing patients to follow one of these diets without using an intensive intervention to help them do it.
- Overall adherence rates were low (<25%).
- Attrition: participants who did not complete the study at months 2, 6, and 12 were 34 (21%), 61 (38%), and 67 (42%), respectively. At 1 year, there was a nonsignificant trend ($P = 0.08$) toward a difference in discontinuation rates between the more extreme diets (48% for Atkins and 50% for Ornish) and moderate diets (35% for Zone and 35% for Weight Watchers).
- The most common reasons cited for discontinuation of the study were that the assigned diet was too hard to follow or not yielding enough weight loss.
- Measurements of dietary intake and adherence relied on self-reporting and are therefore subjective.
- This trial is limited in its ability to exclude long-term safety risks or occasional dangerous adverse effects resulting from the diets.

Strengths

There are a number of popular diets available to patients; however, there have been few rigorous comparative effectiveness studies. Though in practice the interventions were not of sufficient intensity to realistically produce adherence (see above in Limitations), the goal of this study was to provide evidence for comparative effectiveness of different diets, a novel contribution.

Key conclusions

- All four diets resulted in modest weight loss at 1 year, with no statistically significant differences between diets.
- Adherence, not diet type, largely determined treatment effects and weight loss.

Significance for lifestyle medicine

Adherence to any particular dietary program may be more important than the type of diet consumed (Figure K.2), since the more adherent subjects showed greater improvements in weight and cardiac parameters. Thus, the intensity of the intervention may be more important than the specific diet for weight loss.

Figure K.2 One-year Changes in Body Weight as a Function of Diet Group and Dietary Adherence Level

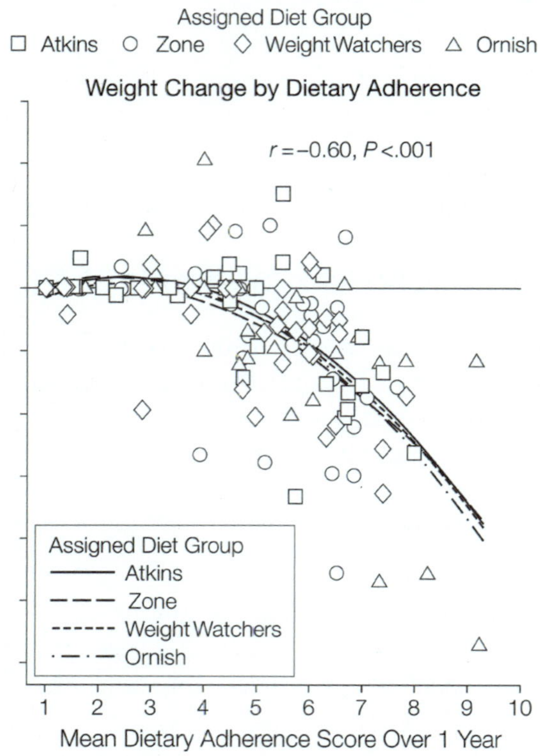

Questions

1. **The most accurate conclusion from this study would be:**
   - **A.** The type of diet was associated with weight loss but not with adherence.
   - **B.** Adherence levels were associated with weight loss but not with the type of diet.
   - **C.** Both adherence and the type of diet were important predictors of weight loss.
   - **D.** Adherence largely determined treatment effects and weight loss.

2. **The amount of variability in the weight loss achieved by the participants in this study demonstrates that one of the major take home messages from this trial is:**
   - **A.** Dietary changes are not useful for weight loss.
   - **B.** The effects of dietary changes reduce the longer a subject is on the diet.
   - **C.** It's important to match the right individual to the right lifestyle modification program.
   - **D.** The intensity of the intervention may be more important than the specific diet for weight loss.

Answers to Questions

1. **Answer: D.** Figure K.2 demonstrates that as adherence scores increase, weight loss increases regardless of the dietary program the participants are following. This indicates that a level of adherence is more important that the type of dietary program the participants are following.

2. **Answer: D.** Weight loss was more strongly associated with adherence level than with the specific diet in this study. The intensity of the treatment is directly related to adherence; thus, intensity may be more important than diet type for weight loss.

The GEMINAL Study: Gene Expression Modulation by Intervention with Nutrition and Lifestyle

Citation: Ornish D., Magbanua M. J. M., Weidner G., et al. Changes in prostate gene expression in men undergoing an intensive nutrition and lifestyle intervention. *Proc Natl Acad Sci USA.* 2008;105(24):8369-8374.

Objective

A pilot study to determine changes in prostate gene expression in a population of men with low-risk prostate cancer undergoing an intensive nutrition and lifestyle intervention.

Study design

Three-month prospective single-arm pilot clinical intervention study in men with indolent low-risk prostate cancer, comprising a 3-day intensive residential retreat, followed by an outpatient phase of weekly telephone contact

Sample population

N = 30 men with low-risk prostate cancer

Location/venue

Not included

Intervention

All subjects participated in an intensive nutrition and lifestyle intervention while undergoing careful surveillance for tumor progression. They had all declined immediate surgery, hormonal therapy, or radiation.

Control

N/A

Outcome(s) of interest

Significant improvements in weight, abdominal obesity, blood pressure, and lipid profile were observed ($P < 0.05$). Gene expression profiles were obtained from the 30 participants, pairing messenger RNA (mRNA) samples from a control prostate needle biopsy taken before the intervention to mRNA samples taken from the same patient 3-months post-intervention.

Summary of methods

N = 30 men with low-risk prostate cancer. A 3-month comprehensive lifestyle modification was used, comprised of a 3-day intensive residential retreat followed by an outpatient phase where participants were in weekly telephone contact with a study nurse.

Gene expression profiles were obtained from participants, pairing mRNA samples from a control prostate needle biopsy taken before the intervention to mRNA samples taken from the same patient 3-months post-intervention, (all within 95% CI). Lifestyle modifications included:

- A low-fat (10% of calories from fat), whole food plant-based diet
- Participants were provided with all of their food during the intervention period.
- The diet was supplemented with soy (a daily serving of tofu, plus 58 grams of a fortified soy protein powdered beverage), fish oil (3 grams daily), vitamin E (100 units daily), selenium (200 mg daily), and vitamin C (2 grams daily).
- Stress management included 60 minutes per day of gentle yoga-based stretching, breathing, meditation, imagery, or progressive relaxation.

- Moderate aerobic exercise of walking 30 minutes per day for 6 days per week
- A 1-hour group support session per week.

Key results

- Patients were able to adhere closely to the lifestyle recommendations. After 3 months, they reported consuming 11.6% (SD = 3.0) of fat calories per day, exercising 3.6 hours per week (SD = 1.5), and practicing stress management 4.5 hours per week (SD = 2.0).
- Significant improvements in weight, abdominal obesity, blood pressure, and lipid profile were observed ($P < 0.05$).

Limitations

- Only 30% of biopsy samples contained tumor tissue.
- Because of the microfocal nature of low-risk prostate tumors and the limitations of ultrasound biopsy guidance, researchers were unable to precisely match pre- and post-intervention tumor samples for individuals in the cohort.
- This study was a small pilot study. This is because it was not feasible to conduct a randomized trial in the absence of data first demonstrating that diet and lifestyle intervention may modulate gene expression.
- 273 men were screened, 96 declined to participate, 146 did not meet inclusion criteria, and 31 were enrolled.

Strengths

The study was safe, with no adverse events observed. The study identified numerous genes previously unknown to be associated with prostate cancer growth and remission.

Key conclusions

Intensive nutrition and lifestyle changes may modulate gene expression in the prostate. Understanding the mechanisms of how comprehensive lifestyle changes affect transcriptional regulation may strengthen efforts to develop effective prevention and treatment strategies for prostate cancer. Larger randomized controlled clinical trials are now warranted to confirm and extend the hypotheses generated by the results of this pilot study and to better understand the relative contribution of each component of the intervention.

Significance for lifestyle medicine

The study showed that intensive nutrition and lifestyle changes may modulate gene expression in the prostate.

Questions

1. **The GEMINAL study is a pivotal study demonstrating the effect of lifestyle modification at the genetic level. Which of the following is the most prominent limitation of this study?**
   - **A.** Short follow-up time
   - **B.** Small sample size
   - **C.** Absence of a comparison group
   - **D.** Number of genes studied was too large, reducing the possibility for multiple comparisons.
2. **Among the biopsies used in the GEMINAL study, only 30% contained tumor tissue, so the results demonstrating changes in gene expression profiles are largely based on normal tissue. Which of the following is an appropriate statement?**
   - **A.** Since the results are based on mainly normal tissue, these results indicate that the impact of lifestyle modification is not restricted to prostate cancer.

B. Since the results are based on mainly normal tissue, these results are questionable.
C. Since the results are based on mainly normal tissue, these results indicate that the impact of lifestyle modification does not impact prostate cancer.
D. Since the results are based on mainly normal tissue, these results apply more to men without prostate cancer than with it.

Answers to questions

1. **Answer: C.** The most significant limitation of the GEMINAL study is the absence of a comparison group. Absence of a control group prevents us from definitively saying that the gene expression changes are due to the comprehensive lifestyle modification and not due to normal changes in gene expression. The GEMINAL study presents high-quality preliminary data that can be used to design future clinical trials that have appropriate control groups. Although multiple comparisons are always a concern when a large number of data points are being analyzed, this was corrected for using a Bonferroni correction. Small sample size and short follow-up are not major limitations, especially given the fact that the results are statistically significant, as this indicates to us that the effect size is large enough to overcome the negatives associated with small sample size and short follow-up.

2. **Answer: A.** Since only 30% of the biopsies had tumor tissue, these results are mainly based on normal tissue from men with prostate cancer. This indicates to us that lifestyle modification can affect both cancer and normal tissue, and thus the benefits of lifestyle modification has a wide applicability and is not restricted to genes associated with prostate cancer. That the findings are based largely on normal tissue does not invalidate the findings. Although the results are largely based on normal tissue in men with prostate cancer, that doesn't mean these results indicate that lifestyle modification does not apply to prostate cancer.

Reversal of Type 2 Diabetes: Normalisation of Beta Cell Function in Association with Decreased Pancreas and Liver Triacylglycerol

Citation: Lim E. L., Hollingsworth K. G., Aribisala B. S., Chen M. J., Mathers J. C., Taylor R. Reversal of type 2 diabetes: normalisation of beta cell function in association with decreased pancreas and liver triacylglycerol. *Diabetologia.* 2011;54(10):2506-2514.

Objectives

1. To test the hypothesis that both beta cell failure and insulin resistance can be reversed by dietary restriction of energy intake.
2. To test the hypothesis that acute negative energy balance alone reverses type 2 diabetes by normalizing both beta cell function and insulin sensitivity.

Study design

Intervention study with matched control group

Sample population

N = 11 people with type 2 diabetes (49.5 ± 2.5 years, BMI 33.6 ± 1.2 kg/m^2, nine male and two female).

Location/venue

Abbott Diabetes Care in Maidenhead, UK

Intervention group

N = 11 Individuals with type 2 diabetes (age 35–65 years, HbA1c 6.5–9.0% [48–75 mmol/L], diabetes duration <4 years, stable body mass index [BMI] 25–45 kg/m^2). Participants were asked to continue their habitual pattern of eating until the start of the study. Assessments of beta cell function, insulin sensitivity, liver and pancreatic fat content and total body fat were carried out at baseline immediately prior to dietary intervention (day −1), and after 1, 4, and 8 weeks of the very-low-energy diet.

Control group

N = 9 participants matched for weight, age, and sex were also studied (seven male, two female, age 49.7 ± 2.5 years

Outcome(s) of interest

Dietary energy restriction alone led to normalization of both beta cell function and hepatic insulin sensitivity in type 2 diabetes. This was accompanied by decreased pancreatic and liver triacylglycerol stores. The study showed that reducing dietary energy intake can reverse the abnormalities underlying type 2 diabetes.

Summary of methods and intervention

N = 11 individuals were studied before and after 1, 4, and 8 weeks on a restricted 600 calorie per day diet. Statin therapy was continued.

Key results

After one week of restricted energy intake

- Fasting plasma glucose normalized in the diabetic group (from 9.2 ± 0.4 mmol/L to 5.9 ± 0.4 mmol/l, or 166 ± 7.22 mg/dL to 106 ± 7.22 mg/dL; P = 0.003).
- Insulin suppression of hepatic glucose output improved from 43 ± 4–74 ± 5% (P = 0.003) versus controls 68 ± 5%.
- Hepatic triacylglycerol content fell from 12.8 ± 2.4% in the diabetic group to 2.9 ± 0.2% by week eight (P = 0.003).
- The first-phase insulin response increased during the study period (0.19 ± 0.02 to 0.46 ± 0.07 nmol min-1 m-2; p<0.001) and approached control values (0.62 ± 0.15 nmol min-1 m-2; p=0.42).
- Maximal insulin response became supranormal at e weeks (1.37 ± 0.27 vs controls 1.15 ± 0.18 nmol min-1 m-2).
- Pancreatic triacylglycerol decreased from 8.0 ± 1.6–6.2 ± 1.1% (P = 0.03).

Limitations

1. Sample size was necessarily small to allow for metabolic investigation and examination by magnetic resonance techniques.
2. Pancreatic fat measurements included intraorgan adipocyte fat content because current methodology precludes the assessment of the more mechanistically important islet intracellular fatty acid content. Animal data suggest that the two variables are linked. Although pancreatic fat content was 30% higher in the diabetic group, the study was powered to demonstrate responses to the dietary intervention rather than to test differences from weight-matched non-diabetic individuals. No correlation was observed between pancreatic fat and BMI within the restricted range of BMI examined in this study.
3. Participants were selected to have had a relatively short duration of type 2 diabetes (up to 4 years), and further studies must establish the extent of reversibility with longer duration type 2 diabetes. In addition, further studies are required to determine the long-term outcome in respect of glucose regulation as the observations made after 12 weeks of return to a normal diet were necessarily limited.

4. Raised liver fat levels despite metabolic normality in some controls can be considered in light of the recent description of the PNPLA3 gene. The G allele of this gene determines high liver fat levels, but in a form that is not associated with metabolic abnormality. This provides a clear genetic basis for the observed individual variation in susceptibility to insulin resistance despite raised liver fat content, and offers a partial explanation of the overlapping hepatic fat levels in type 2 diabetic and control groups. It is likely that other genetic factors yet to be defined underlie the differing individual levels of susceptibility to pancreatic fat accumulation in terms of inhibition of glucose-dependent insulin secretion.

Strengths

This new insight allows an understanding of the causality of type 2 diabetes in individuals as well as in populations. The greatest strength of this study is that it demonstrated for the first time that normal blood glucose levels without medication are achievable in 1 week with a very low energy diet, and was accompanied by reversal of hepatic and pancreatic triacylglycerol in the subsequent 3–4 weeks.

Key conclusions

Normalization of both beta cell function and hepatic insulin sensitivity in type 2 diabetes was achieved by dietary energy restriction alone. This was associated with decreased pancreatic and liver triacylglycerol stores. The abnormalities underlying type 2 diabetes are reversible by reducing dietary energy intake.

Significance for lifestyle medicine

Maximal insulin sensitivity improved, to exceed that of the controls, with dietary caloric restriction. Both beta cell function and insulin sensitivity improved. Both fatty liver and fatty pancreas improved. Beta cell function and insulin sensitivity both improved in the first week.

Questions

1. **Which of the following statements about this study is true?**
   - **A.** This study used a randomized control design with matching controls.
   - **B.** The intervention included a very low-calorie diet of 1,200 calories per day.
   - **C.** The primary outcomes were beta cell function and insulin sensitivity.
   - **D.** Most of the improvement occurred in the final 4 weeks of the study.

2. **Which of the following statements most accurately describes the findings of this study?**
   - **A.** Maximal insulin sensitivity improved to almost equal that of the non-diabetic controls.
   - **B.** Insulin sensitivity improved, but beta cell function remained unchanged.
   - **C.** First-phase insulin response improved to almost equal that of the non-diabetic controls, while maximal insulin response improved and exceeded that of the controls.
   - **D.** Beta cell function improved in one week, but insulin sensitivity only changed after 8 weeks.

Answers to questions

1. **Answer: C.** The study used a case-control design with non-diabetic controls (matched for age, gender, and weight). The intervention consisted of a total energy intake of ~600 calories per day. This included 510 calories per day liquid diet formula (comprised of 46.4% carbohydrate, 32.5% protein, and 20.1% fat; vitamins, minerals, and trace elements) supplemented with three portions of non-starchy vegetables. The hypothesis tested was that beta cell failure and insulin sensitivity can be reversed with dietary restriction. Most of the improvement occurred in the first week (not the last 4 weeks).

2. **Answer: C.** The first-phase insulin response improved to almost equal that of the matched controls, but the maximal insulin response improved and exceeded that of the controls.

The DIETFITS Randomized Clinical Trial

Citation: Gardner C. D., Trepanowski J. F., Del Gobbo L. C., et al. Effect of low-fat vs low-carbohydrate diet on 12-month weight loss in overweight adults and the association with genotype pattern or insulin secretion: the DIETFITS randomized clinical trial. *JAMA.* 2018;319(7):667-679.

Objective

To determine the effect of a healthy low-fat diet versus a healthy low-carbohydrate diet on weight change, and to determine whether genotype pattern or insulin secretion are related to the dietary effects on weight loss.

Study design

12-month randomized clinical trial

Sample population

N = 609 adults (18–50 years old) without diabetes with a body mass index (BMI) of 28–40.

Location/venue

Not specified

Intervention

Health educators delivered the behavior modification intervention to the healthy low-fat participants, (N = 305) and the healthy low-carbohydrate participants, (N = 304) via 22 diet-specific small group sessions administered over 1 year.

Control group

N/A

Outcome(s) of interest

- Effects of a healthy low-fat diet vs a healthy low-carbohydrate diet on weight change
- Relationship of genotype pattern or insulin secretion to dietary effects on weight loss

Summary of methods and intervention

N = 609 overweight adults. Participants were randomized to the 12-month healthy low-fat (HLF); (N = 305) or healthy low-carbohydrate (HLC); (N = 304), diet.

Key results

- Among 609 participants, 244 (40%) had a low-fat genotype; 180 (30%) had a low-carbohydrate genotype; mean baseline INS-30, 93 μIU/ml.
- For the healthy low-fat versus healthy low-carbohydrate diets, respectively:
    - The mean 12-month macronutrient distributions were: 48% vs 30% for carbohydrates; 29% vs 45% for fat; and 21% vs 23% for protein.
    - Weight change at 12 months was −5.3 kg (−11.7 lbs) for the healthy low-fat diet versus −6.0 kg (−13.2 lbs) for the healthy low-carbohydrate diet (mean between-group difference, 0.7 kg [95% CI, −0.2 to 1.6 kg], or 1.5 lbs [95% CI, −0.4 to 3.5 lbs]). This difference in weight loss was not statistically significant.
    - No significant diet-genotype pattern interaction (P = 0.20) or diet-insulin secretion (INS-30) interaction (P = 0.47) with 12-month weight loss.
    - Eighteen adverse or serious adverse events were evenly distributed across the two diet groups.

Limitations

- 481 (79%) completed the trial.
- These results are inconsistent with similar analyses of other dietary weight loss intervention cohorts, and it seems implausible there is no interaction between genotype and weight loss with different macronutrient dietary patterns. It is possible there were confounding factors. For instance, it could be that for the range of macronutrients consumed in this study there is no difference in the interaction, or that the study was underpowered and therefore unable to detect a small difference.
- It is impossible to identify the effect of a gene (genotype) without measuring the epigenetic state and knowing if the gene is active or quiescent. The epigenome was not assessed in this study, a major limitation in any genotype association study.

Strengths

Health educators delivered the behavior modification intervention to both groups via 22 diet-specific small group sessions administered over 1 year. The sessions emphasized diet quality and focused on ways to achieve the lowest fat or carbohydrate intake that could be maintained long-term.

Key conclusions

There is considerable scientific interest in identifying the genetic variants that help explain inter-individual differences in weight loss success in response to diet interventions, particularly diets with varying macronutrient compositions. In this 12-month weight loss diet study, there was no significant difference in weight change between a healthy low-fat diet versus a healthy low-carbohydrate diet. Also, neither genotype pattern nor baseline insulin secretion was associated with the dietary effects on weight loss. In the context of these two common weight loss diet approaches, neither of the two hypothesized predisposing factors was helpful in identifying which diet was better for whom.

Significance for lifestyle medicine

Dietary modification remains key for successful weight loss, yet no one dietary strategy is consistently superior to another for the general population. Previous research suggests genotype or insulin-glucose dynamics may modify the effects of diets. This study demonstrates that epigenetics must be part of the measures assessed in lifestyle diet intervention studies. Diet determines the expression of many genes.

Questions

1. **Which of the following statements about this study is true?**
   - **A.** This study used a case-control parallel design.
   - **B.** The intervention sought to reduce caloric intake to 500–600 calories per day.
   - **C.** The primary outcome was weight loss at 12 months.
   - **D.** Weight loss was not statistically different between the two dietary patterns.
2. **Which of the following statements most accurately describes the findings of this study?**
   - **A.** Weight loss was about the same for both dietary patterns, and there was no interaction between dietary pattern and genotype or insulin level 30 minutes after glucose ingestion.
   - **B.** There was a slight interaction between genotype and insulin level 30 minutes after glucose ingestion, but it was not statistically significant.
   - **C.** Subjects with metabolic syndrome were found to lose more weight on the healthy low-carbohydrate diet.
   - **D.** Weight loss was greater for the low-fat dietary pattern.

Answers

1. **Answer: D.** The study used a randomized parallel design. The intervention did not stipulate any specific caloric intake, but both groups consumed ~500–600 calories per day fewer calories than at baseline. The primary outcomes were weight loss at 12 months and diet interactions with genotype or serum insulin level 30 minutes after glucose ingestion. Weight loss was not significantly different for the low-fat or low-carbohydrate diet. No statistically significant interactions were detected.

2. **Answer: A.** Weight loss was about the same for both dietary patterns (−5.3 kg versus −6.0 kg [−11.7 lbs versus −13.2 lbs] P >0.05), and there was no interaction between dietary pattern and genotype or insulin level 30 minutes after glucose ingestion. There could be no interaction between genotype and insulin level 30 minutes after glucose ingestion because neither of these are outcome variables (interactions modify outcomes, not independent variables). Subjects with metabolic syndrome were excluded from the study and were not included in the analyses. The null hypotheses could not be rejected and the study had "negative" findings.

DiRECT

Citation: Lean M. E., Leslie W. S., Barnes A. C., et al. Primary care-led weight management for remission of type 2 diabetes (DiRECT): an open-label, cluster-randomised trial. *Lancet.* 2018;391(10120):541-551.

Objective

To assess whether intensive weight management within routine primary care would achieve remission of type 2 diabetes, and to provide either a weight management program (intervention) or best-practice care by guidelines (control).

Study design

Open-label, cluster-randomized control trial, randomized by practice group

Sample population

N = 306 individuals aged 20–65 years who had been diagnosed with type 2 diabetes within the past 6 years, with body-mass index (BMI) of 27–45 kg/m^2, and not receiving insulin.

Location/venue

49 primary care practices in Scotland and in the Tyneside region of England

Intervention

N = 149 participants received:

1. Withdrawal of antidiabetic and antihypertensive medications
2. Total diet replacement (825–853 calories per day formula diet for 3–5 months) with a goal to achieve 15 kg weight loss
3. Stepped food reintroduction over a period of 2–8 weeks
4. Structured support for long-term weight loss maintenance

Control

N = 149 participants given evidence-based clinical guidelines for type 2 diabetes from the National Institute of Health and Care Excellence in England, and the Scottish Intercollegiate Guidelines Network in Scotland. To help balance the incentive of the intervention itself, participants in the control group were offered a £50 Amazon voucher.

Outcome(s) of interest

The dual primary outcomes were weight loss of 15 kg (33 lbs) or more, and remission of diabetes defined as hemoglobin A1c (HbA1c) of less than 6.5% (<48 mmol/mol) after ≥2 months off all antidiabetic medications, during the 12-month study period.

Summary of methods

N = 306 individuals from 49 intervention (N = 23) and control (N = 26) general practices, with 149 participants per group in the intention-to-treat population and no participants in the control group.

Key results

At 12 months, the results showed:

- Weight loss of ≥15 kg (33 lbs) was achieved in 36 participants (24%) in the intervention group but in no participants in the control group (P <0.0001).
- Diabetes remission was achieved in 68 participants (46%) in the intervention group and in six participants (4%) in the control group (odds ratio [OR] 19.7, 95% CI 7.8–49.8; P <0.0001).
- Remission was achieved in:
    - None of the 76 participants who gained weight;
    - Six (7%) of the 89 participants who maintained 0–5 kg (0–11 lbs) of weight loss
    - 19 (34%) of the 56 participants with 5–10 kg (11–22 lbs) weight loss
    - 16 (57%) of 28 participants with a 10–15 kg (22–33 lbs) loss
    - 31 (86%) of 36 participants who lost ≥15 kg (≥33 lbs)
- Mean body weight fell by 10 kg (SD 8.0) in the intervention group and by 1 kg (3.7) in the control group (adjusted difference −8.8 kg, 95% CI −10.3 to −7.3; P <0.0001).
- Quality of life measured by the EuroQol 5 Dimensions visual analogue scale improved by 7.2 points (SD 21.3) in the intervention group and decreased by 2.9 points (15.5) in the control group (adjusted difference 6.4 points, 95% CI 2.5–10.3; P = 0.0012).
- Nine serious adverse events were reported by seven (4%) of 157 participants in the intervention group. Two events were reported by two participants (1%) in the control group (RR 4.0). No adverse events led to withdrawal from the study.

Limitations

- 32 (21%) participants withdrew prematurely from the intervention program.
- 23 (8%) participants were lost to follow-up at 12 months, with 128 (86%) participants in the intervention group and 147 (99%) participants in the control group attending the 12-month study assessment.
- The dropout rate of 25% in the intervention group was an indication of non-acceptability for this proportion but should be considered in relation to the overall effectiveness of the program for a much greater proportion.
- Four participants in the intervention group who had diabetes remission had received a short rescue plan in the total diet replacement phase because of weight regain within 60 days of their 12-month assessment. Two of the 12 participants who received rescue plans within 60 days of their 12-month assessment achieved more than 15 kg weight loss.
- The study design stipulated data collection from the control group only at baseline and 12 months, so intercurrent adverse events could not be assessed.
- The data for physical activity should be viewed with caution because they were based on around half of all participants in each group for whom the data were complete.
- We cannot exclude a carryover acute effect of the rescue plans suppressing HbA1c in these participants, but believe any such effect would have been very small and unlikely to affect the study conclusions.

- Racial and ethnic characteristics, while typical of the populations of Scotland and Tyneside, do not allow for unqualified extrapolation to other groups, such as South Asians, who tend to develop diabetes with less weight gain.
- Due to limitations in the data, detailed body composition was not assessed.
- Due to the nature of the lifestyle intervention being examined, participants, caregivers, and research assistants who collected outcome data were aware of group allocation; however, allocation was concealed from the study statistician in charge of developing and conducting the statistical analysis program.
- The conclusions reported here apply to people with type 2 diabetes diagnosed within the previous 6 years, and existing evidence has shown that remission is less likely with longer durations of disease.

Strengths

- A well-defined evidence-based intervention and a robust cluster-randomized study design, managed by a well-established clinical trials unit.
- The sample size exceeded the need for statistical power, and the mean remission rate of 46% greatly exceeded the level of 22% considered clinically important. Hence, the results are robust for the patient group under study.
- The sample had characteristics very similar to the general population of people with type 2 diabetes, so the results are likely to be generalizable.
- In contrast to LookAHEAD, the DiRECT study concluded that remission of type 2 diabetes is a practical treatment goal for primary care. The difference appears to be dosing strength—the LookAHEAD "intensive" lifestyle intervention (1,200–1,800 calories per day) was not strong enough to induce remission, whereas the more intensive DiRECT intervention (825–853 calories per day) was.
- Subsequent analyses might be able to examine routinely collected primary care data from both groups, including all prescriptions.

Key conclusions

The findings show that at 12 months, almost half of participants (46%) achieved remission to a non-diabetic state and off antidiabetic drugs.

- Remission of type 2 diabetes is a practical target for primary care.
- Remission was associated with weight loss for the entire study population.

Significance for lifestyle medicine

Remission of diabetes was strongly associated with weight loss in a dose-response relationship. Average remission rate was 46% in the DiRECT study with a more intense dietary change than the 11.5% and 2% rates for the LookAHEAD study. This is the first large rigorous trial to show such success in remission of diabetes in a clinical practice setting.

Questions

1. **Which of the following statements about this study is true?**
    - **A.** This study used a randomized case-control design.
    - **B.** The intervention used a dietary replacement to reduce caloric intake to ~1,500 calories per day for 3 months.
    - **C.** The primary outcomes were ≥15 kg (33 lbs) weight loss, and remission of diabetes (HbA1c <6.5% off all antidiabetic medications).
    - **D.** Weight loss was weakly predictive of diabetes remission but demonstrated a dose-response relationship.

2. **Which of the following statements most accurately describes the findings of this study?**
   - **A.** Weight loss was the same for the experimental and control groups, but the experimental group showed greater remission of diabetes.
   - **B.** There was a very weak interaction between weight loss and diabetes remission, just as there was in the LookAHEAD study.
   - **C.** 46% of the experimental subjects experienced remission of their diabetes, 86% of subjects with ≥15 kg (33 lbs) weight loss experienced remission, but none of those who gained weight experienced remission.
   - **D.** Beta cell function improved in association with weight loss during the total dietary replacement phase.

Answers

1. **Answer: C.** The study used a randomization stratified by area and practice size. The intervention included a total diet replacement phase with ~850 calories per day. The primary outcomes were ≥15 kg (33 lbs) weight loss and remission of diabetes (HbA1c <6.5% off all antidiabetic medications). Remission of diabetes was strongly associated with weight loss in a dose-response relationship.

2. **Answer: C.** Weight loss was much greater in the experimental group than in the controls (−10 kg vs −1 kg (−22 lbs vs −2.2 lbs). There was a strong correlation between weight loss and diabetes remission in this study, but not in the LookAHEAD study. Beta cell function was not measured and was not an outcome in this study. 46% of the experimental subjects experienced remission, 86% of those who lost ≥15 kg (33 lbs) experienced remission, and none of those who gained weight experienced remission.

Fasting-Mimicking Diet Promotes Ngn3-Driven β-Cell Regeneration to Reverse Diabetes

Citation: Cheng C. W., Villani V., Buono R., et al. Fasting-Mimicking Diet Promotes Ngn3-Driven β-Cell Regeneration to Reverse Diabetes. *Cell.* 2017;168(5):775-788.e712.

Objective
To determine if a short-term diet that mimics periodic fasting modulates beta cell number and promotes insulin secretion and glucose homeostasis with implications for both type 1 diabetes (T1D) and type 2 diabetes (T2D). To also provide an example of a potent and coordinated dietary regulation of cell fate-determination with the potential to serve as a therapeutic intervention to treat diabetes and other degenerative diseases.

Study design
Two crossover single-arm intervention designs, one animal and one human, with similar interventions.

Sample population
N = 102 humans: subjects in this study are at age 49.1 ± 6.9, with heights of 166.7 ± 4.7 cm, with body weights of 63.32 ± 4.8 kg at baseline and 61.36 ± 4.3 at the end of a Fasting-Mimicking Diet (FMD). The fasting mimicking conditions that affect Ngn3 expression and beta cell functions in human pancreatic cells were performed ex vivo using primary human pancreatic islets. IGF-1, glucose, and ketone bodies and treated human pancreatic islets were measured.

Mice: Leptin receptor deficient (Leprdb/db) mice, and age-matched healthy wild-type littermates.

Location/venue

Davis School of Gerontology and University of Southern California (USC), California, US. Study design approved by both the Institutional Review Board of USC and its Institutional Animal Care and Use Committee.

Intervention

Serum from N = 6–8 healthy subjects from enrollment pool of 102 human subjects. N = 102 subjects enrolled in a clinical trial (NCT02158897) testing the effects of a low-protein and low-calorie FMD lasting 5 days. Participant numbers divided into control and intervention groups not specified.

Pancreatic islets from T1D subjects were cultured.

Humans were fed a propriety formulation belonging to L-Nutra (http://l-nutra.com/prolon/). It is a plant-based diet designed to attain fasting-like effects on the serum levels of IGF-I, IGFBP1, glucose, and ketone bodies while providing both macro- and micronutrients to minimize the burden of fasting and adverse effects

Mice: N = 6 mice fed the FMD. To investigate whether the FMD causes de novo expression of Ngn3 and whether Ngn3+ cells may contribute to FMD-induced beta cell regeneration, Ngn3-CreER;tdTomato^{LSL}-reporter mice were generated.

Humans and mice received a low-calorie, low-protein, and low-carbohydrate but high-fat 4-day FMD, which causes changes in the levels of specific growth factors, glucose, and ketone bodies similar to those caused by fasting.

Control group

Humans: Each subject served as their own control for pancreatic function and content, which were compared before and after the FMD intervention. Pancreatic islets from healthy subjects were cultured.

Mice: N = 6 wild mice fed ad libitum

Outcome(s) of interest

- FMD induces prenatal-development gene expression in adult pancreas
- FMD promotes Ngn3 expression to generate insulin-producing beta cells
- Cycles of FMD reverse beta cell failure and rescue mice from T1D and T2D
- Inhibition of PKA or mTOR promote Ngn3-driven beta cell regeneration in human T1D islets

Summary of methods

In mice, a 4-day FMD induces a stepwise expression of SOX17 and PDX-1, resembling that observed during pancreatic development, followed by Ngn3-driven generation of insulin-producing beta cells, to restore insulin secretion and glucose homeostasis in both T2D and T1D.

Human study participants received a suggested FMD meal plan that explained what to eat for each meal. The version of the FMD is a propriety formulation belonging to L-Nutra: a plant-based diet designed to attain fasting-like effects on the serum levels of IGF-I, IGFBP1, glucose, and ketone bodies while providing both macro and micronutrients to minimize the burden of fasting and adverse effects. Day 1 of the FMD supplies ~4600 kJ (11% protein, 46% fat, 43% carbohydrate), whereas days 2–5 provide ~3000 kJ (9% protein, 44% fat, 47% carbohydrate) per day. The mouse version of the FMD is a 4-day regimen using ingredients similar to those used for the human FMD.

Key results

In mice, both T1D and T2D were reversed by the intervention (not just T2D). Among mice with T1D and T2D, a FMD followed by re-feeding was shown to induce expression of factors that resulted in beta cell genesis and insulin production.

The FMD did result in activation of multiple epigenetic factors which re-programmed pancreatic support cells into functioning beta cells by inducing a stepwise expression of SOX17 and PDX-1, followed by Ngn3-driven generation of insulin-producing beta cells. The primary outcome was beta cell genesis and insulin production, not weight loss.

Limitations

The in vivo beta cell neogenesis was done in mice and was not tested in humans yet. The FMD used is a proprietary formulation. (However, the dietary components are described in supplemental materials.)

Strengths

The study results indicate that a FMD promotes the reprogramming of pancreatic cells to restore insulin generation in islets from T1D patients, and reverses both T1D and T2D phenotypes in mouse models.

The study was able to trace the stepwise reprogramming process in mice that produced new beta cells, and show that a similar process appears to occur in human beta cells.

Key conclusions

A low-calorie, low-protein, and low-carbohydrate but high-fat 4-day FMD which causes changes in the levels of specific growth factors, glucose, and ketone bodies are similar to those caused by fasting. Cycles of the FMD are able to promote the generation of functional, stable, and insulin-producing beta cells and investigate the mechanisms responsible for these effects.

Results indicate that a FMD promotes the reprogramming of pancreatic cells to restore insulin generation in islets from T1D patients, and the diet reverses T1D and T2D phenotypes in mouse models.

Significance for lifestyle medicine

The study demonstrates the power of dietary interventions may include reprogramming of tissues to restore lost metabolic function, such as beta cells in the pancreas. If confirmed in humans, this could elevate lifestyle medicine intervention as a primary modality for T2D treatment. Also, should this treatment cause beta cell neogenesis in humans, it could make T1D reversible with lifestyle medicine.

Questions

1. **Which of the following statements about this study is true?**
   - **A.** The intervention was a series of 4-day complete fasts followed by 3 days of re-feeding.
   - **B.** The intervention resulted in activation of multiple epigenetic factors that reprogrammed pancreatic support cells into functioning beta cells producing insulin.
   - **C.** Weight loss was a primary outcome in the study.
   - **D.** The stepwise epigenetic reprogramming process was shown to be the same in humans as in mice.
2. **Which of the following statements most accurately describes the findings of this study?**
   - **A.** T2D was improved by the FMD after re-feeding, but T1D was unaffected.
   - **B.** No epigenetic changes were involved in the beta cell genesis and restoration of insulin production in the study.
   - **C.** Beta cell function was restored by the FMD but stopped upon re-feeding.
   - **D.** Among mice with T1D and T2D, a fasting mimicking diet followed by re-feeding was shown to induce expression of factors that resulted in beta cell genesis and insulin production.

Answers

1. **Answer: B.** The study was not a randomized controlled trial. Each subject did serve as their own control for pancreatic function and content, which were compared before and after the FMD intervention. The intervention consisted of a series of 4-day FMD followed by 3 days of re-feeding. Complete fast was not used. The FMD did result in activation of multiple epigenetic factors which reprogrammed pancreatic support cells into functioning beta cells by inducing a stepwise expression of SOX17 and PDX-1, followed by Ngn3-driven generation of insulin-producing beta cells in mice, but this was not demonstrated in humans. The primary outcome was beta cell genesis and insulin production, not weight loss.

2. **Answer: D.** Both T1D and T2D were reversed by the intervention (not just T2D). Epigenetic factors were integral to the cellular changes induced by the intervention. Beta cell generation and insulin production were restored by the intervention in both T1D and T2D with re-feeding, and the restoration did not end with re-feeding. Among mice with T1D and T2D, the FMD followed by re-feeding did induce expression of epigenetic factors, resulting in beta cell genesis with insulin production.

From Diabetes Care to Diabetes Cure—The Integration of Systems Biology, eHealth, and Behavioral Change

Citation: van Ommen B., Wopereis S., van Empelen P., et al. From diabetes care to diabetes cure—the integration of systems biology, eHealth, and behavioral change. *Front Endocrinol.* 2017;8:381.

Thesis/objective of the review

This article reviews the state of the art in all areas involved in a diabetes cure–focused therapy and discusses the scientific and technological advancements that need to be integrated into a systems-approach, sustainable lifestyle-based healthcare system and economy.

The healthcare approach toward lifestyle-related diseases needs to change. Huge health and economic profits could be achieved if everyone would adopt an "optimal" lifestyle. This article presents abundant scientific evidence that lifestyle interventions can lead to major reductions in obesity, type 2 diabetes, and cardiovascular disease. The (economic) benefits of a lifestyle-based therapy for type 2 diabetes have been demonstrated by a 10-year study, yet the introduction of a new healthcare system for preventing and treating lifestyle-related diseases has not materialized for a number of reasons, as discussed in this article.

Major reasons lifestyle measures aren't used in clinical practice:

1. Difficulty for patients to sustain the changes. In the short term, or in a setting where the lifestyle choices are rigidly imposed, lifestyle change can be achieved, but in the long term, changes fade away due to a lack of support and the many counteracting stimuli from environmental pressures.
2. Lifestyle as medicine has failed to take hold due to the lack of economic benefits within the context of our current healthcare system. A major reason is the failure to take a systems approach instead of making reductionistic changes.

Thus, the theory and practice differ and we face a multifactorial challenge that requires removing economic, social, psychological, and biological barriers.

Significance for lifestyle medicine

The authors provide evidence for the reversibility of insulin resistance and the remission of type 2 diabetes with diet and lifestyle, asserting that complete cure may be achieved if beta cell function is still adequate and complications have not yet occurred. They demonstrate that type 2 diabetes is a "systems disease" with multiple organs and processes involved, and assert that the disease deserves to be treated in a personalized manner and, as needed, in a "personalized lifestyle–personalized medicine combination."

Compliance to lifestyle changes has been a major obstacle for implementation in healthcare, but the advancements in behavioral change technologies, eHealth, health literacy, and personal health data valorization may now allow for a switch from a research setting to real-life socioeconomic implementation. We have the tools available to:

1. Implement a lifestyle-based therapy for type 2 diabetes and other food-related lifestyle diseases
2. Extend this to a prevention and optimal health-focused healthcare

Also, there will be an enormous economic gain in implementing a lifestyle-based healthcare system, which will, in turn, finance healthcare system and economic changes that support lifestyle-based approaches for optimal health and prevention. Since stakeholders, losses, and profits in this new economy will be substantially different from the current situation, the present healthcare industry will transition slowly toward this new system.

Description of scope and methods

A reorientation of health research and care is needed, starting with:

- Re-defining health and its underlying mechanisms
- Realizing that integrated, participatory, and personalized health optimization strategies are needed
- Redesigning the methods to quantify health toward the development of a new generation of health biomarkers, lifestyle interventions, support tools, and economic values.

All of these changes need to be focused on self-empowerment, as listed below.

1. Refocusing on flexibility as a core characteristic of human physiology, as chronic disease is reversible.
2. Diagnosis has to quantify much more than the medical condition. A 360° diagnosis is needed to determine all the relevant biological, sociological, psychological, and contextual conditions of the patient. The trajectory toward disease needs to be identified and quantified to empower the individual to achieve a sustainable and perceivable lifestyle change.
3. Interventions will need to span all relevant bio-socio-psycho-economic factors and thus change from reductionist to systemic, and from generic to fine-tuned toward personal goals.
4. Motivational tools are required in the form of personal coaching as well as information and communications technology (ICT) support.
5. Health literacy needs to be improved as part of personal health empowerment.
6. Personal health data handling needs to completely refocus in order to empower the citizen/patient to valorize their health data for personal health and research.
7. Together, the points above need to lay the foundation of a new approach in lifestyle-related health science and a new health economy.

Key conclusions

Creative ways to implement lifestyle interventions need to be explored. Ultimately, health data cooperatives may become the basis and drivers for this change, but this will take some time to develop into an economic reality. In the meantime, creative new "ecosystems" need to be explored that combine all the necessary instruments for specific type 2 diabetes populations to be really effective. The goal would be to demonstrate its therapeutic efficacy but also—and possibly more importantly—to demonstrate that a new health economy that provides the necessary support services can become profitable while significantly reducing net healthcare costs. Those services would include coaching, ICT, foods, diagnostics, and medication, all of which should be personalized and integrated.

Questions

1. **Which of the following statements about this article is true?**
   - **A.** This paper is a presentation and summary of the evidence from multiple randomized trials that type 2 diabetes can be reversed and prevented with a lifestyle medicine approach.
   - **B.** The paper recommends an approach involving piecemeal change at the local level, rather than an incremental global approach to implement the paradigm change.
   - **C.** The profit incentives are strong and compelling for existing stakeholders to embrace the new approach to "cure rather than care."
   - **D.** The economic incentives for society and governments to change are strong and compelling, since this approach would save both money and lives.

2. **Which of the following statements most accurately describes the conclusion and recommendations of this paper?**
   - **A.** Although the evidence reveals that type 2 diabetes can be reversed and prevented with lifestyle and diet changes, the cost of changing the system from care to cure outweighs any economic benefits and therefore this should not be attempted.
   - **B.** Evidence from multiple disciplines reveals that type 2 diabetes involves a lifestyle-genetic interaction in susceptible individuals and thus it can be avoided and reversed with the proper lifestyle and dietary changes. Although changing to a completely different approach will disrupt the present stakeholders, if the change is made it will save lives and increase profits by reducing expenses for avoidable care.
   - **C.** The concept of curing type 2 diabetes is being promoted by unscientific change agents seeking to disrupt the present system, which has successfully developed a standard of care second to none.
   - **D.** The profit incentives are strong and compelling for existing stakeholders to embrace the new approach to "cure rather than care."

Answers

1. **Answer: D.** The paper is a call for a total system change, and it presents the science from multiple disciplines that type 2 diabetes is reversible and preventable with lifestyle and dietary changes. The authors recommend making the change at the regional level where all the pieces are available, such as in the South Side Chicago example. Existing profit incentives are strong and compelling for the present stakeholders NOT to embrace the new approach. However, the economic and health incentives for society and government to adopt the new approach are strong and compelling, because we cannot afford to continue the present approach.

2. **Answer: B.** The costs of implementing the new "cure" approach do not outweigh the savings. The concept of "curing" diabetes is not being promoted by unscientific disrupters; rather it's being proved through the best science we have, and from many disciplines. The present "care" approach to diabetes is not working; it is breaking the system.

APPENDIX
Overweight and Obesity

Objective 1 Assess for the presence of overweight or obesity **362**

Objective 2 Describe the treatment recommendations for obesity **364**

Objective 3 Describe weight loss goals and expectations. **366**

Obesity Appendix References **367**

OBJECTIVE 1

Assess for the presence of overweight or obesity

1) **Obesity is defined as excess accumulation and storage of body fat.[1]**

   a) The percentage of people who are overweight or obese has sharply risen over the last several decades.[2]

   b) In the US, the incidence of overweight and obesity (body mass index [BMI] ≥30) in 2017–2018 was 42.4% among adults with no significant differences between ages or gender. Extreme obesity (BMI ≥40) was higher in women (11.5%) than in men (6.9%).[3]

2) **BMI which describes weight in kilograms relative to height in meters squared (kg/m^2) is a well-established measure of overweight and obesity.[1]**

   a) BMI equation: weight (kg)/height (m^2)

   b) Strengths: BMI calculation is easy to use and inexpensive. It provides well defined cutoff points for normal weight, overweight, and obesity. BMI highly correlates with risk of chronic disease and premature death.[4] All adults with a BMI ≥25 are at increased risk of developing cardiovascular diseases, insulin resistance and diabetes, osteoarthritis, obstructive sleep apnea, and increased risk of some cancers.[1]

   c) Limitations: BMI calculation cannot differentiate between body fat and lean body mass; at the same BMI, women typically have a higher percentage of body fat than men and Asians than Caucasians. It is also less accurate in the elderly.[4]

   d) Ranges

      1. Underweight: <18.5 kg/m^2
      2. Normal weight: 18.5–24.9 kg/m^2
      3. Overweight: 25.0–29.9 kg/m^2
      4. Obesity: ≥30.0 kg/m^2
         a. Class 1: 30.0–34.9 kg/m^2
         b. Class 2: 35.0–39.9 kg/m^2
         c. Class 3: ≥40.0 kg/m^2

3) **Percent body fat**

   a) Can be measured through a variety of methods, including:[4]

      1. Bioelectric impedance (BIA)
         a. Strengths: easy to use, inexpensive, portable, and safe
         b. Limitations: less accurate than other body fat measures and more difficult to calibrate. Also, the accuracy decreases as the ratio between body water to body fat changes, such as in states of dehydration, weight loss, or illness.
      2. Densitometry (underwater weighing)
         a. Strengths: more accurate than BIA testing
         b. Limitations: difficult to perform as individuals must be submerged underwater

3. Air-displacement plethysmography ("Bod Pod")
    a. Strengths: accurate, safe, and easier to complete than densitometry
    b. Limitations: relatively expensive
4. DEXA Scans, CTs, and MRIs can also be used and are accurate, but relatively expensive and not portable.

b) Ranges of percent body fat (see Table A.1)[5]

1. Normal
    a. Male <25%
    b. Female <32%
2. Obese
    a. Male ≥25%
    b. Female ≥32%

Table A.1 Ranges for Percent Body-Fat[5]

	Women	Men
Essential Fat	10–12%	2–4%
Athletes	14–20%	6–13%
Fitness	21–24%	14–17%
Acceptable	25–31%	18–25%
Obese	32% plus	26% plus

4) Waist circumference[4]

a) Waist circumference correlates with abdominal fat, which is an independent risk factor for cardiometabolic risk, cardiovascular events, and mortality beyond an elevated BMI.[1,6]

b) A debate remains as to the best location for measurement. Waist measurement can be taken at the umbilicus, the narrowest part of the waist, or just above the iliac crests. The World Health Organization recommends measuring at the midpoint between the lowest rib and iliac crest.[7]

c) Strengths: waist circumference is easy to measure, inexpensive, and strongly correlated with percent body fat and development of chronic disease and premature death.

d) Limitations: though easy to perform, waist measurement techniques have not been standardized. It may be less accurate in individuals with a BMI greater than 35 kg/m^2.

e) Normal

1. Male <40 in (<102 cm)
2. Female <35 in (<88 cm)

f) Obese

1. Male ≥40 in (≥102 cm)
2. Female ≥35 in (≥88 cm)

5) Edmonton obesity staging (see Table A.2)[8,9]

a) A way of staging obesity according to functional status and morbidity associated with excess weight.

b) Stages are from Stage 0 (no loss of function or noted morbidity) to Stage 4 (severe loss of function and/or severe obesity-related morbidities).

Table A.2 Edmonton Obesity Staging System[9]

Stage	Description	Management
0	**No** obesity-related comorbidities **No** physical or functional limitations, or impairment of well-being	Identify of factors contributing to increased weight. Provide lifestyle change counseling to prevent future weight gain.
1	**Mild** obesity-related diseases **Mild** physical symptoms and functional limitations, and impairment of well-being	Investigate other causes of obesity-related illnesses. Offer more intense lifestyle interventions. Monitor risk factors and health status.
2	**Confirmed** obesity-related chronic diseases **Moderate** physical symptoms, functional limitations, and impairment of well-being	Treat obesity with lifestyle, pharmacological, or surgical treatment options with close monitoring and management.
3	**End-organ damage** from obesity-related chronic diseases **Significant** physical symptoms, functional limitations, and impairment of well-being	Pursue intensive obesity treatment and aggressive management of comorbidities.
4	**End stage organ failure** from obesity-related chronic diseases **Severe or disabling** physical symptoms, functional limitations, and impairment of well-being	Pursue as aggressive obesity management as tolerated as well as palliative care.

OBJECTIVE 2

Describe the treatment recommendations for obesity

1) **US Preventive Services Task Force recommends:[10]**
   a) All adults should be screened for obesity and clinicians should offer or refer patients with a body mass index (BMI) of 30 kg/m^2 or higher to intensive, multicomponent behavioral interventions.
      1. These are Grade 'B' recommendations, meaning the benefit is moderate to substantial.

2) **The Centers for Medicare and Medicaid Services states:[11]**
   a) Treatment with intensive behavioral therapy is reasonable and necessary for the prevention and early detection of illness or disability in individuals diagnosed with obesity, defined as a BMI of ≥30 kg/m^2.

3) **American College of Cardiology/American Heart Association/The Obesity Society (ACA/AHA/TOS) 2013 Obesity Guidelines[12]**
   a) Individuals who should be referred to a comprehensive lifestyle intervention program
      1. Patients with BMI ≥25 with cardiovascular disease risk factors
      2. Patients with BMI ≥30
   b) Comprehensive lifestyle interventions
      1. Most effective programs are in person, high-intensity (≥14 sessions in 6 months), individual or group based, and are led by trained interventionists or nutrition professionals.
      2. Programs will include caloric restriction, increased physical activity, and behavioral strategies to facilitate lifestyle changes.

3. If intensive programs are not available, patients should be offered less effective weight loss alternatives, such as counseling via electronic sources (web or phone), commercial programs, and/or food replacement programs.

4) Weight loss recommendations[12]

a) Calorie reduction

1. An energy deficit is created by reducing calories, which can lead to weight loss. To lose 1 pound over the course of the week by caloric restriction, a patient should eat approximately 3,500 calories less per week.
    a. Women are recommended to reduce calories by 500 calories per day with a goal total calorie intake of 1,200–1,500 calories per day.
    b. Men are recommended to reduce calories by 750 calories per day with goal total calorie intake of 1,500–1,800 calories per day.

b) Non-resting energy expenditure should be increased.

1. The total energy expenditure (TEE) over 24 hours is the sum of the follow three types of energy expenditures:
    a. Resting energy expenditure (REE), approximately 60% of TEE
    b. Thermic effect of eeeding (TEF), approximately 5–10% of TEE
    c. Non-resting energy expenditure (NREE), approximately 30–40% of TEE
        (1) NREE can be increased through physical activity.
2. Weight loss is usually difficult to accomplish with exercise alone.[13]
    a. In order to lose 1 pound per week, an individual would have to burn about 500 extra calories per day, the equivalent of walking 5 miles a day or 35 miles per week.

c) Optimal diets have been debated: high-protein diet, low-fat, versus low-carbohydrate.[14] No particular diet has been found to be superior.[15,16]

d) Different patients may be able to adhere to different diets better than others, however, the diet must be hypocaloric regardless of macronutrient composition.[14,17,18] Eating a whole food plant-based diet may be helpful for weight loss due caloric density, particularly being high in fiber.[19,20]

5) Referral to bariatric surgery[12,21]

a) BMI ≥40, or

b) BMI ≥35 with at least one obesity-associated comorbid condition

c) Must also be motivated to lose weight, without sufficient response to lifestyle interventions alone

1. The American College of Lifestyle Medicine, in agreement with the AHA/ACC/TOS 2013 Obesity Guidelines, strongly encourages any patient who needs to lose weight be referred to a comprehensive lifestyle intervention, preferably run by a trained interventionalist or nutritionist. Though the AHA/ACC/TOS guidelines do not recommend a specific amount of time, it is reasonable to treat with lifestyle change for at least 6 months before initiating more invasive treatment for obesity. 6 months should be considered a minimum time for lifestyle treatment, not the "ideal" or optimal period for making lifestyle change. Lifestyle change treatments should not be considered to have failed without trying an intensive lifestyle immersion program or the patient having declined it.

OBJECTIVE 3

Describe weight loss goals and expectations

1) **Weight loss goal for overweight or obese patients**

   a) 5–10% of initial body weight

      1. Average weight loss in intensive lifestyle intervention is ~8 kg (17 lbs) within 6 months.

   b) In overweight or obese with cardiovascular disease risk factors:

      1. Weight loss of 3–5% is clinically meaningful by improving glucose, hemoglobin A1c (HbA1c), triglycerides, and reducing progression to diabetes.
      2. Weight loss above 5% can improve hypertension, dyslipidemia, and allow for medication reduction.

2) **Managing expectations of patient weight loss**

   a) The pathophysiology of weight gain at its most basic level appears straightforward, with caloric intake exceeding the calories expended. Nevertheless, obesity as a disease is far more complex than passive accumulation and storage of body fat. The risk of obesity depends on factors such as energy homeostasis, hormonal regulation, genetic predisposition, developmental exposures, environmental or social influences, and toxins such as endocrine disrupting chemicals.[22]

   b) BMI and weight loss associated goals from patients who come to obesity specialty clinics often do not align with predicted weight loss from lifestyle changes (~8 kg or 17 lbs) or what is necessary to improve clinical outcomes (3–5% weight loss).

      1. Patient expectations for weight loss[23]
         a. Dream = 24.8 BMI (30.9% loss)
         b. Happy = 27.1 BMI (25.2% loss)
         c. Acceptable = 29.3 BMI (19.7% loss)
         d. Disappointed = 33.0 BMI (10.4% loss)
      2. Weight loss needed to achieve clinical outcomes[12]
         a. A weight loss of 3–5% can lead to improvements in triglycerides, glucose, HbA1c, and lower the risk of developing diabetes.
         b. A weight loss of more than 5% can improve hypertension, dyslipidemia, and reduce need for medications even in patients with diabetes.

   c) Managing the plateau phenomenon[24]

      1. When 10% or greater weight loss occurs, a person's non-resting energy expenditure decreases by about 30% because of changes in lean mass and fat mass. Individuals must compensate for this reduction in total energy expenditure by eating 10–15% less calories than expected for a person of his same height and weight but who has not lost weight. This effect can persist for several months to several years.
      2. In addition, structural changes occur to the hypothalamus with weight gain and the brain must readapt for sustained body weight control.[25]

OBESITY APPENDIX REFERENCES

1. Clinical Guidelines on the Identification, Evaluation, and Treatment of Overweight and Obesity in Adults–The Evidence Report. National Institutes of Health. *Obes Res.* 1998;6 Suppl 2:51s-209s.
2. World Health Organization. Obesity and overweight. Updated April 1, 2020. https://www.who.int/news-room/fact-sheets/detail/obesity-and-overweight. Accessed January 23, 2021.
3. Hales C. M., Carroll M. D., Fryar C. D., Ogden C. L. *Prevalence of Obesity and Severe Obesity Among Adults: United States, 2017–2018.* NCHS Data Brief, no 360. Hyattsville, MD: National Center for Health Statistics; 2020. https://www.cdc.gov/nchs/products/databriefs/db360.htm.
4. Harvard T. H. Chan School of Public Health. Measuring Obesity. *Obesity Prevention Source.* December 17, 2018. https://www.hsph.harvard.edu/obesity-prevention-source/obesity-definition/how-to-measure-body-fatness/.
5. Muth N. D. What are the guidelines for percentage of body fat loss? 2018. https://www.acefitness.org/education-and-resources/lifestyle/blog/112/what-are-the-guidelines-for-percentage-of-body-fat-loss.
6. Ness-Abramof R., Apovian C. M. Waist circumference measurement in clinical practice. *Nutr Clin Pract.* 2008;23(4):397-404.
7. Serviente C., Sforzo G. A. A simple yet complicated tool: measuring waist circumference to determine cardiometabolic risk. *ACSMs Health Fitness J.* 2013;17(6):29-34. https://journals.lww.com/acsm-healthfitness/Fulltext/2013/11000/A_Simple_Yet_Complicated_Tool__Measuring_Waist.7.aspx.
8. Carretero G. J., Arevalo L. J. C., Gomez H. R., et al. Prevalence of obesity according to Edmonton staging in the Internal Medicine consultations. Results of the OBEMI study. *Revista clinica espanola.* 2017;217(2):71-78.
9. Sharma A. M., Kushner R. F. A proposed clinical staging system for obesity. *Int J Obes (Lond).* 2009;33(3):289-295. https://pubmed.ncbi.nlm.nih.gov/19188927/.
10. US Preventive Services Task Force. Obesity in adults: screening and management. *Recommendations for Primary Care Practice.* 2012;2018. https://www.uspreventiveservicestaskforce.org/uspstf/recommendation/obesity-in-adults-screening-and-management.
11. Centers for Medicare and Medicaid Services. *Decision Memo for Intensive Behavioral Therapy for Obesity.* Baltimore, MD: Centers for Medicare and Medicaid Services; 2011. https://www.cms.gov/medicare-coverage-database/details/nca-decision-memo.aspx?&NcaName=Intensive%20Behavioral%20Therapy%20for%20Obesity&bc=ACAAAAAAIAAA&NCAId=253.
12. Jensen M. D., Ryan D. H., Apovian C. M., et al. 2013 AHA/ACC/TOS Guideline for the management of overweight and obesity in adults: a report of the American College of Cardiology/American Heart Association Task Force on Practice Guidelines and The Obesity Society. *Circulation.* 2014;129(25 Suppl 2):S102-138.
13. Wadden T. A., Webb V. L., Moran C. H., Bailer B. A. Lifestyle modification for obesity: new developments in diet, physical activity, and behavior therapy. *Circulation.* 2012;125(9):1157-1170. https://www.ncbi.nlm.nih.gov/pubmed/22392863.
14. Thom G., Lean M. Is there an optimal diet for weight management and metabolic health? *Gastroenterology.* 2017;152(7):1739-1751.
15. Sacks F. M., Bray G. A., Carey V. J., et al. Comparison of weight-loss diets with different compositions of fat, protein, and carbohydrates. *N Engl J Med.* 2009;360(9):859-873.
16. Moore W. J., McGrievy M. E., Turner-McGrievy G. M. Dietary adherence and acceptability of five different diets, including vegan and vegetarian diets, for weight loss: the New DIETs study. *Eat Behav.* 2015;19:33-38.
17. Dansinger M. L., Gleason J. A., Griffith J. L., Selker H. P., Schaefer E. J. Comparison of the Atkins, Ornish, Weight Watchers, and Zone diets for weight loss and heart disease risk reduction: a randomized trial. *JAMA.* 2005;293(1):43-53.
18. Nordmann A. J., Nordmann A., Briel M., et al. Effects of low-carbohydrate vs low-fat diets on weight loss and cardiovascular risk factors: a meta-analysis of randomized controlled trials. *Arch Intern Med.* 2006;166(3):285-293.
19. Kahleova H., Dort S., Holubkov R., Barnard N. D. A plant-based high-carbohydrate, low-fat diet in overweight individuals in a 16-week randomized clinical trial: the role of carbohydrates. *Nutrients.* 2018;10(9).
20. Sylvetsky A. C., Edelstein S. L., Walford G., et al. A high-carbohydrate, high-fiber, low-fat diet results in weight loss among adults at high risk of type 2 diabetes. *J Nutr.* 2017;147(11):2060-2066.
21. American Society for Metabolic and Bariatric Surgery. Who is a candidate for bariatric surgery? 2018. https://asmbs.org/patients/who-is-a-candidate-for-bariatric-surgery.
22. Schwartz M. W., Seeley R. J., Zeltser L. M., et al. Obesity pathogenesis: an endocrine society scientific statement. *Endocr Rev.* 2017;38(4):267-296. https://pubmed.ncbi.nlm.nih.gov/28898979/.
23. Dutton G. R., Perri M. G., Dancer-Brown M., Goble M., Van Vessem N. Weight loss goals of patients in a health maintenance organization. *Eat Behav.* 2010;11(2):74-78. https://www.ncbi.nlm.nih.gov/pubmed/20188289.
24. Rosenbaum M., Leibel R. L. Adaptive thermogenesis in humans. *Int J Obes (Lond).* 2010;34 Suppl 1:S47-55. https://www.ncbi.nlm.nih.gov/pubmed/20935667.
25. Sumithran P., Proietto J. The defence of body weight: a physiological basis for weight regain after weight loss. *Clin Sci (Lond).* 2013;124(4):231-241. https://pubmed.ncbi.nlm.nih.gov/23126426/.

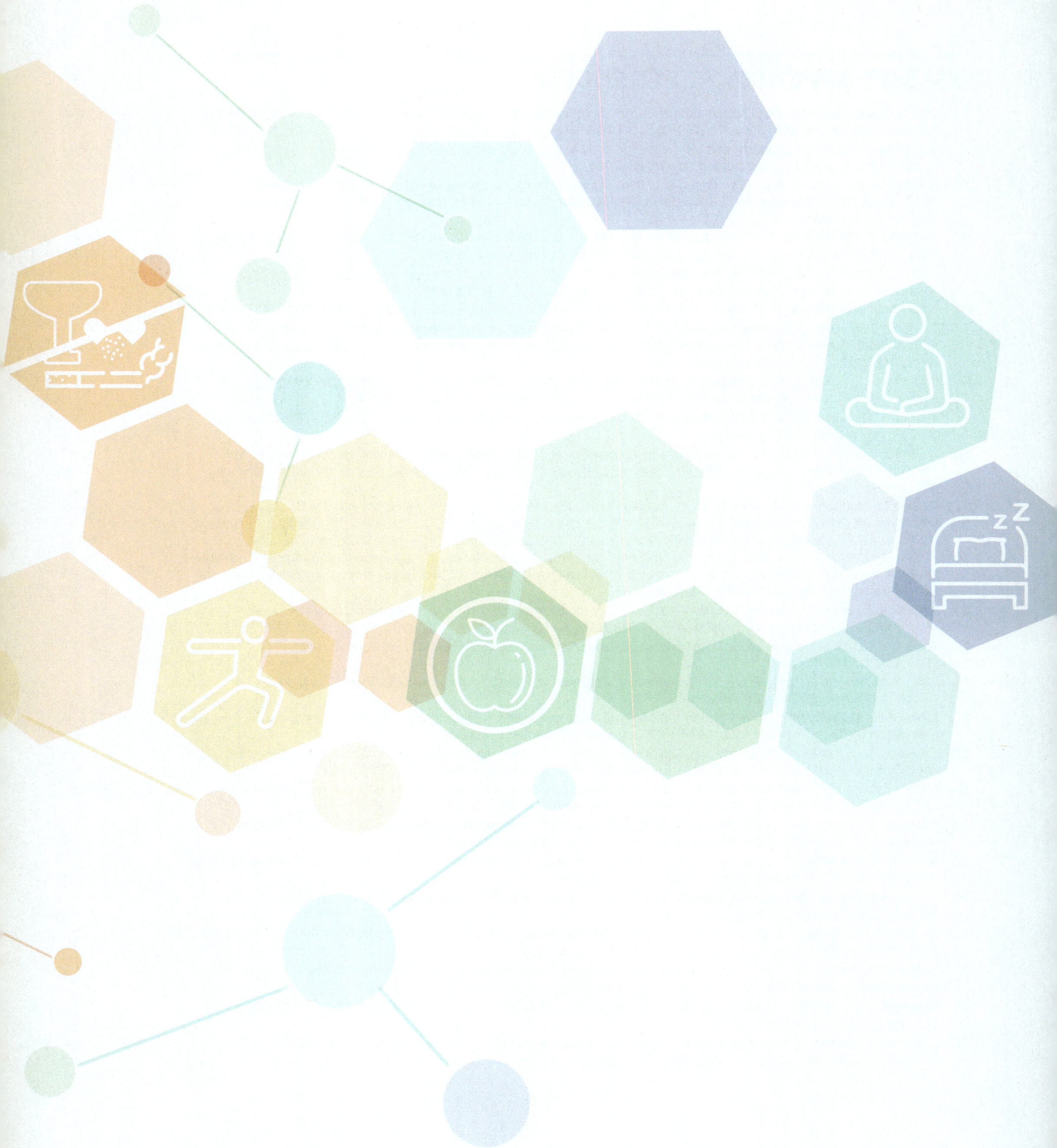

INDEX

Note: Page numbers followed by *t* refer to tables. Page numbers followed by *f* refer to figures.

A

A1c. *See* hemoglobin A1c
ABC (antecedent/behavior/consequence) chart, 214
ABCDE model of behavioral change, 30, 32
ABCD nutrition assessment, 116
abdominal aortic aneurysm, 66
abdominal breathing, 241
abdominal obesity, 13, 345–346
abnormal platelet adherence, 240
Academy of Nutrition and Dietetics, 72, 115
acamprosate, 314
accident, 11*t*
accomplishment, 326
ACCORD (Action to Control Cardiovascular Risk in Diabetes) study, 152
accountability, 42, 46, 48, 76
accountable care organization, 78
acid/base balance, 66
action plan
  coaching process, 46
  emotional well-being, 241, 246
  goal, 36
  maintenance, 37
  management skill, 9
  relapse prevention planning, 41–42
  review question/answers and summaries, 52, 54, 100–101
  stage of change treatment prescription, 33–35, 96
action stage, 27, 29, 34*t*–35*t*, 39, 47, 53, 212
Activity Counseling Trial (ACT), 210–211
activity level, 117
acupuncture, 71, 302
acute myeloid leukemia, 282
acute myocardial infarction (AMI), 12–13
added salt, 132
added sugar, 106–107, 112, 125–126, 132
addiction, 238–239, 252
addiction counseling, 309
addiction specialist, 314
addiction to distraction, 254
adenosine level, 277
adequate intake (AI), 120*t*
adhesion molecule, 154
adipocyte cell, 152–154
adiponectin, 153, 161
adipose tissue, 152
adiposity, 149, 192*t*
administrative assistant, 76–77
adolescent, 302–303, 322, 324, 328
adrenal gland, 270, 271*f*
adrenaline, 235
advanced glycation end products (AGEs), 127–129, 164, 168, 281
Adventist Health Study 2, 15, 158, 166, 170
adverse childhood event, 11
advise, 43, 212, 303*t*, 304
aerobic exercise
  activity guideline, 194, 218
  benefits of, 188
  defined, 223
  exercise types, 187
  Lifestyle Heart Trial, 114, 144
  maximum amount, 200
  PAV interpretation, 202
  physician health behavior, 196
  pregnancy and postpartum guidelines, 219
  review question/answers and summaries, 225, 228
  strength training comparison, 189*t*
Aerobics Center Longitudinal Study, 185, 227
affirmation, 29
Affordable Care Act, 10
aflatoxin, 127
African American population, 64, 134
African population, 142
Agency for Healthcare Research and Quality (AHRQ), 77–78, 80
AGEs (advanced glycation end products). *See* advanced glycation end products (AGEs)
aggressive therapeutic lifestyle change, 136
aging, 149*f*, 154
Agouti mice research, 149
agree, 43, 212, 303*t*
air-displacement plethysmography ("Bod Pod"), 65, 363
air pollution, 12
Alaska, 308
Alaska Native population, 151
albumin, 117
albuminuria, 140
alcohol
  abuse, 11
  consumption, 9–10, 13–14, 80, 132*t*, 150, 159*f*, 235, 283, 308–311, 317–318
  consumption vital sign, 62
  hypertension, 134
  misuse intervention, 312–314
  use, heavy, 309
  use disorder model, 41
  use screening, 311–312
"alcoholic", 310
alcoholic beverage, 112, 127
Alcoholics Anonymous, 314
"alcoholism", 310
alcohol-related serious medical illness, 309
alcohol use disorder (AUD), 308–310, 312–315, 317–318
Alcohol Use Disorder Identification Test (AUDIT), 311–312, 314
aldehyde dehydrogenase, 314
aldosterone, 270
alertness, 272, 275, 282
all-cause mortality, 106, 123–124, 157, 185–186, 192*t*, 198–201, 218, 285
allele, 150
allergy, 154
allied health professional, 75–76
allium vegetable, 127
all-or-nothing thinking, 30
Alternative Healthy Eating index, 115
alternative medicine, 17
Alzheimer's disease, 11*t*, 154, 327
amaranth, 135
ambient temperature, 271, 272*f*, 274, 277
American Board of Lifestyle Medicine (ABLM), 7
American College of Cardiology, 64–65, 207
American College of Cardiology/American Heart Association/The Obesity Society (ACA/AHA/TOS) 2013 Obesity Guidelines, 364–365

American College of Lifestyle Medicine (ACLM), 6–8, 63, 365
American College of Preventive Medicine (ACPM), 7
American College of Sports Medicine (ACSM), 72, 197, 206–207, 208*t*, 209, 216
American Council on Exercise (ACE), 216
American Diabetes Association (ADA), 64
American Diabetes Association (ADA) diet, 115, 140, 157–159
American diet, 155–156, 167–168, 171. *See also* Western-style diet
American Heart Association (AHA), 65, 73, 107–108, 134
American Heart Association (AHA) Step 1 diet, 16, 114
American Heart Association (AHA) Step 2 diet, 336–337
American Heart Association's Life's Simple 7 Questionnaire, 63
American Indian population, 64, 151. *See also* Native American population
American Institute for Cancer Research, 113
American Journal of Clinical Nutrition, 155, 163
American Journal of Lifestyle Medicine, 44
American Medical Association (AMA) Foundation, 7
American Medical Association Code of Ethics, 254
American Medical Association Code of Medical Ethics: "Physician Health and Wellness", 95
American Planning Association, 99
American Psychiatric Association, *Diagnostic and Statistical Manual* (DSM-5), 237–238, 242, 309–311
American Public Health Association, 99
amino acid, 121, 128
amplified reflection, 46
amputation, 221
amygdala, 251, 282, 327
Anderson, J.W., 140, 166
angina, 66, 144
"Angina Pectoris and Atherosclerotic Risk Factors in the Multisite Cardiac Lifestyle Intervention Program" study, 144
angiogenesis, 154, 161, 270*f*
animal fat, 140
animal food, 109
animal product, 60–61, 107, 125, 128, 132, 134, 136, 141
animal protein, 121–122, 132*t*, 140, 158
anthropometric data, 116
antibiotic, 152
anticoagulant, 218
antidepressant medication, 253, 313, 322
antihypertensive medication, 140
anti-inflammatory diet, 243
anti-inflammatory food, 126
anti-inflammatory molecule, 126
antioxidant, 112, 126, 132, 141, 154, 239
antioxidant-rich food, 136, 161
antiplatelet therapy, 218
anti-relapse medications (ARMs), 309, 314–315, 317–318
anxiety, 192*t*, 193, 237, 240–245, 251–253, 290, 292, 322–325, 328
anxiety disorder, 238–239
aortic dissection, 208
aortic stenosis, 208
apnea, 279
apnea-hypopnea index (AHI), 279
apoptosis, 270*f*, 282
appendicitis, 137
appetite, 276
apple, 122*t*
arachidonic acid, 123, 239, 324
Aribisala, B.S., 347–349
arrange, 43, 303*t*, 304
arrhythmia, 208
arsenic, 239
arthritis, 11, 154, 188
artificial sweetener, 135
ASCVD Risk Estimator Plus, 64
Asian, non-Hispanic population, 151
Asian American population, 64, 68
Asian Indian young adult, 157
Asian population, 18, 65, 308
ask, 303*t*, 304
Ask the Dietitian, 118
aspirin therapy, 64
assess, 43, 96, 212, 303*t*, 304
assessment skill, 8
assist, 43, 213, 303*t*, 304
asthma, 12, 154, 306*t*
atherosclerosis, 128, 141, 143, 154, 236, 337
atherosclerotic cardiovascular disease (ASCVD), 13–14, 64
athlete, 123
Atkins diet, 342–344
ATP synthesis, 273
at-risk behavior, 9
at-risk drinking, 309
at-risk patient, 9
attention deficit hyperactivity disorder (ADHD), 193*t*
attitude, 38
AUDIT-C (The Alcohol Use Disorders Identification Test-Concise), 62
Australian government type 2 diabetes risk assessment tool, 64
Australian women, 323
autogenic training, 277
autoimmune disease, 149*f*, 154, 239
autonomic nervous system, 270
autonomous motivation, 40, 45, 48, 53
avocado, 108, 135
awareness, 46, 248, 250, 254–255
Azimuth test, 63

B

balance, 188, 196, 202, 219, 222–223
banana, 122*t*
bariatric surgery, 119, 365
Barnard, Neal, *Dr. Neal Barnard's Program for Reversing Diabetes*, 136
Barnard, Tom, *Defeating Diabetes*, 136
Barnes, A.C., 352–355
baroreceptor sensitivity, 273
Basal Energy Expenditure: Harris-Benedict Equation calculator, 118
basic disease process, 120–129
Baylor Cardiovascular Institute, 143
bean, 60, 134–135, 145
Beck Anxiety Inventory (BAI), 237
Beck Depression Index (BDI), 244
Beck Depression Inventory (BDI-II), 236
beef, 108, 122*t*
beer, 323
behavior
  assessment, 8
  change, 9, 33, 41, 46, 76, 129, 214–217, 303*t*
  change intervention, 72
  change process, 29–32, 37, 38*t*, 39
  change theory, 37–38
  change therapy, 326
  change "working" groups, 33
  contract, 41
  healthy, 37
behavioral
  capability, 38
  change, 36, 358–360
  determinant, 10–11
  health disorder, 278
  health provider, 242
  health specialist, 29
  intention, 38
  intervention, 313, 364
  method, 284
  principle, 6
  therapy, 243
behaviorally induced insufficient sleep syndrome (BIISS), 278
belief, 40
Benjamin, Regina, 10
benzene, 127
benzodiazepine, 277, 284
berry, 126
beta-carotene, 136
beta cell, 152–154, 161, 355–358
beta cell apoptosis, 155

beta cell function, 67, 84, 157, 347–349, 359
beta-cell regeneration, 157
bibliotherapy, 241–242
Billings, J. H., 336–337
"binge" drinking, 309
biochemical body function, 17
biochemical data, 116–117
biochemical treatment, 19
bioelectric impedance (BIA), 65, 116, 362
biofeedback, 17, 302
biological predisposition, 8, 10–11
biomarker, 120
biometric assessment, 76
bioterrorism, 17
bipolar disorder, 244, 278, 282, 301, 324
birth defect, 302
Black, non-Hispanic population, 151
Black population, 68, 151, 308. *See also* African American population
bladder cancer, 192*t*
"blissful immersion", 325
Block Dietary Fat Screener, 118
blood count, 66
blood glucose level, 45, 63, 66, 120*t*, 125, 152–153, 156–157, 186
blood glucose management, 152
blood glucose normalization, 156
blood glucose regulation, 140
blood osmolality, 277, 289
blood pressure. *See also* diastolic blood pressure; hypertension; systolic blood pressure
  American Heart Association's Life's Simple 7 Questionnaire, 63
  blue light, 275
  collaborative and chronic care models, 76
  DASH diet, 113–114, 147
  dose-dependent, 166, 170
  exercise, 218
  The GEMINAL Study, 345–346
  Mediterranean diet, 146
  physical activity, 193*t*
  physician competencies, 8
  sleep, 273, 281
  2017 Guideline for the Prevention, Detection, Evaluation, and Management of High Blood Pressure in Adults (American College of Cardiology and American Heart Association), 65–66
  vasodilation, 272
  water-only fasting, 135
  whole food plant-based diet, 140
blood protein, 66
blood vessel, 154
blue light, 275, 289
blue light spectra, 291–292
Blue Zones Project, 98
BMI Percentile Calculator, 118
BodPod, 65, 363
body
  composition, 116, 187, 189*t*, 205, 223
  fat, 135, 188, 189*t*, 362–363
  frame, 118
  weight, 13*t*, 121. *See also* weight
body mass index (BMI). *See also* BMI Percentile Calculator
  adolescent, 324
  Adventist Health Study 2, 15
  Asian population, 65
  assessment skill, 9
  diabetes testing, 68
  dietary assessment tool, 118
  health and wellness coach, 44
  low-fat whole food plant-based diet, 147
  Nurses' Health Study, 14
  nutrition assessment, 116
  obesity, 362, 366
  physical activity, 193*t*
  physician personal behavior, 95
  plant-based diet, 139
  red meat replacement, 159*f*
  sleep, 281, 283
  vital sign, 63
bone fracture, 297
bone health, 105, 122, 187, 192*t*, 193
bone mineral density, 188, 189*t*
Borg category-ratio scale, 203
Borg scale of perceived exertion, 203, 223
brain
  break, 256
  carbohydrate, 120*t*
  connectivity, 252
  energy, 255
  executive function, 193
  health, 192*t*
  neuroplasticity, 251
  serotonin, 239
brain-derived neurotrophic factor (BDNF), 244, 282
brain reward (dopamine) pathway, 300*f*
Braman, Marc, 7
breast cancer
  Mediterranean diet, 146
  nutrition prescription, 136, 139
  physical activity, 192*t*–193*t*, 218, 221
  physician competencies, 8
  review question/answers and summaries, 166, 169–170
  sleep, 282
breastfeeding, 150
broccoli, 122*t*
Brussels sprout, 122*t*
Buono, R., 355–358
bupropion, 300–302
Burkitt, Dennis
  "The Development of the Concept of Dietary Fiber", 138
  "The Etiological Significance of Related Diseases", 137
  "Western Diseases and Their Emergence Related to Diet", 138
burnout syndrome, 95, 237, 253
Buse, J.B., 156
Butler, C.
  Health Behavior Change: A Guide for Practitioners, 36*t*
  Motivational Interviewing in Health Care: Helping Patient Change Behavior, 36*t*
butyrate, 152, 161

C

caffeine, 134, 283, 290, 292
calcium
  biochemical data, 117
  bone health, 122
  colon cancer, 137
  dietary risk factor, 138*f*
  hypertension, 134
  micronutrient, 127
  nutrient deficiency and mood, 245, 323
  underconsumed nutrient, 60, 109–110
calcium-rich food, 105
Caldwell B. Esselstyn Jr. Cleveland Clinic, 7
California Health Interview Survey (CHIS), 60
California Smokers' Helpline (1-800-NO-BUTTS), 73
caloric burn, 276
caloric intake, 161–162, 198
calorie, 7, 107–108, 112, 120*t*, 121, 135, 152–153, 155, 198
Calorie King, 119
calorie reduction, 365
Campbell, T. Colin, "Diet, Lifestyle and Etiology of Coronary Artery Disease", 142
Canadian Cardiovascular Society (CCS), 339–340
cancer. *See also under specific type*
  Adventist Health Study 2, 15
  adverse childhood event, 11
  alcohol consumption, 308
  angiogenesis, 154
  body mass index, 63
  depression, 240
  depression/anxiety assessment, 239
  epigenetics, 149*f*
  insulin dosing, 152
  motivational interviewing, 306*t*

NF-kß, 154
nutrition assessment, 119
nutrition prescription, 131–137, 139
physical activity, 192*t*, 221
physician competencies, 8
review question/answers and summaries, 164, 169
risk factor, 164, 169
smoking and, 296
treatment failure rate, 297
vegetarian diet, 146
cancer-causing chemical, 302
carbohydrate, 7, 120*t*, 125, 132*t*, 135, 239, 276–277, 281, 324
carcinogen, 127, 296
cardiac disease, 206, 240
cardiac event, 114
cardiac mortality, 106
cardiac risk factor, 13
cardiac stenosis, 7
cardiometabolic condition, 192*t*
cardiometabolic risk factor profile, 146
cardiorespiratory endurance, 223
cardiorespiratory fitness (CRF), 185, 187, 192*t*
cardiorespiratory fitness test, 204
cardiovascular
disorder, 281
event, 147
exercise, 59
fitness, 187
function, 235
health, 146, 198
incidence, 192*t*
mortality, 193*t*
risk factor, 141, 143, 192*t*, 281, 366
risk factor calculator, 64
system, 201
cardiovascular disease (CVD)
Adventist Health Study 2, 15
ASCVD Risk Estimator Plus, 64
behavioral determinant, 11
cholesterol, 106
dairy, 105, 124, 134
DASH diet, 147
death, 281
diabetes cure-focused therapy, 358–360
diabetes testing, 68
dietary pattern, 123
dietary risk factor, 138*f*
exercise preparticipation health screening recommendation, 208*t*, 209
high sensitivity c-reactive protein, 67
hypertension, 66
intensive medication management, 152
job characteristic, 235
Life's Simple 7 Questionnaire, 63
lifestyle intervention, 145
(MRFIT) Study, 14
nicotine replacement therapy, 301
nutrition in preventing and treating, 137, 141
obesity, 201
physical activity, 193*t*
prevention and treatment practices, 10
registered dietitian, 119
risk, 199–200
saturated fat, 143
Western-style diet, 142
care-seeking behavior, 12
carnitine, 158
carotenoid, 126–127
cataract, 140, 278
catecholamine production, 236
Caucasian American population, 142
cause and effect diagram, 83
CBT for insomnia (CBT-I), 284
cell, 120*t*, 121, 136
Cell, 355–358
cell cycle, 270*f*, 282
cell damage, 128
cell death, 124
cell membrane fluidity, 244
cell signaling, 120*t*
cellular metabolism, 17
Centers for Disease Control and Prevention (CDC), 64, 118, 160, 296, 302
Centers for Disease Control and Prevention National Diabetes Prevention Program, 73
Centers for Medicare and Medicaid Services, 145, 364
central oscillator, 269, 271*f*, 289
central sulcus, 270*f*
ceramide (CER), 153
cerclage, 219
cerebellum, 270*f*, 300*f*
cerebral cortex, 270*f*
cerebral palsey, 221
cerebrovascular disease, 206
Certified Clinical Exercise Physiologist, 72
certified exercise physiologist, 71
certified health coach, 6
Certified Medical Fitness facilities, 72
Certified Personal Trainer, 72
cervical cancer, 136
cervix, 219
character strength, 248, 326
cheese, 105–108, 122*t*
chef/food service, 76–77
chemical food contaminant, 150
Chen, M.J., 347–349
Cheng, C.W., Fasting-Mimicking Diet Promotes Ngn3- Driven β-Cell Regeneration to Reverse Diabetes, 355–358
chest pain, 208
Chicago Heart Association Detection Project in Industry, 13
chicken, 122*t*
chickpea, 122*t*
childhood event, 11
child nutrition, 150
children, 123, 149–150
Chilean college students, 325
Chinese population, 65, 142, 150
"CHIP Lifestyle Program at Vanderbilt University Demonstrates an Early ROI for a Diabetic Cohort in a Workplace Setting" (Shurney, Hyde, Hulsey, et al.), 19
chiropractic, DC, 71
cholesterol
all-cause mortality, 185*t*
American Heart Association's Life's Simple 7 Questionnaire, 63
ASCVD Risk Estimator Plus, 64
cardiovascular disease, 141
DASH diet, 113
egg, 106
fasting lipid, 67
fiber, 125
heart disease risk factor, 142–143
hyperlipidemia, 132
Jenkin's Portfolio diet, 18
kidney disease, 140
lifestyle change, 13*t*
Lifestyle Heart Trial, 144
Mediterranean diet, 146
overconsumed nutrient, 107
physical activity, 188
physician health behavior, 95
choline, 109, 158
chromatin, 149*f*
chromosome, 149*f*
chronic care management, 309
chronic care model, 75–80, 84, 86, 88
Chronic Care Model, 78–79
chronic disease. *See also under specific type*
aerobic exercise, 194–195
AGEs (advanced glycation end products), 128
alcohol consumption, 308–311
American College of Lifestyle Medicine, 6
chronic care model, 77
Complete Health Improvement Program (CHIP), 7
control, 18–19
dietary pattern, 123
diet vital sign, 60
management, 74
mental illness, 239–240
nicotine replacement therapies, 301
nutrition prescription, 115
physical activity, 187
positive emotion, 326

prevention and treatment practice, 137
registered dietitian, 119
review question/answers and summaries, 85, 87
risk factor, 115
self-management, 75
sleep role in, 278–282
tobacco cessation, 297–298
tobacco use, 298
whole food plant-based diet, 161
chronic illness medication, 27
chronic illness somatic symptom, 237
chronic inflammation, 67
chronic insomnia, 279, 284
chronic kidney disease, 63, 141
chronic lower respiratory disease, 11*t*
chronic obstructive pulmonary disease (COPD), 140, 297, 306*t*
chronic pain, 252
chronic stress, 150
cigarette, 296
cigarette fading, 302
circadian biomarker, 270*f*
circadian oscillator, 269, 289
circadian physiology, 269–277, 291–292
circadian regulation, 283
circadian rhythm, 239, 269–273, 276, 284, 289–290, 292
circadian system, 271
Circulation, 338–341
cleft lip, 297
cleft palate, 297
Cleveland Clinic, 7, 296
clinical assessment, 116–117
clinical depression, 238–239
clinical expert (MD/DO), 78
clinical information system, 79
clonidine, 301
coach, 44, 49, 51, 71, 120, 215, 259–260. *See also* health and wellness coach
Coaching Psychology Manual (Moore, M.), 36*t*
coal-tar, 127
cocaine, 300*f*
coffee creamer, 124
cognition, 193*t*, 281
cognitive
agility, 254–255
behavioral technique, 29–30, 40, 48, 241
behavior therapy technique, 131
distortion, 30
function, 192*t*
impairment, 327
processing, 282, 322
restructuring, 131, 246, 284
Cognitive Behavioral Techniques: A Practitioner's Guide (Leahy, R. L.), 42*t*
cognitive behavioral therapy (CBT), 29–30, 240–241, 243, 252–253, 284, 323. *See also* CBT for insomnia (CBT-I)
review question/answers and summaries, 259–260
colitis, 154
collaborative care, 34–35, 43–44, 74–76, 131, 255
Collaborative Care Manager Model, 77–78
collaborative communication, 28
collaborative nutrition assessment, 119
Collings, Cate, 7
colon cancer, 125, 127, 136–137, 192*t*, 218, 221
colonic disease, 125
colonic function, 144
colorectal cancer, 124, 127, 193*t*, 282
"combination diet", 113–114
commercially prepared food, 108, 124
communication strategy, 160
community
advocacy, 97–98
design, 99
and employee program, 40
factor, 40
resource, 33, 70, 77–79, 131, 242
support, 9–10, 72, 84
system, 98
community-based exercise program, 77
comorbid disease, 161
Comparison of the Atkins, Ornish, Weight Watchers, and Zone diets for weight loss and heart disease risk reduction: a randomized trial (Dansinger, Gleason, Griffith, et al.), 342–344
compassion, 253, 255, 259–260
competence motivation, 40
complementary medicine, 17
Complete Health Improvement Program (CHIP), 6–7, 114, 148
complete protein, 121
complex carbohydrate, 125–126, 132, 286
comprehensive group medical visit, 74
computerized intervention, 242
condition management nurse, 6, 69
confidence scale, 35, 96, 130
confidentiality release, 75
connectedness, 7, 16, 328
connection, 329
conscious thought, 251
constipation, 125
contemplation stage, 27, 29, 34*t*–35*t*, 39, 47, 212
content, 254
contentment, 247
continuity of care, 76
conventional health care, 19
conventional medicine, 17, 21–22
cooking method, 128
coping skill, 325
core body temperature (CBT), 270*f*, 272*f*, 273, 274*f*, 275–277, 281
corn, 122*t*
corneal opacity, 278
coronary artery disease (CAD), 18, 125, 142–145, 163, 168, 240, 337–341
coronary artery stenosis, 114
coronary calcium score, 64
coronary heart disease (CHD)
Chinese rural male population, 142
fiber, 120*t*
Health Professionals Follow-Up Study, 15
Lifestyle Heart Trial, 114, 336–337
Lyon Diet Heart Study, 16
MESA risk score, 64
Nurses' Health Study, 14–15
physical activity, 217–218, 220
plant-based diet, 15
saturated fatty acids, 124
tobacco cessation, 297
coronary thrombosis, 142
coronary vascular disease (CVD), 124
corpus callosum, 270*f*
cortical function, 327
cortisol, 157, 236, 272–273, 275, 277, 280
cost, 74–75, 141, 151–152, 162, 187, 268, 296
cost savings analysis, 69
counseling
alcohol consumption, 314
interdisciplinary team, 72–73
nutritional, 131
physical activity, 210–213
physician personal behavior, 94–95, 196
review question/answers and summaries, 226
tobacco cessation, 298–299, 301, 303
courage, 248
C-peptide measurement, 67, 84
C-reactive protein (CRP), 327, 342–343
Creative Placemaking, 99
creative pursuit, 241, 245, 256
Crohn's disease, 140
Cronometer, 119
cruciferous vegetable, 126
CRY protein, 271–272
CT (computed tomography) scan, 363
cultural background, 33, 119, 268
cultural factor, 238
cultural interpretation, 237
cultural restriction, 119
curcumin, 324
cutaneous blood flow, 272
cutaneous fat store, 271–272
cutaneous vasodilation, 273
cytochrome P-450 drug, 284
cytokine, 153–155, 282

D

daily reference value (DRV), 110
dairy, 60, 105, 107, 113, 124, 128, 134, 145, 159
Danish population, 150
Dansinger, M. L., Comparison of the Atkins, Ornish, Weight Watchers, and Zone diets for weight loss and heart disease risk reduction: a randomized trial, 342–344
DASH diet. *See* Dietary Approaches to Stop Hypertension (DASH) diet
Davis, Brenda, *Defeating Diabetes*, 136
daylight, 275
Dean Ornish Preventive Medicine Research Center, 7
death, 11, 308. *See also* mortality
Deci, E.L., 327
decision-maker, 97–98
decision support technology, 9, 79
deconditioning, 187, 223
Defeating Diabetes (Davis and Barnard), 136
Del Gobbo, L.C., 350–352
delivery system design, 79
dementia, 192*t*–193*t*, 221
densitometry, 205, 362
Department of Health and Human Services (HHS), 105
depression
  adiponectin, 153
  arachidonic acid, 324
  InterSTROKE Study, 13
  major depressive disorder, 237
  meditation, 251
  mental health referral, 242
  mindfulness, 252, 325
  nicotine replacement therapy, 301
  nutrition, 243–245
  pharmacotherapy, 243
  PHQ-4 screening, 238–239
  physical activity, 192*t*, 193, 219, 243
  physician personal behavior, 94
  plant-based diet, 323–324
  review question/answers and summaries, 258, 260, 330–331
  screen and diagnose, 236, 241
  sleep, 290, 292
  sleep intervention, 323
  social media, 328
  therapeutic lifestyle change, 322
Depression and Anxiety Assessment Test (DAAT), 239
dessert, 112
desynchrony, 276
detoxification, 17, 270*f*
development, 149*f*, 239
DEXA bone scan, 65, 363
diabetes. *See also under specific type*
  Adventist Health Study 2, 15
  Agouti mice research, 149
  all-cause mortality, 185*t*
  ASCVD Risk Estimator Plus, 64
  Asian population, 65
  behavioral determinant, 11–12
  body mass index, 63
  cost, 151–152
  dairy, 105
  depression, 239–240
  depression/anxiety assessment, 239
  dietary pattern, 123
  dietary research, 157–160
  Dutch Hunger Winter, 149
  egg, 106
  emotional health and, 240
  epigenetics, 149*f*, 150
  family history, 159*f*
  health and wellness coach, 44
  health literacy, 13
  laboratory testing, 67–68
  lifestyle counseling, 212
  medication, 156
  NF-kß, 154
  nutrition prescription, 131–137
  pathogenesis of, 152–155, 165, 169
  prevention, 217
  registered dietitian, 119
  reversal, 136, 355–358
  review question/answers and summaries, 85, 87
  risk, 125
  risk assessment, 64
  smoking, 296
  statistics, 151–152
  weight loss, 366
diabetes cure-focused therapy, 358–360
Diabetes Prevention Program (DPP), 18, 160–161, 165, 169
Diabetes Prevention Program Outcomes Study, 18
Diabetes Prevention Program Research Group, 217
diacylglycerol, 153
Diagnostic and Statistical Manual DSM-5 (APA), 237–238, 242, 309–311
diastolic blood pressure (DBP), 13*t*, 113, 135, 140
diet
  acute myocardial infarction, 13
  American Heart Association's Life's Simple 7 Questionnaire, 63
  anxiety, 322
  cardiovascular disease, 141
  depression, 322
  diabetes, 151
  Dutch Hunger Winter, 149
  epigenetic influencer, 149–151
  insulin resistance, 153
  lifestyle medicine, 6–7
  lifestyle vital sign, 9
  maternal, 149
  mindfulness, 254
  premature death, 11
  Prescription for Health model, 80
  score, 14
  sleep, 283, 285–286
  unhealthy, 235
  vital sign, 60
"Diet, Lifestyle and Etiology of Coronary Artery Disease" (Campbell, T. Colin), 142
"Diet, nutrition, and the prevention of chronic diseases" (WHO), 7
dietary
  assessment, 60, 116–119
  change, 129–131, 160
  cholesterol, 113
  needs, 119
  pattern, 123, 125, 243, 323
  preference, 124
  recommendation, 120, 125
  risk factor, 138, 141, 150
Dietary Approaches to Stop Hypertension (DASH) diet, 113–114, 134, 146–147, 167, 171
Dietary Guidelines Advisory Committee (DGAC), 105, 113
Dietary Guidelines Advisory Committee Report, 109
Dietary Guidelines for Alcohol Consumption (DGAC), 309
Dietary Guidelines for Americans (DGA), 105–106
Dietary Guidelines for Americans, 2020–2025 (USDA), 60
dietary portfolio for treatment of hypercholesterolemia, 113–115
Dietary Screener Questionnaire (DSQ), 60
"diet-derived metabolic acidosis", 122*t*
DIETFITS randomized clinical trial, 350–352
diet induced thermogenesis, 59
dietitian, 60, 75, 85, 87. *See also* registered dietitian
diffusion of innovation theory, 40
digestive function, 17, 125
digital resource, 131
digital technology, 41–42
dihomo-γ-linolenic acid, 123
direct-to-consumer marketing, 19
discrepancy, 306*t*
disease-focused approach, 17
disease pathophysiology, 18–19
disease prevention, 7, 119
disease reversal, 7, 18, 20, 119
disqualifying the positive, 31
distraction, 255
Disulfiram, 314
diuretic, 218
diurnal insulin secretion, 135
diverticular disease, 137

DNA (deoxyribonucleic acid), 149*f*, 271
DNA-methylation, 12, 148, 149*f*, 150, 282
DNA remodeling and repair, 273
DNA repair, 270*f*, 282
DNA sequence, 11–12
Doody, R.S., 144
dopamine, 239, 244, 300*f*, 324
dopamine reward system, 162, 300*f*
dorsal striatum, 300*f*
dose-response relationship, 299
double-sided reflection, 46, 49–50, 53
dough, 124
Dr. Esselstyn's Prevent & Reverse Heart Disease Program, 147–148
Dr. Neal Barnard's Program for Reversing Diabetes (Barnard, Neal), 136
drop-in group medical appointments (DIGMAs), 75, 84
drug abuse, 11
drug intervention, 217–218
drug metabolism, 270*f*
drug/pharmaceutical, 149*f*
drug reaction, 21–22
drug therapy, 144
Dundee Stress State Questionnaire (DSSQ), 62
Dutch Hunger Winter, 149
dysbiosis, 135, 152
Dysinger, Wayne, 7–8
dyslipidemia, 11, 154–155, 281
dyspnea, 208

E

ear infection, 306*t*
earthquake, 12
eastward travel, 276
Eating at Americas Table Study (EATS), 60
eating pattern, 6, 60, 131, 162, 324–325
e-cigarette, 302–303
e-cigarette or vaping product use-associated lung injury (EVALI), 302, 315
economic factor, 238
ectopic pregnancy, 297
ectopic tissue, 153
Edison, Thomas, 7
Edmonton obesity staging, 363, 364*t*
education, 45, 62, 73, 75–76, 120, 162
effective inhibition, 255
"Effectiveness of Physical Activity Advice and Prescription by Physicians in Routine Primary Care: A Cluster Randomized Trial", (Grandes, Sanchez, Sanchez-Pinilla, et al.), 115, 211
Effect of low-fat vs low-carbohydrate diet on 12-month weight loss in overweight adults and the association with genotype pattern or insulin secretion: the DIETFITS randomized clinical trial (Gardner, Trepanowski, Del Gobbo, et al.), 350–352
"Effects of a Dietary Portfolio of Cholesterol-Lowering Foods Versus Lovastatin on Serum Lipids and C-Reactive Protein" (Jenkins, et al.), 133
"Effects of a Dietary Portfolio of Cholesterol-Lowering Foods Versus Lovastatin on Serum Lipids and Hypercholesterolemia" (Jenkins, et al.), 163
"The Effects of Stress Management Training and Dietary Changes in Treating Ischemic Heart Disease" (Ornish, Scherwitz, Doody, et al.), 144
egg, 60, 106, 108, 122*t*, 158
Egger, Gary, Lifestyle Medicine textbook, 6
eHealth, 358–360
e-hookah, 302
eicosanoid, 120*t*
elderly population, 118, 123, 134, 192*t*, 193, 218–219, 278, 322, 327
electroencephalogram (EEG), 273
electrolyte, 66
electronic device, 271
electronic medical records (EMRs), 69, 73, 79
electronic nicotine delivery systems, 302
Electronic Preventive Services Selector (ePSS), 80
Ellis, Albert, 32
emotion, 31–32, 45, 119
emotional
  distress, 238–240, 282
  energy, 255
  exhaustion, 95
  fitness, 63
  health, 240
  reasoning, 31
  regulation, 273
  well-being, 6, 9, 16, 235–238, 241–242, 245–246, 322, 324–328, 330–331
  well-being vital sign, 62
empathy, 29, 44–45, 252–253, 306*t*
The End of Diabetes (Fuhrman, Joel), 136
endogenous oscillator, 271, 272*f*, 289
endometrial cancer, 137, 192*t*, 282
endothelial cell, 150
endothelial cell damage, 124, 154–155, 161
endothelial dysfunction, 240, 281
endothelial injury, 281
endothelium, 153
end-stage organ damage, 152
end-stage renal disease, 152
endurance exercise, 187, 223
energy expenditure, 186
engagement, 325–326
entrainment, 269, 271, 276, 289
environmental
  chemical contaminant, 149*f*, 151
  factor, 12, 149–150, 238
  hazard, 238
  influence, 40, 45
  principle, 6
  quality, 10
  toxicant, 112
enzyme, 120*t*
EPIC study, 158
epigenetic, 11–12, 148–151, 161, 351
"Epigenetic differences arise during the lifetime of monozygotic twins" study, 12
epinephrine, 270
epithelium-derived factor, 154
Epworth Sleepiness Scale (ESS), 62, 287–288
erectile dysfunction, 297
ergospirometry, 341*t*
esophagus cancer, 192*t*
Esselstyn, Caldwell Jr.
  "Introduction: More Than Coronary Artery Disease,", 143
  "Is the Present Therapy for Coronary Artery Disease the Radical Mastectomy of the Twenty-First Century?", 142
  "Updating a 12-year Experience with Arrest and Reversal Therapy for Coronary Heart Disease (an Overdue Requiem for Palliative Cardiology)", 145
Esselstyn diet, 167, 171
Esselstyn plant-based diet for coronary artery disease, 114, 167, 171
estrogen, 272
eudaimonia, 327, 329
eudemonic feeling, 324
European population, 150
EuroQol 5 Dimensions visual analogue scale, 353
evidence-based complementary modalities, 17
evidence-based lifestyle therapeutic intervention, 6
evidence-based psychological treatment (EBT), 284
Excellence in Medicine Award, 7
exercise. *See also* physical activity
  angina, 144
  as a medication, 217–218
  circadian physiology, 274
  components of, 187–188
  coronary heart disease, 14*t*

defined, 186–187, 223
depression, 322
electrocardiography testing, 207
epigenetic aspect of, 150–151
ergospirometry result, 341*t*
health and wellness coach, 44
heart disease, 13*t*
intensity assessment tool, 202–203
journal, 131
levels of, 199–201
lifestyle medicine, 7, 18
lifestyle prescription, 36*t*
medical screening, 206–210
mental health and, 243
mortality, 217–218
Ornish lifestyle intervention, 114
Ornish Spectrum program, 76
physician competencies, 8
physician personal behavior, 94–95
physiologist, 76, 215
prescription, 115–116, 189–191
review question/answers and summaries, 258, 260
screening, 226, 228
sleep, 277, 283, 285
stress testing, 207–208
training progression for the sedentary low-risk participants, 210*t*
type 2 diabetes, 156
weight, impact on, 197–198
weight loss, 365
Exercise is Medicine, 202, 216
exercise preparticipation health screening recommendation, 208*t*
exercise tolerance test (ETT), 223
expectation, 39
external motivation, 45
eye, 128

F

falls, 192*t*, 193, 196, 219–220
family, 33, 63, 119, 141, 245, 247, 308, 324
famine, 12, 149
fast food, 244, 323
fasting, 135
fasting blood glucose, 156*f*, 158
fasting-mimicking diet (FMD), 157, 355–358
Fasting-Mimicking Diet Promotes Ngn3- Driven β-Cell Regeneration to Reverse Diabetes (Cheng, Villani, Buono, et al.), 355–358
fasting serum glucose, 67–68
fasting serum insulin, 67
fat, 7, 108, 113–114, 120*t*, 121, 123, 127, 135, 156, 244
fat-free body mass, 116
fat tissue, 116
fatty acid, 153, 273, 323–324
fatty liver, 153
FDA (Food and Drug Administration), 109, 124, 300, 302
fear extinguishing, 281–282
Federation of Chiropractic Licensing Boards (FCLB), 71
feeding pattern, 270*f*–271*f*
Ferriss, David, 8
ferritin, 117, 280
fertility, 149
fetal harm, 306*t*
fiber, 14, 60, 109–110, 120*t*, 125, 132, 135–138, 140, 161
finance, 247
financial reimbursement, 68–69, 145
financial resource, 119
fingerprint alteration, 149
Finnish Diabetes Association, 64
fish, 107–108, 159*f*
fish oil, 323
fitness
coach, 215
collaboration, 77
components, 204
defined, 187, 223
device, 217
instruction, 77
measurement, 66, 69
physician competencies, 8
review question/answers and summaries, 258, 260
safety and principles, 76
testing option, 66
trainer, 71
fitness registry and the importance of exercise national database (FRIEND), 204
F.I.T.T., 191*t*
FITT-VP cardiovascular exercise prescription, 191, 223–225, 227–228
5 A's
defined, 223
office visit, 43*f*
physical activity, 212
review question/answers and summaries, 50, 53, 226, 228, 316, 318
tobacco cessation, 303*t*, 304
flavonoid, 113
flaxseed, 324
flexibility, 187–188, 190, 195, 202, 205, 219, 223
fluid, 271, 272*f*, 274, 277, 283
focus, 254–255
folate, 14, 60, 137, 239, 243–245, 323
folic acid, 245
follow-up, 42, 68–70, 76, 131, 137, 213, 305
food. *See also under specific type*
addiction, 162
brain reward (dopamine) pathway, 300*f*
canned, 134
carbohydrate, 276–277
circadian physiology, 274
component, 106–107
desert, 12
endogenous oscillator, 271
health-promoting, 111–113
healthy, 96
industry influence, 105
journal, 131
label, 106–107
package, 112, 123
pattern, 120–129
preparation, 120–129, 136
processed, 60–61, 105, 112, 125, 128, 132, 134, 136
type, 120–129
"food family", 126
food-related disease, 119
food-seeking behavior, 272, 280
formaldehyde, 127
fortune telling thinking, 30, 53
foundation diet, 132
Four Points: economic vitality, design, promotion, and organization, 99
Framingham Heart Study, 13–14
free fatty acid, 155
free thyroxine, 67
frenzy, 255
Friedewald equation, 67
fried food, 60, 112, 124, 244, 323
friend, 33, 245
"From diabetes care to diabetes cure—the integration of systems biology, eHealth, and behavioral change" (van Ommen, Wopereis, van Empelen, et al.), 358–360
frontal lobe, 239, 270*f*, 300*f*
fructose, 135
fruit. *See also under specific type*
adolescent, 324
behavioral determinant, 11
breast cancer, 139
carbohydrate, 125
cardiovascular disease, 145
Chilean college students, 325
chronic obstructive pulmonary disease, 140
concentrate, 135
DASH diet, 113
dietary risk factor, 138*f*
diet vital sign, 60–61
emotional well-being, 324
gastric cancer, 137
heart disease, 13*t*
hypertension, 134
micronutrient, 126–127
nutrient, 111

nutrition prescription, 132–133
physician personal behavior, 95
Fruit and Vegetable Intake Screener, 60
fruit/vegetable/fiber screener, 118
frustration tolerance, 241
Fuhrman, Joel, *The End of Diabetes*, 136
functional capacity, 203–204
functional medicine, 17
functional performance, 272
functional status, 45, 119

G

Gabapentin, 314
gallbladder surgery, 137
gamma-glutamyl transferase (GGT), 314
gamma radiation, 127
Gardner, C.D., Effect of low-fat vs low-carbohydrate diet on 12-month weight loss in overweight adults and the association with genotype pattern or insulin secretion: the DIETFITS randomized clinical trial, 350–352
garlic, 135
gastric bypass surgery, 157
gastric cancer, 137
gastrointestinal disorder, 119, 154
The GEMINAL Study: Gene Expression Modulation by Intervention with Nutrition and Lifestyle (Ornish, Magbanua, Weidner, et al.), 345–347
gender interpretation, 237
gene mutation, 136
general anxiety disorder, (GAD), 237, 240
general anxiety disorder 2-question screening tool (GAD-2), 237
general anxiety disorder 7-question screening tool (GAD-7), 237
genetic factor, 149
genetic inheritance, 148
genetic predisposition, 11–12
genetics, 115, 238–239
gene transcription, 282
gestational diabetes, 68, 153, 192*t*, 219
ghrelin secretion, 273
Gleason, J.A., 342–344
Global Burden of Disease, 138
glucocorticoid, 270, 271*f*
gluconeogenesis, 152
glucose, 117, 135, 150, 240, 281, 355–356, 366. *See also under* blood glucose
glucose control, 188
glucose homeostasis, 355
glucose metabolism, 189*t*
glucose tolerance, 188
glucosinolate, 126
glucotoxicity, 155
GLUT-4 receptor, 150–151
glutamate neurotransmission, 314
glutathione, 244
glycemic control, 150, 161
glycemic index, 162
glycemic load, 162
goal, 36, 41, 46, 119, 129–131
Goodbye Diabetes (Youngberg, Wes), 136
grain, refined, 61
grain product, 107–109
Grandes, G., 115, 211
gratitude journal, 245
gray matter density, 251
"Greater Survival After Breast Cancer in Physically Active Women with High Vegetable-Fruit Intake Regardless of Obesity" (Piece, et al.), 139, 166, 170
greens, 134
Griffith, J. L., 342–344
group support, 77
group support specialist, 76–77
group visit, 73–75, 86–87
growth hormone, 273, 281
growth hormone IGF-1 (insulin-like growth factor1), 139
guided mindfulness meditation practice, 249
gut health, 125
Guthrie, George, 7
gut microbiota, 135, 150
gym, 217

H

hallucination, 323
Hambrecht, R., Percutaneous coronary angioplasty compared with exercise training in patients with stable coronary artery disease: a randomized trial, 338–341
Hamilton anxiety scale (HAM-A), 237
Hamilton depression scale (HAM-D), 236
Hans Diehl Coronary Health Improvement Project (CHIP). *See* Complete Health Improvement Program
Harvard School of Public Health, 113
Hawaii, 308
hazard ratio (HR), 220
HDL cholesterol, 67, 117, 123, 133*f*, 144, 189*t*, 339, 342–343
head concussion, 239
health
behavior change, 44–45
behavior change counseling, 325–326
behavior model, 40
challenge, 96
club, 217
counseling, 43
educator, 71, 76
fields, 21–22
habit, 10
indicator, 9–10
literacy, 12
maintenance, 137
outcome, 10–13, 44–45, 75
promotion, 326
promotion clinic, 215
risk assessment tool, 9
Health and Retirement Study, 327
health and wellness coach, 16, 27–28, 34, 44–47, 53, 76, 130, 215
Health Behavior Change: A Guide for Practitioners (Rollnick, Mason, and Butler), 36*t*
health belief model (HBM), 37–38, 51, 53
health care
access, 10
cost, 187
delivery model, 80
engagement, 10
financing, 19
professional, 74
professional referral, 9
provider, 6, 9–10, 12, 71–72, 75, 206, 241–242, 259–260, 325–326
quality, 12, 81–83, 86
services, 71–72, 81
system, 10, 78–79, 84
Healthcare Effectiveness Data and Information Set (HEDIS), 68–69
Health Professionals Follow Up Study (HPFS), 15, 157–158, 160
Healthwatch 360, 119
healthy behavior, 326–327
Healthy Body Calculator, 118
healthy eating behavior, 76, 131
Healthy People 2020, 9
heart attack, 8, 11, 13*t*, 16, 281, 297, 306*t*, 327
heart disease. *See also* coronary heart disease
Agouti mice research, 149
Chicago Heart Association Detection Project in Industry, 13
dairy, 134
death, leading causes of, 11*t*
exercise during pregnancy, 219
exercise stress testing, 208
hypertension, 66
Nathan Pritikin Longevity Center, 7
review question/answers and summaries, 165, 169
risk, 123–124
risk factor, 142, 235
tobacco cessation, 297
heart failure, 66, 208, 217, 220

heart muscle function, 188
heart rate, 235, 240, 275
heart rate reserve (HRR), 203, 209–210, 223
heat stress, 219
Heber, D., *Primary Care Nutrition: Writing the Nutrition Prescription*, 115
hedonia, 327, 329–331
height, 116
hematocrit, 117
heme iron, 154
hemoglobin, 117
hemoglobin A1c
  biochemical data, 117
  diabetes, 153, 158
  electronic medical records, 69
  health and wellness coach, 44
  physical activity, 193*t*
  plant-based diet, 159, 161
  prediabetes lab test, 68
  screening and diagnostic test, 67–68
  type 2 diabetes, 18, 140, 156–157
  weight loss, 366
hemorrhoid, 138
hepatic steatosis, 188
hepatitis B virus, 127
hepatitis C virus, 127
herb, 111
hiatus hernia, 138
high-density muscle and bone mass, 116
higher education, 12
high-fiber diet, 144
high glycemic index food, 135
high intensity interval training (HIIT), 201, 223
high nutrient density diet, 140
high-protein, low-carbohydrate diet, 157
high risk patient, 69, 85
high-sensitivity CRP (c-reactive protein), 64, 67
high-tech/high-touch counseling, 41
hip fracture, 106
hippocampus, 153, 244, 251
Hippocrates, 7
Hispanic population, 64, 151
histone acetylation, 148, 149*f*
histone micro-RNA, 150
histone remodeling, 282
HIV/AIDS, 12, 119
Hollingsworth, K.G., 347–349
home-based exercise program, 77
homeostasis, 126
homeostatic model assessment for insulin resistance (HOMA-IR), 67, 84
homicidal ideation, 242
hope, 247
hormonal rhythm, 270*f*
hormone, 17, 120*t*, 159*f*, 235
hospital admission, 12
House, Franklin, *The 30-Day Diabetes Miracle*, 136
humanity, 248
human papilloma virus, 136
human services, referrals, and information, 73
humility, 255
humor, 241
hydration, 117, 219
hydrochloric acid, 121
hydrostatic underwater weighing (hydrodensitometry), 65, 117
hypercholesterolemia, 124, 141, 143, 159*f*, 163, 165, 168–169
hypercoagulability, 236
hyperglycemia, 150, 154–155
hyperlipidemia, 131–137
hypertension. *See also* blood pressure
  alcohol consumption, 308
  ASCVD Risk Estimator Plus, 64
  behavioral determinant, 10
  cardiovascular disease, 141
  dairy, 105
  DASH diet, 113
  diabetes, 68
  exercise during pregnancy, 212
  Interheart Study, 13
  job characteristic, 235
  lifestyle medicine, 66
  nutrition prescription, 131–137
  nutrition role in, 140
  patient-provider relationship, 45
  physical activity, 185*t*, 192*t*–193*t*
  plant-based diet, 132*t*
  pregnancy induced, 220
  red meat replacement, 159*f*
  review question/answers and summaries, 164, 169
  type 2 diabetes risk factor, 152
  vegetarian diet, 15
hypertensive emergency, 208
hypervitaminosis, 67
hypnosis, 17, 302
hypnotic medication, 284–285
hypopnea, 279
hypothalamic-pituitary-adrenal cortex axis, 240
hypothalamus, 270, 270*f*, 300*f*, 366
hypothyroidism, 239

I

ice cream, 122*t*
IL-1Beta, 155
imagination, 255
immersion program, 6
immune function, 125, 140, 297
immune system, 115, 126, 136, 235–236, 282, 297
immunization, 10, 17
impaired glucose tolerance (IGT), 151
importance scale, 35
impotence, 306*t*
inclusive environment, 28
income level, 62
incomplete protein, 121
indole-3-carbinol, 126
induction phase, 7, 9
industrial revolution, 138
infection, 151, 208
infertility, 297, 306*t*
inflammation
  advanced glycation end products, 128
  angiogenesis, 154
  cardiovascular disease, 235
  dairy, 106
  diabetes, 153
  lung cancer, 136
  micronutrient, 126–127
  mindfulness, 252
  nutrition prescription, 120–129
  omega-6 fatty acid, 123
  plant-based diet, 141
  plant food, 112
  subclinical, 240
  weight loss, 157
  whole food plant-based diet, 161
inflammatory mediator, 152–153
inflammatory process, 136
inflammatory protein, 150
influenza, 11*t*
information sharing, 69–70
injury, 10, 308
Innovative Care for Chronic Conditions (ICCC), 77
input, 269, 271–272, 274, 289
insoluble fiber, 125
insomnia, 237, 268, 274*f*, 279, 284, 323
Institute of Medicine, 220
institutional factor, 40
instruction, 72
insular cortex grey matter, 327
insulin
  depression, 240
  intensive medication management, 152
  level, 186, 189*t*
  production, 67, 84, 153–154
  receptor, 152
  reduction, 166, 170
  response, 189*t*
  secretion, 153, 240, 350–352, 355
  sensitivity, 67, 84, 125, 150, 157, 161, 189*t*, 239–240, 280, 348–349
  sleep, 273
  type 2 diabetes, 140
  weight loss, 342–343

insulin-dependent type 2 diabetes, 157. *See also* type 2 diabetes (T2D)
insulin-like growth factor 1 (IGF-1), 355–356
insulin resistance, 68, 124–125, 152–154, 156, 276, 347, 359
insurance, private, 307
integrative medicine, 17
integrative medicine practitioner, 71
intellectual disability, 221
intensive behavioral health nutrition counseling, 115
intensive behavioral therapy, 364
intensive cardiac rehab program, 76
Intensive lifestyle changes for reversal of coronary heart disease (Ornish, Scherwitz, Billings, et al.), 144, 336–337
intensive lifestyle intervention, 73, 145, 157, 243
intensive medication management, 152
intensive therapeutic lifestyle change (ITLC) program, 6–7, 20, 69, 71
intentional self-harm (suicide), 11*t*
Interactive Dietary Reference Intake (DRI) Calculator for Healthcare Professionals, 118
interdisciplinary team, 72, 75–76, 78, 85, 87, 119
interest, 247
Interheart Study, 12–13
interleukin-6 (IL-6), 327
internal dialogue, 30
internal motivation, 45
International Association for Obesity, 65
International Board of Lifestyle Medicine (IBLM), 8
International Lifestyle Medicine, 8
internet modality, 19
interpersonal factor, 40
interpersonal therapy, 243
InterSTROKE Study, 13
interthalamic adhesion, 270*f*
intervention program, 9, 33, 336–337
intestinal bacteria, 125
intestinal barrier, 125
intramyocellular fat accumulation, 152
intrapersonal factor, 40
intra-treatment support, 305
intrauterine growth restriction, 302
"Introduction: More Than Coronary Artery Disease," (Esselstyn), 143
iron, 109, 117, 245, 323
ischemic heart disease, 15, 137, 146, 208, 220, 240
ischemic threshold, 341*t*
Israeli Health Study, 196
"Is the Present Therapy for Coronary Artery Disease the Radical Mastectomy of the Twenty-First Century?" (Esselstyn), 142
Italian population, 150

J

Japanese population, 65, 150, 323
Jenkins, D.J., 133, 163
Jenkin's Portfolio Diet, 18
jetlag mitigation, 284–286
JNK pathway, 154–155, 161
John McDougall Program, 7
Johnson, Mark, "Physician Competencies for Prescribing Lifestyle Medicine", 7
joint, 188
Journal of the American Medical Association, 7, 59, 336–337, 342–344, 350–352
joy, 247
justice, 248
"Juuling", 302

K

Kabat-Zinn, Jon, 249
Kaiser Permanente, 99, 113, 202
Katz, David, 7
Kelly, John, 7
kelvin color, 275
ketone, 355–356
kidney, 66, 157
kidney cancer, 192*t*
kidney disease, 128, 140
kinetic activity, 272
knowledge, 8, 248
Korean population, 65, 150

L

labeling/mislabeling thinking, 31
laboratory testing, 67–68, 117, 160
lacto-ovo-vegetarian, 139, 146
lacto-vegetarian, 144
Lancet, 352–355
Lancet Psychiatry Journal, 244
lapse, 41, 49
Larimer, M. E., Relapse Prevention: an overview of Marlatt's cognitive behavioral model, 42*t*
Latino, English speaking, 237
Latino, Spanish speaking, 237
Latino population, 68. *See also* Hispanic population
lauric acid, 123
laxation, 120*t*
LDL cholesterol
  aerobic and strength training comparison, 189*t*
  biochemical data, 117
  cardiovascular disease, 143–144
  egg, 106
  exercise, 339
  hypercholesterolemia, 113
  Lifestyle Heart Trial, 337
  monounsaturated fat, 123
  plant-based diet, 159
  popular diet comparison study, 342–343
  portfolio diet, 133
  screening and diagnostic test, 67
lead, 239
leadership, 8
Leahy, R. L., *Cognitive Behavioral Techniques: A Practitioner's Guide*, 42*t*
leaky gut, 125
Lean, M.E., Primary care-led weight management for remission of type 2 diabetes (DiRECT): an open-label, cluster-randomized trial, 352–355
lean body mass, 189*t*
learning, 282
legume, 60–61, 111, 113, 125, 132–134, 138*f*, 145
leisure time, 247
leptin, 152–155, 161, 273, 276, 280–281
Leslie, W.S, 352–355
Let's Move, 216
lettuce, 122*t*
Li, Z., *Primary Care Nutrition: Writing the Nutrition Prescription*, 115
Lianov, Liana, 7–8
life expectancy, 14, 198
life purpose, 327
life satisfaction, 247
Life's Simple 7 Questionnaire, 63
lifestyle
  cause, 239
  change, 7–8, 16, 33, 42, 139, 149, 157, 160, 240
  choice, 12
  counseling, 212
  disease, 9–10
  education, 9
  health impact, 258, 260
  influencer, 150–151
  intervention, 9, 28, 81, 86, 165, 167, 169, 171, 322, 358–360
  intervention program, 364–366
  measure, 69
  modification, 10, 72, 74–75, 77–80, 147, 210, 217, 242
  practices, 10
  prescription, 9, 34–35, 86, 88, 115, 282
  therapy, 18
  vital sign, 9, 82
Lifestyle Assessment Long Form, 63
Lifestyle Assessment Short Form, 63
lifestyle-based healthcare system, 358–360
Lifestyle Heart Trial, 7, 144, 147, 162, 336–338
Lifestyle Medicine (Egger, Garry), 6

lifestyle medicine (LM)
advocacy, 97–98, 100–101
comparison, 16–17
core competencies, 8, 21–22
cost, 16, 18–19
defined, 6
elements and intervention modalities, 16
history of, 6–7
intervention, 71–72, 165, 169
pioneers of, 6–7
prescription, 141
prevention and treatment, 18
provider, 21–22
tracking, 68–69
visit, 85, 87
vital sign, 69, 72, 86, 88
Lifestyle Medicine (Rippe, James), 7, 94
Lifestyle Medicine Certification Exam, 8
Lifestyle Medicine Trailblazer Award, 7
lifestyle-related condition, 9–11
lifestyle-related disease, 6, 9, 66
lifestyle-related health problem, 6
light, 270–271, 272*f*, 274–276
light exposure, 238, 278, 283, 285–286
light spectra, 275
light therapy, 241–242
Lim, E.L., Reversal of Type 2 Diabetes: Normalisation of Beta Cell Function in Association with Decreased Pancreas and Liver Triacylglycerol, 347–349
limb amputation, 221
limb movement, 280
linguistic barrier, 12
linolenic acid, 123
lipid
aerobic and strength training comparison, 189*t*
core competencies, 8
fasting, 67
The GEMINAL Study, 345–346
hyperlipidemia, 132
Interheart Study, 13
omega-6 fatty acid, 120*t*
plant-based diet, 144
review question/answers and summaries, 163, 168
type 2 diabetes, 193*t*
lipid lowering medication, 143
lipolysis, 153
lipoprotein, 189*t*
lipotoxic mediator, 152–153
literacy level, 33
liver, 66, 152–153, 156–157, 347–349
liver disease, 119
L-Nutra, 356
Loma Linda University, 63
longevity, 327–328
long-term disability, 306*t*
LookAHEAD "intensive" lifestyle intervention, 354
LoseIt, 119
lovastatin, 113, 133, 163, 168
love, 247
low birth-weight infant, 219, 297, 306*t*
low-carbohydrate diet, 350–352
low-density lipoprotein, 154
lower-fat foods prescription, 124
low-fat dairy, 159*f*
low-fat diet, 144, 350–352
low-fat vegan diet, 158
low-fat vegetarian diet, 7
low-fat whole food plant-based diet, 147
low-level physical activity, 206
lung, 8
lung adenocarcinoma, 296
lung cancer, 136, 192*t*, 296–298, 306*t*
lung-damaging chemical, 302
lung disease, 207, 219
lycopene, 136
Lyon Diet Heart Study, 16, 114
lysine, 121

M

MacColl Institute, 78
macronutrient, 113, 120–129, 135, 141
macrophage recruitment, 153–154
macrovascular complication, 150
macular degeneration, 297
Magbanua, M.J., 345–347
magnesium, 60, 109–110, 127, 135, 243, 280
magnification/minimization thinking, 30
Mainstreet America, 99
maintenance stage, 27, 29, 34*t*–35*t*, 37, 39, 48, 212
major depression, 253, 282, 322–323
major depressive disorder (MDD), 237, 240, 278*t*
malt, 135
management skill, 9
marijuana use, 94, 302
marital issues, 253
marketing recruiter, 76–77
Marlatt, A., Relapse Prevention: an overview of Marlatt's cognitive behavioral model, 42*t*
Mason, P., *Health Behavior Change: A Guide for Practitioners*, 36*t*
massage therapy, 71, 241
maternal depression, 244
maternal diet, 149
maternal nutrition, 150
Mathers, J.C., 347–349
maximal heart rate percentage, 203
maximum heart rate (MHR), 210
meal composition and timing, 285–286
meal schedule, 119, 131
meaning, 326
meat, 60, 107, 112, 124, 127, 132, 135, 145, 158–159
mechanism of action, 300, 324
mechanistic target of rapamycin (mTOR), 356
Medicaid, 307
medical
assessment, 28, 33
assistant, 77
cause, 239
expert, 16, 27–28, 34, 53
fitness collaboration, 77
history, 117
intervention, 208
mobility impairment, 221
nutrition therapy, 120
principle, 6
Medicare, 13, 75, 99, 307
medication. *See also under specific type*
conventional, 17
depression, 240
Depression and Anxiety Assessment Test, 239
diabetes, 140, 156
exercise as a, 217–218
gastric bypass surgery, 157
hypertension, 68
lifestyle medicine, 18
low-fat whole food plant-based diet, 147
management, 152
plant-based diet, 159
tobacco cessation, 298–299
meditation, 17, 245, 251, 277, 283, 325
Mediterranean-DASH Diet Intervention for Neurodegenerative Delay (MIND) diet score, 60
Mediterranean diet, 16, 114, 145–146, 157
medula, 270*f*
melanopsin, 270
melatonin, 270, 272–273, 274*f*, 275–276, 278, 282, 284–286, 289
memory, 273, 282
menopausal status, 159*f*
mental disorder, 149*f*, 322
mental down time, 254
mental filter thinking, 30
mental health, 10, 243, 245, 258, 260, 322–324, 328, 330–331
mental health disorder, 252
mental health professional, 242
mental health provider, 242, 326
mental health score, 244
mental illness, 11, 221, 238–240, 246, 301

mercury, 239
mesocortical pathway, 300*f*
mesolimbic pathway, 300*f*
messenger RNA (mRNA), 345
MET (metabolic equivalent of a task). *See* metabolic equivalent of a task (MET)
metabolic
complication, 65
disease, 208*t*, 209
disorder, 280–281
function, 235
panel, 66
syndrome, 10, 15, 105, 149, 281
metabolic equivalent of a task (MET), 196–197, 199, 203, 223
metabolite, 17
metastasis, 154
metformin, 18, 165, 169, 217
methionine, 121
methylation, 149
methyl group, 149, 244
microbiome, 161
micro-moment of connection, 329
micronutrient, 113, 120–129, 164, 169
Micro-RNA, 148
midwifery, CPM, 71
milk, 105, 107–108, 122*t*, 138*f*. *See also* dairy
Miller, W., *Motivational Interviewing in Health Care: Helping Patient Change Behavior*, 36*t*
Million Hearts Initiative, 73
mind-body medicine, 17
mind-body technique, 76
mindful eating, 131
mindfulness, 241–242, 250, 254–257, 259–260, 325
mindfulness-based stress reduction (MBSR), 249–253, 258, 260, 283
Mindfulness Center, University of Virginia School of Medicine, 249
mindfulness meditation program, 251
mind reading thinking, 30
mineral, 126
Mini Nutritional Assessment (MNA), 118
mini sleep assessment, 286, 291–292
mobile app, 73, 96, 119
Möbius-Winkler, S., 338–341
molecular change, 148
monoamine oxidase inhibitors (MAOs), 243
monosaccharide, 128
monounsaturated fat, 108, 123, 244, 323
monozygous twins, 12
mood, 244–245, 281, 322–324, 328
mood disorder, 236, 241–242, 323–324
moonlight, 275
Moore, M., *Coaching Psychology Manual*, 36*t*
moral judgement, 282
morbidity, 17, 66, 187, 296, 316, 318
mortality. *See also* all-cause mortality
Adventist Health Study 2, 15
cardiometabolic condition, 192*t*
deconditioning, 187
dietary risk factor, 138*f*
exercise, 199, 217–218
hypertension, 66
Multiple Risk Factor Intervention Trial (MRFIT) Study, 14
physical inactivity, 185
prevention and treatment practices, 10
preventative medicine, 17
review question/answers and summaries, 316, 318
sedative medication, 284
sleep, 281
tobacco use, 296
motivation, 40, 43, 119, 255
motivational interviewing (MI), 28–30, 137, 299, 305, 306*t*, 325–326
Motivational Interviewing in Health Care: Helping Patient Change Behavior (Rollnick, Miller and Butler), 36*t*
motivational principle, 6
Motorola's wellness program, 216
motor skill, 272
MRI (magnetic resonance imaging), 363
Multicenter Cardiac Lifestyle Intervention Program, 147
multidisciplinary care team, 119
Multifactor Screener, 60
multi-modality team, 6
Multiple Risk Factor Intervention Trial (MRFIT) Study, 14
multiple sclerosis, 141, 193*t*, 221
Multisite Cardiac Lifestyle Intervention Program, 147
multi-tasking, 254
mu-opioid receptor, 314
murine model, 157
muscle, 152–153, 156, 187, 189–190, 198, 219, 297
muscle strength, 222
muscular dystrophy, 221
muscular endurance, 205
muscular fitness, 192*t*, 204–205
musculoskeletal disorder, 63
My Fitness Pal, 119
myocardial infarction (MI), 12, 64, 66–67, 114, 142, 206, 208, 301
MyPlate, 105
MyPlate Calorie Counter, 119, 160
myristic acid, 124

N

N-acetyl cysteine (NAC), 244
Naltrexone, 313–314
narcolepsy, 62, 280
Nathan Pritikin Longevity Center, 7
National Academies of Sciences, Engineering, and Medicine, 105
National Academy of Medicine (NAM), 95
National Academy of Sports Medicine (NASM), 216
National Association of Nutrition Professionals, 72
National Board-certified Health & Wellness Coaches (NBC-HWC), 28
National Board for Health & Wellness Coaching (NBHWC), 28
National Board of Medical Examiners, 28
National Cancer Institute's Automated Self-Administered 24-Hour Dietary Assessment Tool (ASA24), 117
National Certification Board for Therapeutic Massage and Bodywork (NCBTMB), 71
National Certification Commission for Acupuncture and Oriental Medicine (NCCAOM), 71
National Complete Streets Coalition, 99
National Diabetes Education Program, 73
National Endowment of the Arts, 99
National Health and Nutritional Examination Survey (NHANES), 60
National Health Interview Survey (NHIS) Cancer Control Supplements (CCS), 60
National Institute on Alcohol Abuse and Alcoholism (NIAAA), 309, 315
National Institutes of Health (NIH), 60, 159, 308, 311, 313
National Physical Activity Plan, 216
National Prevention Strategy, "America's plan for better health and wellness", 10
national quitline network, 305
National Strength and Conditioning Association (NSCA), 216
National Weight Control Registry (NWCR), 198
Native American population, 68. *See also* American Indian population
natural disaster, 12
natural killer cell, 136
naturopathic medicine, ND, 71
negative prescription, 124, 129
neoplasm, 138*f*
nephritis, 11*t*
nephropathy, 152
nephrosis, 11*t*
nephrotic syndrome, 11*t*
neurogenesis, 244

neurological development and growth, 120*t*
neuromotor exercise, 196
neuronal tract, 270
neuropeptide, 235
neuroscience, 251
neurotransmitter modulation, 244
neurotransmitter serotonin, 239
Newman, Ian Blake, *The 30-Day Diabetes Miracle*, 136
newsletter, 131
New York School of Medicine, 296
NF-kß p65 promoter unit, 150
NF-kß pathway, 154–155, 161
Ngn3 expression, 355–358
nicotine, 297, 303, 315
nicotine liquid, 302
nicotine replacement inhaler or nasal spray, 300
nicotine replacement therapies (NRTs), 300–301, 315–316, 318
nicotinic receptor, 300
nigrostriatal pathway, 300*f*
nitric oxide, 272
nonadherence behavior, 27
non-alcoholic fatty liver disease (NAFLD), 152, 188
nondairy food, 105
nondairy milk, 134
non-DNA sequence component, 148
non-exercise activity thermogenesis (NEAT), 186, 198–199
non-Hispanic white population, 64
non-insulin dependent diabetes, 158
nonproductive thinking, 30–32, 50, 53
non-resting energy expenditure (NREE), 365–366
non-screen activities, 245
non-vegetarian diet, 15, 132, 134, 139
norepinephrine, 239, 244, 270, 300
North American Board of Naturopathic Examiners (NABNE), 71
North American Registry of Midwives (NARM), 71
nortriptyline, 301
Norwegian women, 323
Novick, Jeff, 109
nuclear myocardial perfusion test, 208
nucleosome, 149*f*
number needed to treat (NNT), 211
nurse, 71, 76, 115
nurse practitioner (NP), 78
Nurses' Health Study, 14–15, 158, 160, 166, 170, 199
Nurses' Health Study 2, 15
nut
    advanced glycation end products, 128
    dietary risk factor, 138*f*
    fiber, 125
    hyperlipidemia, 133
    magnesium, 135
    mood, 324
    nutrition prescription, 132
    plant protein, 122*t*
    saturated fat, 108
    SOS-Free (salt/oil/sugar-free) Diet Screener, 61
    type 2 diabetes, 159
    vitamin E, 111
    whole plant food, 113
nutrient, 60, 112, 118, 323–324
nutrient-based supplement, 244
nutrient deficiency, 245
nutrient dense food, 111–113
nutrition
    assessment, 116–120
    calculator, 118
    counseling, 77, 131, 164, 168
    Depression and Anxiety Assessment Test, 239
    health and wellness coach, 44
    history, 117
    intervention, 145–148
    knowledge, 119
    label, 109
    mental health, 243
    mental illness, 238
    physician personal behavior, 95
    prescription, 113–116, 129–137, 164, 168
    status, 116–117, 120
    study, 113–115
"Nutritional medicine as mainstream in psychiatry" (Sarris, Logan, Akbaraly, et al.), 244
nutrition counseling, 164, 168
nutritionist, 78
nutrition prescription, 164, 168

O

oat, 122*t*
obesity
    acute myocardial infarction, 13
    Agouti mice research, 149
    all-cause mortality, 185*t*
    Asian population, 65
    assessment, 362–365
    body mass index, 63
    breast cancer, 136
    cancer, 139
    cardiovascular disease, 141
    dairy, 106
    DASH diet, 147
    diabetes cure-focused therapy, 358
    diet vital sign, 60
    Dutch Hunger Winter, 149
    dyslipidemia, 155
    exercise, 197, 219
    health and wellness coach, 44
    job characteristic, 235
    leptin, 153
    lifestyle influencer, 151
    lifestyle medicine, 9–10
    lifestyle prescription, 68
    pathophysiology of, 366
    patient-provider relationship, 28
    physical activity, 185–186, 201
    physician personal behavior, 94–95
    pregnancy, 220
    review question/answers and summaries, 164, 168
    skinfold measurement, 117
    sleep, 281
    social support, 40
    sugar intake, 156*f*
    treatment recommendation, 364–365
    vegetarian diet, 146
    weight loss goal, 366
    Western-style diet, 138
observational learning (modeling), 38
Observing Protein and Energy Nutrition (OPEN) study, 60
obsessive-compulsive disorder (OCD), 253
obstructive sleep apnea, 279
occipital lobe, 270*f*
occupational therapist, 71
office staff, 9, 115
office systems, 68–70, 82
office tool, 68–70
office visit, 43, 72
office workflow, 70, 72
oil, 61, 108, 133, 145
omega-3 fatty acid, 14, 120*t*, 123, 132*t*, 133, 138*f*, 239, 243–245, 323–324
omega-6 fatty acid, 120*t*, 123, 132
omnivore diet, 140
Omron scale, 65
online resource, 131, 242
open-ended question, 29, 46
operator, 272
ophthalmologist, 78
optimism, 324–325
oral glucose tolerance test (OGTT), 67, 153
oral survey, 311
organ, 270*f*
organ damage, 235
organ meat, 107
organosulfur, 127
oriental medicine, 71
Ornish, Dean, 99, 144, 149–150, 165, 169
    "The Effects of Stress Management Training and Dietary Changes in Treating Ischemic Heart Disease", 144
    The GEMINAL Study: Gene Expression Modulation by Intervention with Nutrition and Lifestyle, 345–347

Intensive lifestyle changes for reversal of coronary heart disease, 336–337
Ornish Diet, 167, 171
Ornish lifestyle intervention (Lifestyle Heart Trial) for coronary artery disease (CAD), 114
Ornish lifestyle intervention for prostate cancer, 114, 167, 171
Ornish program, 6
Ornish Program for Reversing Heart Disease, 147
Ornish Spectrum program, 76, 145, 342–344
orthostatic hypotension, 240
osteoarthritis, 193*t*
osteoporosis, 11, 106, 306*t*
outcome tracking, 9, 314
output, 272, 289
ovarian cancer, 137
overconsumed nutrient, 111–113, 119, 163, 168
overgeneralization thinking, 30
over-the-counter medication, 284, 298
overweight
Asian population, 65
assessment, 362–365
body mass index, 63
cancer, 139
dairy, 106
DASH diet, 147
diabetes, 68
diet vital sign, 60
lifestyle medicine, 9
nutrition prescription, 115
physical activity, 185–186
physician personal behavior, 94
review question/answers and summaries, 164, 168
skinfold measurement, 117
weight loss goal, 366
overweight/obesity classification, 65t
oxidation, 120–129
oxidative stress, 17, 112, 127–128, 155, 161
oxidized fat, 127

P

Pacific Islander population, 68
packaged food, 60
pain, 193*t*, 251
"palliative cardiology", 145
Palmer, R, S., Relapse Prevention: an overview of Marlatt's cognitive behavioral model, 42*t*
palmitic acid, 124
pancreas, 153–154, 157, 347–349
pancreatic cancer, 127, 137
pancreatic cell, 355
pancreatic islet, 355
panic disorder, 253
Papua highlanders (New Guinea), 142
paranoia, 323
parasympathetic nervous system, 328
parasympathetic system, 270*f*
parietal lobe, 270*f*
parieto-occipital sulcus, 270*f*
park and recreation services, 73, 217
Parkinson's disease, 193*t*, 221–222
partially hydrogenated oil, 124
pathogen, 17
patient
behavior, 10–11, 196
communication, 19
education, 19
empowerment, 28
engagement and responsibility, 16, 75, 129
gatherings, 131
history, 59–66
outcome, 94–95
portal system, 69, 73
referral, 70–71, 73
registry, 73
risk factor, 85, 87, 119
satisfaction, 74
self-assessment, 63
self-care, 78
self-efficacy, 28–29
support, 10, 137
patient-centered approach to care, 43
patient-centered medical homes, 78
patient-facing material, 131
patient health questionnaire four question screening tool (PHQ-4), 238
patient health questionnaire nine question screening tool (PHQ-9), 236
patient health questionnaire two question screening tool (PHQ-2), 236, 241
patient-provider relationship, 245, 253
patient-readiness assessment, 27–28
pea, 122*t*
pedometer, 96
peer modeling strategy, 33
peer to peer program, 33
people-first language, 28
pepper, green, 122*t*
peptide synthesis, 273
perceived behavioral control, 38
perceived power, 38
perceived stress scale assessment, 61, 236*t*
%Daily Value, 110–111
Percentage of Energy from Fat Screener, 60
perception, 38*t*
Percutaneous coronary angioplasty compared with exercise training in patients with stable coronary artery disease: a randomized trial (Hambrecht, Walther, Möbius-Winkler, et al.), 338–341
percutaneous coronary intervention (PCI), 338–342
performance metric, 68
perinatal infection, 238
peripheral artery disease (PAD), 66
peripheral cutaneous vasodilation, 282
peripheral neuropathy, 161–162
peripheral oscillator, 269, 271, 289
peripheral perfusion, 281
peripheral vascular disease, 206, 220, 297
PERMA model, 330–331
PER protein, 271–272
personal
action plan, 96, 100. *See also* action plan
behavior, 196
behavior change plan, 43*f*
belief, 37
freedom, 247
growth, 45
readiness assessment, 96, 100
trainer, 72, 216
well-being, 322
personality disorder, 253
personalization and blame thinking, 31
person-to-person treatment, 299
pesco-vegetarian diet, 139, 146
pharmaceutical, 19
pharmacist, 6, 71, 78
pharmacotherapy, 243, 302, 322
phase shift, 276
Phillips, Eddie, 8
PHQ-2 screening, 259–260
physical
energy, 255
examination, 59–66, 117, 119
exercise, 254
fitness, 63, 76, 187, 193*t*, 223–225, 227–228
function, 192*t*
health, 247
inactivity, 13, 68, 80, 134, 185–186, 223, 235
therapist, 6, 71, 85, 87, 115, 215
vital sign, 69
work capacity, 341*t*
physical activity. *See also* exercise
adolescent, 324
American Heart Association's Life's Simple 7 Questionnaire, 63
anxiety, 322
assessment tool, 118, 201–205
benefits of, 224, 227
childhood, 322
Chilean college students, 325
components of, 188–190
counseling, 210–213
defined, 186–187, 223
depression, 241–242, 322
Diabetes Prevention Program, 160

disability and, 221–222
emotional well-being, 322
health and, 185–186
lifestyle influencer, 150
lifestyle medicine, 6–7, 16
lifestyle vital sign, 9
medical screening, 206–210
Nurses' Health Study, 14
nutrition prescription, 115–116
office culture, 96
patient-physician collaboration, 210–213
physician personal behavior, 94–95
premature death, 11, 200*f*, 200*t*
protective gear and equipment, 194
recommendations, 218–222
red meat replacement, 159*f*
related health benefits, 192*t*–193*t*
sleep, 283, 285
type 2 diabetes, 50
US guidelines for Americans, 191, 193–196
vigorous intensity, 201
vital sign, 59
weight loss, 197–198, 365
young adult, 322
Physical Activity Guidelines for Americans (PAGA), 191, 192*t*, 193–196
Physical Activity Readiness Questionnaire (PAR-Q) assessment, 76
Physical Activity Readiness Questionnaire for Everyone (PAR-Q+), 207
physical activity vital sign (PAVS), 202, 223
physical shared medical appointments, 75, 84
physician, 8, 12, 76, 94–95, 100–101, 196, 253–254. *See also* health care provider
physician assistant (PA), 78
"Physician competencies for prescribing lifestyle medicine" (Lianov and Johnson), 7, 59
physician-patient relationship, 10, 27–28, 32, 42, 44–45
physiological feedback, 302
physiologic body function, 17
phytochemical, 126, 162
phytonutrient, 112, 154
phytosterol, 126
Pierce, J.P., 166
pillars of positive psychology (PERMA), 325–326
pineal gland, 270
pineal melatonin secretion, 273
Pittsburgh Sleep Quality Index (PSQI), 288
pituitary gland, 270*f*, 300*f*
PKA, 356
place and health connection, 99
placenta previa, 219
places of longevity, 98
Plan4Health initiative, 99
Plan-Do-Study-Act (PDSA) cycle, 81–84, 88
plant-based cardiac rehabilitation program, 99
plant-based diet
amino acid profile, 122
angina, 144
cancer, 136, 139
chronic disease, 137
coronary heart disease, 15
dairy, 134
defined, 20
emotional well-being, 323–325
Esselstyn plant-based diet for coronary artery disease, 114
fasting-mimicking diet, 356
fiber, 110
foundation diet, 132
insulin use discontinuation/ reduction, 166, 170
lifestyle change program, 7
lipid, 144
mental health, 243
National Institutes of Health (NIH) funded study, 159
physician competencies, 8
physiologic impact, 161–162
review question/answers and summaries, 166, 170, 330–331
type 2 diabetes, 135, 140
vegetarian, 146
plant-based dietary pattern, 132*t*
plant-based fat, 134
plant-based food, 147, 160
plant food, 105, 112–113, 132*t*, 136, 324
plant-only diet, 126
plant protein, 121, 124, 141
plant protein content as % Energy, 122*t*
plant stanol, 133
plant sterol, 113, 133
plaque stenosis, 144
plasma FFA, 153
plateau phenomenon, 366
pneumonia, 11*t*
pneumonia vaccine, 140
pneumonic TAF, 129
podiatrist, 78
policymaker, 97–98
political factor, 238
Pollan, Michael, 112
polycystic ovary syndrome, 68
polyphenol, 126
polysomnography, 279
polyunsaturated fat, 105, 108, 123–124, 132, 134, 138*f*, 163, 168, 244, 323
pons, 270*f*, 300*f*
population-based intervention, 17
pork, 122*t*
portfolio diet, 133, 163, 167–168, 171
positive affect, 329
positive emotion, 247–248, 255, 257, 326
positive prescription, 129
positive psychology, 7, 16, 32, 35, 37, 45, 161, 246–248, 257, 325–330
positive psychology technique, 29–30
positive relationship, 242
positive resonance, 329
postpartum, 194, 219
postpartum depression, 192*t*, 236
postsynaptic neuron, 300
post-traumatic stress disorder (PTSD), 244, 282
potassium, 60, 109–110, 117, 127, 134
potato, 122*t*, 134–135
poultry, 107, 159*f*
practical counseling, 299
practice-based research networks (PBRNs), 80
precaution adoption model, 40
precontemplation stage, 27, 29, 34t–35t, 39, 47, 53, 212
prediabetes, 64, 68, 119, 151–153, 160, 217
Prediabetes Risk Test, 64
preeclampsia, 219–220
prefrontal cortex, 251, 254, 259–260
pregnancy, 123, 149–150, 192*t*, 194, 219–220, 236, 244, 301, 306*t*, 324
premature birth, 302
premature death, 200*f*, 200*t*
premature labor, 219
premenstrual dysphoria, 245
premenstrual syndrome (PMS), 282
preparation stage, 27, 29, 34*t*–35*t*, 39, 47, 212
prescribed treatment, 27–28, 46
"Prescription for Health" model, 80
prescription-strength medication, 284, 298
presentation, 8
The President's Challenge, 216
preterm birth, 219
preterm delivery stillbirth, 297
preventative measure, 37
preventative medicine, 17
pride, 247
primary care, 76, 115
Primary care-led weight management for remission of type 2 diabetes (DiRECT): an open-label, cluster-randomized trial (Lean, Leslie, Barnes, et al.), 352–355
Primary Care Nutrition: Writing the Nutrition Prescription (Heber and Li), 115
Pritikin Longevity Program, 147
Pritikin program, 6, 145, 147

proactive electronic medical records, 9
probiotic, 324
problematic social media use (PSMU), 328
problem-solving, 29, 31, 46–48, 214, 241
process and outcome tracking, 9
processed carbohydrate, 125
processed food, 60–61, 105, 112, 125, 128, 132, 134, 136
processed grain, 127, 135
processed meat, 108, 112, 127, 136–137, 138*f*, 154, 158
process mapping, 81–82
productivity, 324
program director, 76
pro-inflammatory food, 161
Project for Public Spaces, 99
prostate cancer, 8, 114, 127, 136, 149–150, 193*t*, 282, 345–347
Prostate Cancer Lifestyle Trial, 139
prostate gene expression, 345
protease enzyme, 121
protein, 7, 120*t*, 121, 122*t*, 132*t*, 136
provider satisfaction, 74
pseudo grain, 132
psychiatric patient, 308
psychiatric screening, 242
psychological predisposition, 8, 10–11
psychological stress, 13, 251
psychological support, 114
psychological treatment, 242
psychological well-being, 251
psychologist, 71, 78, 115
psychosis, 244, 323
psychosocial factor, 119
psychosocial risk factor, 13
psychosocial support, 144
psychotherapy, 240, 243, 252, 322
PTCA (percutaneous transluminal coronary angioplasty), 18
public policy factor, 40
pulmonary disease, 207
pulse, 65
pupillary reflex, 271, 272*f*
putamen, 300*f*

Q

QT prolongation, 240
quality metric, 68
quality of life, 13, 147, 192*t*, 193, 251, 297, 324, 353
quinoa, 122*t*, 135

R

race/ethnicity, 12, 62, 64, 116, 151, 159*f*, 354
radiation, 127
"RAIN" of compassion, 253
range of motion, 190
rapid eye movement (REM), 273, 281
rating of perceived exertion (RPE), 203
reaction time, 223
readiness assessment, 96, 100, 119
readiness scale, 35
reciprocal determinism, 38
recommended dietary allowance (RDA), 120*t*, 121
recreation, 254
rectum cancer, 137
red meat, 127, 136–137, 138*f*, 154–155, 159
reference daily intake (RDI), 110
referral resource, 9, 70–72
refined carbohydrate, 125
refined grain, 244, 323
reflection, 29, 46
reframing, 47–50, 53
Registered Clinical Exercise Physiologist, 72
registered dietitian (RD), 6, 71, 76–77, 115–120, 130
registered nurse, 76
reinforcement, 39, 131
relapse, 49
Relapse Prevention: an overview of Marlatt's cognitive behavioral model (Larimer, Palmer and Marlatt), 42*t*
relapse prevention planning, 41–42, 214–215, 241, 246
relapse stage, 212–213
relatedness motivation, 40
relationship building, 252, 325
relaxation, 17, 245
relaxation training therapy, 284
relevance, 306*t*
religious restriction, 119
renal disease, 119, 208*t*, 209
renin-angiotensin dysfunction, 280
repetition, 306*t*
reproduction, 297
resident, 78
residential program, 6
resilience, 247
resistance, 29, 306*t*
resistance training, 188–189, 194–195, 197, 202, 203*t*, 218, 225, 227
resource
  action plan, 36*t*
  alcohol consumption, 313
  dietary change, 131
  emotional well-being, 62, 242
  healthy lifestyle, 73
  lifestyle medicine, 98
  online referral, 72
  physical activity, 212
  relapse prevention planning, 42*t*
  risk assessment tool, 64
  tobacco cessation, 305
respiratory disease, 11
respiratory infection, 306*t*
respiratory rate, 203
rest-activity rhythm, 270*f*
resting energy expenditure (REE), 59, 365
resting heart rate (RHR), 210, 341*t*
restless leg syndrome (RLS), 279–280
restricted environmental stimulation therapy, 302
resveratrol, 136
"Rethinking Drinking" (NIH), 313
reticular activating system, 270*f*
retina, 270, 278
retinal ganglion cells (RGC), 270–271, 289
retinol-binding protein, 154
retinopathy, 152, 162
Reversal of Type 2 Diabetes: Normalisation of Beta Cell Function in Association with Decreased Pancreas and Liver Triacylglycerol (Lim, Hollingsworth, Aribisala, et al.), 347–349
reward, 131, 306*t*, 327
Reynold's risk score, 64
rheumatoid arthritis, 296
Rippe, James, *Lifestyle Medicine*, 7, 94
risk condition, 12–13
risk factor calculator, 64
risk factor measurement, 63–64
roadblock to quitting, 306*t*
road crash injury, 308
Roberts, W. C., 143
Robert Wood Johnson Foundation, 80
Robert Wood Johnson Foundation: "Creating a Culture of Health", 98
Rockport fitness walking test, 204
Rollnick, S.
  Health Behavior Change: A Guide for Practitioners, 36*t*
  Motivational Interviewing in Health Care: Helping Patient Change Behavior, 36*t*
root cause analysis, 82–84
Ryan, R.M., 327

S

S-adenosyl methionine (SAMe), 244
saffron, 245, 324
salt, 7, 61
Sanchez, A., 115, 211
Sanchez-Pinilla, R.O., 115, 211
sandwich, 112
Sarathi, V., 18
Sarris, J., "Nutritional medicine as mainstream in psychiatry", 244
satiety, 120*t*, 125, 154
Satisfaction with Life Scale (SWLS), 62
saturated fat
  American diet, 167, 171
  behavioral determinant, 11

cancer, 136
cardiovascular disease, 141, 143
DASH diet, 113
diabetes, 135
food groups to avoid, 112
hypertension, 134
multiple sclerosis, 141
nutrition prescription, 121, 123–124
overconsumed nutrient, 108
portfolio diet, 133
processed dairy product, 105
review question/answers and summaries, 167, 171
saturated fatty acids (SFAs), 124
Schaefer, E.J., 342–344
Scherwitz, L.W., 144, 336–337
schizophrenia, 149, 193t, 244, 301
screening, 17
screening and diagnostic test, 66
screening frequency, 68–70
seafood, 138*f*
Seale, Stuart, *The 30-Day Diabetes Miracle*, 136
seasonal affective disorder (SAD), 278, 282
seaweed, 122*t*
secondary insomnia, 280
secondhand smoke, 12, 62, 302, 306*t*, 324
sedative medication, 284
sedative/tranquilizer use, 94
sedentary behavior, 185–186, 191, 202, 206, 210*t*, 224, 227, 238
seed, 61, 108, 111, 113, 125, 128, 132, 138*f*
selective serotonin reuptake inhibitors (SSRI), 240, 243
selenium, 136, 245, 323
self-awareness, 131, 251
self-care, 6, 253–254
self-confidence, 45–46
self-determination of goal, 137
self-determination theory, 40
self-efficacy
coaching, 45–46
health behavior model, 40
interdisciplinary team, 72
key construct, 38*t*
lifestyle change, 42
motivational interviewing, 306*t*
nutrition assessment, 119
nutrition prescription, 130
positive psychology, 248
review question/answers and summaries, 52, 54
social cognitive theory, 39
self-harm, 11
self-management, 6, 9, 32, 40–41, 72, 78–80, 241, 245–246
self-monitoring, 42, 46, 48, 131, 214
self-motivation, 45–46
self-talk, 31–32
Selker, H.P., 342–344
semi-vegetarian diet, 139–140, 146
senior center services, 73
sensorimotor disorder, 279
serotonin, 244
serotonin and norepinephrine reuptake inhibitors (SNRIs), 243
"set switches", 149
sexual behavior, 9
Shanghai Women's Health Study, 199
shared medical appointments, 75, 84, 131
shellfish, 107
shifting focus, 47
short-chain fatty acid, 125, 152, 161
"shortfall" nutrient, 109–110
Short Form Food Frequency Questionnaire (SFFFQ), 61
shortness of breath, 306*t*
short physical performance battery (SPPB), 222
short sleep misperception, 280
"Short Stress State Questionnaire", 62
Shurney, Dexter, 7–8
silexan, 245
Silver Sneakers, 216
simple reflection, 46
single nucleotide polymorphisms (SNPs), 271–272
sit and reach test, 205
sitting, 185, 224, 227
Six- Sigma quality management strategies, 72
skeletal muscle, 150, 186, 201, 223, 225, 227
skill power, 41
skin collagen, 128
skinfold measurement, 117
skin-fold thickness testing, 205
skin function, 120*t*
sleep
amount of, 268
anxiety, 322
assessment, 9, 286–288
blue light, 275
brain health, 192*t*
cancer, 282
carbohydrate, 276–277
cardiovascular disease, 235
chronic disease, 278–282
circadian physiology, 269–277
culture, 268
deficiency, 277
delay, 276
depression, 322
dietary behavior, 282–285
disorder, 278–280, 290, 292
disruption, 276, 285, 290, 292
duration, 269*f*, 291–292
emotional well-being, 323
environment behavior, 282–285
epigenetics, 150–151
exercise, 285
fragmentation, 285
health, 278–285
hygiene, 284, 287
lifestyle adjustment, 285–286
lifestyle-based activity, 282–285
lifestyle medicine, 6, 16
light exposure, 278
meal composition and timing, 285–286, 290–292
melatonin secretion, 278
metabolic disorder, 280–281
mindfulness, 242, 254
mood, 281
output, 272
physical activity, 193, 285
physician personal behavior, 94
physiology of, 268–277
poor-quality, 286–288
propensity, 274*f*
restriction, 284
review question/answers and summaries, 290, 292
social media, 328
statistics, 268
stress, 285
vital sign, 62
wakefulness-sleep cycle, 270*f*
slow wound healing, 128
SMART goal
confidence and importance score, 36
defined, 223
nutrition prescription, 123–124, 129–131, 137
personal action plans for providers, 96
physical activity, 213
review question/answers and summaries, 51, 53–54, 164, 168
smoking, 13, 95, 136, 141, 150, 185, 235, 306*t*, 308. *See also* tobacco use
smoking, absence of, 14
smoking cessation, 7–8, 13*t*, 16, 114, 144, 297–298, 316, 318
smoking-related death, 296
smoking status, 63–64, 159*f*
snack, 283, 324
social
connection, 6, 325
cue, 282
factor, 238
fitness, 63
function score, 244
history, 119
interaction, 328
learning theory, 38
media, 42
network, 247, 328
norms, 38, 40

predisposition, 8, 10–11
stress, 239
support, 33, 48, 76, 119, 131, 213, 241–242, 299
support strategy, 40
well-being, 322
worker, 78
social cognitive theory, 38–39
social media use (SMU), 328
socioeconomic status, 12
sodium
biochemical data, 117
dairy, 105
DASH diet, 113–114, 146–147
dietary risk factor, 138*f*
food groups to avoid, 112
hypertension, 132*t*, 134, 272
overconsumed nutrient, 108–109
sleep, 283
solar cycle, 276
soluble fiber, 125
SOS-Free (salt/oil/sugar-free) Diet Screener, 60
South African Bantu, 142
South Asian population, 65
soy, 136
soybean, 121, 122*t*
soy protein, 113
special interest groups, 105
speed of movement, 223
sphingosine (Sph), 153
spice, 111
spinach, 122*t*
spinal cord injury, 221
spiritual fitness, 17, 63, 245
splanchnic nerve, 270
stage-matched intervention, 33, 34*t*, 47–48
stage-matched response, 27–28
stage of change, 8, 33–34, 130
stamina, 272
STAMPEDE (Surgical Treatment and Medications Potentially Eradicate Diabetes Efficiently) trial, 157
standing workstation, 96
starch, 126, 144
State or Area Agency on Aging, 73
statin medication, 18, 64, 348
stearic acid, 123–124
stenoses, 336–337
step testing, 204
stillbirth, 302
stimulus control, 284
stomach cancer, 127, 192*t*
STOP-BANG: brief obstructive sleep apnea (OSA) assessment, 287
strategic thinking, 256
strength, 272, 326
strength training, 59–60, 188–189, 194–197
stress
assessment, 236*t*
epigenetic influencer, 150
hypertension, 134
InterSTROKE Study, 13
level, 9
management, 6–7, 16, 114, 131, 144, 157, 235, 241, 248
management specialist, 76–77
meditation, 245
mental illness, 238
mindfulness, 254, 325
physician personal behavior, 94
plant-based diet, 324
reaction, 248, 250, 257
response, 248, 257
review question/answers and summaries, 258, 260
screening tool, 235
sleep, 283, 285
vital sign, 61–62
stretching, 195, 219
stroke
alcohol consumption, 308
dairy, 105
depression, 240
exercise, 217
hypertension, 66
InterSTROKE Study, 13
life purpose, 327
lifestyle-related death, 11*t*
physical activity, 193*t*, 220–221
physician competencies, 8
smoking, risk of, 306*t*
tobacco cessation, 297
subjective norms, 38
submaximal talk test for ventilatory threshold (VT1), 204
substance abuse, 9, 16, 253
substance avoidance, risky, 6
substantia nigra, 300*f*
sucrose, 135
sudden infant death syndrome (SIDS), 297, 306*t*
suffering, 248–249
sugar, 61, 106–107, 125–126, 135–136, 156*f*, 244, 323
sugar-sweetened beverage, 60, 107, 112, 138*f*
suicidal ideation, 240, 242–243, 247, 301, 324, 326. *See also* suicide
suicide, 11*t*, 308
sulforaphane, 126
sulfur, 121
summary, 29, 37
sunlight, 274, 283, 285
supplement, 19, 126, 136, 284, 324
supplementary material, 305
support, 42, 120, 160
support analysis tool, 33*t*
support group, 33, 40, 245
support staff, 72
support system, 42, 45, 78
suprachiasmic nucleus (SCN), 269–270, 271*f*, 274–276, 289
surgical birth delivery, 219
surgical history, 117
surgical intervention, 17, 208
Swedish Obese Subjects study, 157
sweet snack, 112
swimming, 201
sympathetic nervous system, 240, 270*f*, 328
sympathetic tone, 273, 275, 281
synaptic cleft, 300*f*
synaptic vesicle, 300*f*
syncope, 208
syrup, 135
systems biology, 358–360
systolic blood pressure (SBP), 113, 134–135, 140, 218

T

tachycardia, 65
tai chi, 17, 219, 222, 241
talk test, 202–203, 223, 225, 227
tar, 297
Tarahumara Indians (northern Mexico), 142
taste bud, 162
Taylor, J.C., 347–349
T. Colin Campbell Center for Nutrition Studies, 60
team approach, 9, 72, 74, 131, 215
team characteristics, 73
technology, 96, 275
telehealth counseling, 41
telephone "quitline" counseling, 299
television viewing, 186
telomerase, 154
temperature, 271–274, 274*f*, 277
termination stage, 27, 39
temperance, 248
testosterone level, 281
test result, 68–70
thalamus, 270*f*, 300*f*
THC (tetrahydrocannabinol), 302
"The Aerobics Center Longitudinal Study", 224
"The Development of the Concept of Dietary Fiber" (Burkitt and Trowell), 138
"The Effects of Stress Management Training and Dietary Changes in Treating Ischemic Heart Disease," (Ornish, Scherwitz, Doody, et al.), 144
"The Etiological Significance of Related Diseases" (Burkitt, Dennis), 137
"The National Strategy for Quality Improvement in Health Care" (US Department of Health and Human Services), 10

theory of planned behavior, 38
theory of reasoned action, 38
therapeutic intervention, 6
therapeutic lifestyle change (TLC), 322, 329
thermic effect of feeding (TEF), 365
thermogenesis, 59
Third National Health and Nutrition Examination Survey (NHANES III), 212
36-Item Short Form (SF-36), 62
The 30-Day Diabetes Miracle (House, Seale, and Blake Newman), 136
thought adjustment, 32, 252
3-day food record, 118
thyroid stimulating hormone, 67
time management, 241
time perspective, 248
time zone, 269, 290, 292
tissue damage, 235
TNF-alpha, 153–154
tobacco cessation, 303*t*, 304–305, 306*t*, 307
tobacco use, 9, 11, 62, 69, 80, 127–128, 134, 296–297. *See also* smoking
tomato, 122*t*
tool, 72
Topiramate, 314
total cholesterol (TC), 67, 117, 142, 147, 166, 170–171
total energy expenditure (TEE), 59, 365
toxicity, 239
tracking, 68–70, 120
transcendence, 248
trans fat, 109, 123–124, 127, 132, 135, 138*f*, 143, 155, 244, 323
transport carrier, 120*t*
transtheoretical model (TTM), 39, 47–49, 51, 53, 96
transtheoretical model-stages of change, 27–28, 212
trauma patient, 308
traumatic brain injury (TBI), 282
treadmill desk, 96
treatment compliance, 72, 75
treatment plan, 246
treatment prescription, 33
Trepanowski, J.F, 350–352
triacylglycerol, 152–153, 157, 347–349
trichotillomania, 244
tricyclic antidepressants (TCAs), 240, 243
triglycerides (TG), 67, 117, 132, 135, 144, 146, 153, 189*t*, 366
Trowell, H.C., "The Development of the Concept of Dietary Fiber", 138
trust, 12
tryptophan, 239
tuberculosis, 297
tuberoinfundibular pathway, 300*f*
tumor development, 136
tumor-fighting immune cell, 136
tumorigenesis, 149, 165, 169
tuna, 122*t*
turmeric, 324
12-Item Short Form (SF-12), 62
24-hour recall, 117
two-item exercise vital sign, 59
2018 Lifestyle Medicine Core Competencies, 6
2015 Exercise Screening Guidelines, 206–207
2015 MESA (Multi-Ethnic Study of Atherosclerosis) risk score, 64
2017 American Heart Association and American College of Cardiology guidelines on lifestyle management, 143
2017 Guideline for the Prevention, Detection, Evaluation, and Management of High Blood Pressure in Adults (American College of Cardiology and American Heart Association), 65
2013 Baylor University Conference, 142
type 1 diabetes (T1D), 67, 84, 128, 151, 153, 355–358
type 2 diabetes (T2D)
- advanced glycation end products, 128
- cardiovascular disease, 141
- Complete Health Improvement Program (CHIP), 114–115
- C-peptide measurement, 84
- diabetes cure-focused therapy, 358–360
- diagnosis, 153
- dietary intervention, 156
- dietary risk factor, 138*f*, 155
- DiRECT trial, 352–355
- "disease management" approach, 152
- egg, 106
- epigenetics, 150
- exercise, 156, 218
- fasting-mimicking diet (FMD), 355–358
- flexibility exercise, 190
- gastric bypass surgery, 157
- group visit, 75
- heme iron, 154
- high-protein, low-carbohydrate diet, 157
- insulin sensitivity, 150
- lifestyle change, 157
- lifestyle related risk factor, 155
- Mediterranean diet, 146, 157
- myristic acid, 124
- nutrition prescription, 135–136
- nutrition role in, 139–140
- obesity, 201
- pathogenesis of, 152–155
- physical activity, 192*t*–193*t*, 220–221
- plant-based diet, 132*t*, 160
- preventing, treating, and reversing, nutrition role in, 155–157
- red meat consumption, 159
- remission, 156, 352–355
- reversal, 156–157, 347–349
- risk assessment tool, 64
- sleep, 281
- vegetarian diet, 146
- very-low-calorie diets, 157
- weight loss, 155
- whole food plant-based diet, 157
- work stress, 235

tyrosine, 239

U

Ugandan population, 141–142
ultraviolet B (UV-B) radiation, 111
underconsumed nutrient, 109–113, 119
underlying belief, 32
underserved patient, 74
understanding, 29, 37
United Kingdom, 244, 323
United States (Midwest), 308
United States (Northeast), 308
United States Department of Agriculture Economic Research Service, 155
United States population, 142
unsaturated fat, 132*t*
unstable angina, 208
"Updating a 12-year Experience with Arrest and Reversal Therapy for Coronary Heart Disease..." (Esselstyn), 145
Urban Land Institute, 99
US Army's Global Assessment Tool, 63
US Department for Veterans Affairs Whole Health Personal Health Inventory, 63
US Department of Agriculture (USDA), 105, 113
US Department of Agriculture, *Dietary Guidelines for Americans, 2020–2025*, 60
US Department of Health and Human Services (HHS), 10, 299
US Department of Veterans Affairs hospital system, 80
US Physical Activity Guidelines for Americans, 224, 227
US Preventive Services Task Force (USPSTF), 80, 115, 207, 210, 236–237, 309, 364
US Public Health Service (USPHS) Clinical Practice Guidelines, 298–299
US Registry of Exercise Professionals, 72

V

vaccination, 196
value-based care, 78
valvular disease, 208
van Empelen, P., 358–360
van Ommen, B., From diabetes care to diabetes cure—the integration of systems biology, eHealth, and behavioral change, 358–360
vaping, 302
varenicline, 300–302
varicose vein, 138
vascular disease, 66, 132
vascular dysfunction, 280
vascular repair, 124
vascular tone, 272
vasoconstriction, 272
vasodilation, 272
vasospastic disorder, 281
vegan, 144
vegan diet, 114–115, 132, 134–135, 139–141, 146, 157–158
vegetable
- adolescent, 324
- breast cancer, 139
- carbohydrate, 125–126
- cardiovascular disease, 145
- Chilean college students, 325
- chronic obstructive pulmonary disease, 140
- coronary heart disease, 141
- dietary risk factor, 138*f*
- diet vital sign, 60–61
- emotional well-being, 324
- gastric cancer, 137
- heart disease, 13*t*
- hypertension, 134
- micronutrient, 127
- nutrition prescription, 132
- physician personal behavior, 95
- plant-based diet, 133
- protein, 158
- underconsumed nutrient, 111
- whole plant food, 113

vegetable oil, 133
vegetarian diet, 7, 15, 95, 114, 139–140, 143–144, 146, 159, 324
VEGF (vascular endothelial growth factor), 154
ventral tegmental area, 300
ventricle, fourth, 270*f*
very-high fiber diet, 144
very-low-calorie diets, 157
very low-density lipoprotein, 154
Villani, V, 355–358
violence, 10
virtue, 326
visceral adipose tissue, 188
viscous fiber, 113, 133
visual imagery, 17
visual impairment, 280
visualization, 255
vital sign, 59, 117, 201
vitamin, 60, 109, 113, 126
vitamin A, 109–111
vitamin B6, 284
vitamin B9, 244
vitamin B12, 113, 117, 126, 245, 323
vitamin C, 109, 111, 136, 324
vitamin D, 67, 109, 111, 113, 117, 244, 280
vitamin D (25-hydroxycholecalciferol), 67
vitamin E, 109, 111, 136
volunteer, 241

W

Wagner, Ed, 78, 84
waist circumference, 64, 116, 363
Waist Circumference and Waist-Hip Ratio (WHO), 65
waist-to-hip ratio, 65, 118
walking, 139, 193*t*, 200, 222
"Walk with a Doc", 96, 216
walnut, 122*t*, 324
Walther, C,, 338–341
war, 12
water-only fasting, 135
water supply, 12
"weekend warrior", 200
Weidner, G., 345–347
weight
- change by dietary adherence, 344*f*
- control, 135, 156
- DASH diet, 113
- excess, 134
- exercise impact on, 197–198
- gain, 135, 152–153, 192*t*, 301
- healthy, 11, 187
- history, 117
- maintenance, 147, 188
- management, 63, 147, 352–355
- nutrition assessment, 116
- people-first language, 28
- promoting medication, 119
- reduction, 76, 147
- related disorder, 119
- status, 192*t*

weight loss
- chronic care model, 75
- DIETFITS randomized clinical trial, 350–352
- DiRECT trial, 352–355
- The GEMINAL Study, 345–346
- goals and expectation, 366
- lifestyle intervention, 165
- low-fat whole food plant-based diet, 147
- physical activity, 192*t*, 197–198
- physician personal behavior, 95
- popular diet comparison study, 342–344
- recommendations, 365
- review question/answers and summaries, 44, 166, 169
- social support, 40
- type 2 diabetes, 155, 157–159
- water-only fasting, 135

weight-loss counseling, 165, 169
Weight Watchers diet, 342–344
wellness and disease prevention, 10
wellness program, 216
wellness program for health provider, 95–96, 100–101
"Western Diseases and Their Emergence Related to Diet" (Burkitt, Dennis), 138
Western-style diet, 137, 142, 152
white population, 65, 151, 308
whole-body fat mass, 188
whole food, 112, 120, 122–123, 125–126, 128
whole food plant-based diet, 132
- cancer, 136
- cardiovascular disease, 141, 145
- dietary intervention, 156
- diet vital sign, 60
- John McDougall Program, 7
- lifestyle medicine, 6, 16
- nutrition intervention, 147–148
- physiologic impact, 161–162
- type 2 diabetes, 157
- underconsumed nutrient, 110–111
- weight loss, 365

whole-grain, 60–61, 111, 113, 124–125, 132–133, 138*f*, 141, 145, 159
"Whole Health model" of care, 80
whole-person need, 17
whole plant food, 108–109, 112
wisdom, 248
withdrawal, 314
Women's Health Initiative, 220
Wopereis, S., From diabetes care to diabetes cure—the integration of systems biology, eHealth, and behavioral change, 358–360
working memory, 255
worksite wellness, 70, 216
work situation, 247
work stress, 235
World Health Organization (WHO), 7, 62, 65, 77, 107
wound healing, 297
written screening, 311

X

x-ray, 127

Y

Yale-Griffin Prevention Research Center, 72
yoga, 17, 277
yogurt, 105–106, 122*t*
young adult, 328
Youngberg, Wes, *Goodbye Diabetes*, 136
youth, 157

Z

zinc, 244–245, 323
Zone diet, 342–344